Natural Answers for Women's Health Questions

A Comprehensive
A–Z Guide to Drug-Free
Mind-Body Remedies

D. Lindsey Berkson

A FIRESIDE BOOK
Published by Simon & Schuster
New York   London   Toronto   Sydney   Singapore

FIRESIDE
Rockefeller Center
1230 Avenue of the Americas
New York, NY 10020

FIRESIDE and colophon are registered trademarks
of Simon & Schuster, Inc.

For information about special discounts for bulk purchases,
please contact Simon & Schuster Special Sales:
1-800-456-6798 or business@simonandschuster.com

Designed by Christine Weathersbee

Manufactured in the United States of America

1   3   5   7   9   10   8   6   4   2

Library of Congress Cataloging-in-Publication Data
Berkson, Lindsey.
Natural answers for women's health questions : a comprehensive
A–Z guide to drug-free mind-body remedies / D. Lindsey Berkson.
p.   cm.
1. Women—Health and hygiene.   2. Women—Diseases—
Alternative treatment.   3. Naturopathy.   4. Mind and body.
5. Self-care, Health.   I. Title.
RA 778.B5235   2002
613'.04244—dc21   2001057563

ISBN 0-684-86514-9

This publication contains the opinions and ideas of its author. It is intended to provide helpful and informative material on the subjects addressed in the publication. It is sold with the understanding that the author and publisher are not engaged in rendering medical, health, or any other kind of personal professional services in the book. The reader should consult his or her medical, health, or other competent professional before adopting any of the suggestions in this book or drawing inferences from it.

The author and publisher specifically disclaim all responsibility for any liability, loss, or risk, personal or otherwise, that is incurred as a consequence, directly or indirectly, of the use and application of any of the contents of this book.

I dedicate this book to all my global mothers, sisters, and daughters as well as to my best friend, Janet Steinberg. She always makes me feel lucky.

Acknowledgments

I could not do the work I do and keep the necessary balance in my life without the consistent, skillful assistance of Parvati Markus. Immense thanks goes to her. Also, I want to acknowledge the pioneering work of many doctors and researchers in the field, too many to mention, except for the distinguished efforts of Jonathan V. Wright and Alan R. Gaby. Their lifetime achievements and elbow grease, along with their friendship, add to my message and mental health. Thanks to my agent, Meredith Bernstein, and my very understanding editor at Simon & Schuster, Caroline Sutton, and her assistant, Nicole Diamond. Particular thanks goes to these patient readers who gave of their time, expertise, and energy in the midst of their extremely busy lives: Jonathan V. Wright, M.D., Myron Moorehead, M.D., Christine Green, M.D., Erica Elliot, M.D., Davis Lamson, N.D., and Theo Gerontinos, R.N. I would also like to acknowledge the groundbreaking work of John R. Lee, M.D., in the field of natural hormones.

CONTENTS

14   Contents

Foreword

Who would have ever guessed?

It was one of those long, overwhelming days in medical school working on the hospital wards. As I searched for a patient who was not in his bed, I was shocked to see someone I knew in the next bed—the father of my best friend from grammar and high school. It had been seventeen years since we had seen each other. As I reintroduced myself to Mr. Berkson and recognition began to cross his face, we hugged each other and began to cry, an emotional encounter that would herald a new era of collaboration for me with his daughter, Lindsey.

Back in the days when the two of us were blond models for Clairol, no one ever would have imagined that we would both end up as doctors, especially when I got married right out of high school (Lindsey was a bridesmaid).

As destiny would have it, Lindsey and I were both pushed by our own illnesses and the suffering of our family members into our mutual passion to understand and promote health. I learned most of what I know the hard way—by being chronically ill for the first seventeen years of my life. I took antibiotics as if they were vitamins until it became painfully obvious that was not the answer to my problems. I missed 20–30 percent of high school because of recurrent illness and subsequent fatigue, until my desperation became the inspiration for me to find the path out. While Lindsey struggled with her health problems caused by DES (a powerful synthetic estrogen pharmaceutical) exposure in the womb and I fought my own illnesses, my mother and younger sister both died of premenopausal breast cancer. I was advised to have my breasts removed prophylactically and consider having my ovaries removed before I was forty. Health was a real life-and-death concern.

Ultimately it became perfectly clear to both of us that it was much easier to change lifestyle and dietary habits rather than to remain ill. Knowing how to live, eat, meditate, and be still all lead to authentic health.

Now it is with great pleasure that I get to introduce this exceptional new book that I believe will become the definitive primer on natural answers for women's health.

You don't have to learn the hard way. In this empowering new book, Dr. Berkson gives you the information you need to create the health you desire. You will learn to avoid and eliminate the hidden dangers in your environment and kitchen. You will learn cutting-edge facts on how hormones play a vital role in your symptoms and treatment. Lindsey's information is so up-to-date that many doctors are not aware of it. Her information is based on the thousands of scientific studies she wades through meticulously. Then she combines all that scientific knowledge with her nutritional expertise and makes it accessible to everyone in an easy-to-read way.

You and your loved ones will benefit from the clear guidance she has created. I know I will recommend this powerful book to all my patients.

Jesse L. Hanley, M.D.
Malibu, California
Co-author of *What Your Doctor*
May Not *Tell You About Perimenopause*
(Warner Books, 1999) and *Tired*
of Being Tired (Putnam, 2001)

Preface

Dr. Lindsey Berkson has for many years been a pioneer and leader in the field of women's health. I have personally known Dr. Berkson for decades. We have lectured together, been interviewed on television shows together, and we even practiced together for a short period of time. So I know Berkson's work is powerful and enlightening, a true asset for women wanting to support their health naturally through the use of safe herbal and nutritional remedies.

I was therefore delighted to learn about Lindsey's new book, *Natural Answers for Women's Health Questions*. This wonderful book is a much-needed resource for the many women who are seeking to improve their health and well-being through complementary medicine.

I highly recommend this book to all women who are looking for answers to their health issues and want the information communicated to them in an easy-to-access and useful format.

Susan M. Lark, M.D.
Los Altos, California

Dr. Lark has written eleven books on health and publishes an ongoing newsletter.

Introduction

Living in a woman's body means inhabiting a different universe from the one a man lives in. Any woman can tell you this. Historically, however, most medical research and many medical recommendations have been based on the male anatomy and the way the male body functions. This book is uniquely female. It takes into account women's major hormonal events—puberty, menstruation, pregnancy, peri- and postmenopause—and looks at the ways in which these circumstances affect symptoms and the treatments of various illnesses.

This book is a guide to help you work along with your health allies: the doctors and practitioners who listen to your whole story and figure out how to make you the best and healthiest you can be. The old Chinese proverb holds true: Give a starving woman a fish to eat and soon she will be hungry again, but teach her how to fish and she will be able to feed herself and her whole family. This book is about helping us feed our bodies and souls with facts and guidelines that are uniquely female.

That various medical conditions are affected and often exacerbated by specific phases of the menstrual cycle is a well-recognized phenomenon in medical literature,* but this fact has not yet made the transition into clinical practice. When was the last time a doctor asked you if your asthma or irritable bowel symptoms cycled with your menstrual cycle? Did your doctor consider running a complete evaluation to see if an imbalance of your hormones had anything to do

---

* *Archives of Internal Medicine* 158:1405–12, 1998.

with your recurrent carpal tunnel syndrome, diabetes, or migraine headaches?

You are a soul having a human experience in a female body that ovulates, responds sensitively to hormonal fluxes as well as to the moon, and is a mystery to us all, even doctors. No matter how much anyone seems to have all the answers, you and you alone are responsible for your health. There is such an explosion of information today that no one doctor can know everything that is available or keep up-to-date on the latest studies. That does not make any doctor wrong, bad, or arrogant, nor does it fossilize you into permanent victimhood. It is just the fact. Life is fast and furious, and so is information. Get smart and stretch your mind, lifestyle, nutrition, and options. Let me help you help yourself and your doctors so you can enjoy yourself as fully as possible on this magical mystery tour called life.

Read This First

The information in this book is to be used in conjunction with a physician who monitors your treatment and progress. All your health concerns should be medically supervised. Always tell your doctor everything you are taking, including all nutrients and herbs, especially if you are or will be taking any medication, are planning surgery, or are presently pregnant or planning on becoming pregnant. In dealing with health issues, risk can never be completely ruled out, nor can any guarantees be made.

Dosages in this book are given for adults, and alterations should be made for adults with certain conditions. Most RDAs (recommended dietary allowances) tend to be too low to produce a therapeutic effect. However, never take supplement dosages higher than the RDAs without professional supervision. Certain individuals may experience allergic or other adverse reactions from using a natural dietary supplement or from some substance mixed with it. Call your doctor immediately if any reaction occurs. Do not put off proper medical supervision because you think you can self-medicate based on what you read here; instead, share the information in this book with your doctor or health-care practitioner.

It makes sense to try natural means to heal many problems before using drugs, unless the situation is serious or an emergency. Drugs are not without side effects, some of which require hospitalization. Adverse reactions to drugs account for 3.1–6.2 percent of hospitalizations per year in America, and 0.13–0.21 percent of deaths.* These are only the reactions that are tracked; many reactions don't lead to hospital admission and are therefore not counted. Women, as well as the elderly, more than men, are at risk for hospital admissions due to drug reactions.

How to Use This Book

This book is an A-to-Z guide to health conditions that occur more frequently in women than men, that affect women differently, or that are related to women's hormones. It focuses on simple explanations of what the conditions are, how being female affects both symptoms and treatment, and goes on to give nutritional and other suggestions for improving health.

Many conditions that are not classically thought to be linked to female hormones and menstruation may in fact be closely coupled with our ovaries and their influence. An alarming number of doctors don't realize the extent to which our hormones orchestrate our disease processes, so it is up to you to connect the dots and start explaining this link to your doctors.

Read Part One first. It sets the scene for your basic information and orients you in using this book. Then go on to Part Two, which provides easy access and information for each condition—the dos and don'ts for diet and nutrients along with pertinent ideas to discuss with your doctor. When there is a long list of causes or symptoms, don't be overwhelmed. Read the list and figure out which apply to you.

When there is a long list of nutrients, it is sometimes hard to decide which ones are the most important for you. Discuss this with your doctor and refer to the charts on pages 35–39 to find which nutrients might be best to take for your body. Blood tests are a notoriously unreliable way to recognize nutrient deficiencies until very late in the game.

---

* Shen Li et al., *Chemical Research and Toxicology* 11:94–101, 1998.

HOW TO USE THIS BOOK

1. Read Part One first.

2. Look up your specific health condition in Part Two.

3. Before you take any nutrients, see "How to Take Nutrients" on page 37 and review with your doctor the interactions of nutrients with food, herbs, drugs, and each other in appendices I–L. You don't want to take an inappropriate nutrient. This section is a must!

4. Read whichever hormonal links pertain to you. For example, if your problem is related to excess estrogen, read *Estrogen Dominance* and the section on estrogen under *Hormones*.

5. Check the nutrient charts (pages 35–39) to get an idea of what deficiencies you may have. This will help you decide which nutrients listed under your condition are the best for you to use. Don't use all the nutrients listed.

6. Read the section on digestive enzymes (appendix F) to evaluate whether or not you need them. Taking nutrients and herbs without digesting them is useless.

7. Go to Stress-Reduction Techniques (page 52) for mind-body tools.

8. Check other sections that may be related to your health, such as *Wine and Alcoholic Beverages, Caffeine in Coffee and Tea, Fats and Essential Fatty Acids,* or *Immune Enhancement.*

9. Share with your doctor the information about hormone testing and lab resources in appendix A.

10. If you don't understand a word, look it up in the Glossary.

 Remember, the information in this book is to be used in conjunction with medical supervision and any necessary tests and conventional therapies.

My Story

My interest in women's health is partially destiny. I am a DES (diethylstilbestrol) daughter (my mother was given this synthetic estrogen early in her pregnancy), and this in-utero liability shape-shifted my life. Because I was exposed to such a potent chemical at such a vulnerable age, I have suffered with multiple female hormonal problems, undergone numerous surgeries, and found I couldn't have children. Living through a constant hormonal morass inspired me to investigate women's health with a fervor that has always startled those around me.

I look at it as making hormonal lemonade out of hormonal lemons.

Just out of college, I became an actress with Arena Stage in Washington, D.C., armed with enthusiasm as well as degrees in psychobiology and theater/communications. But I hit a hormonal wall that even surgery couldn't help. I went from doctor to doctor, getting more exhausted and frustrated. Finally, a nutritionist brought about the first relief I had felt from my symptoms. I was astonished at what natural diets and nutrients could do. This led to an extended fast in the mountains of Colorado, where I meditated and prayed for guidance: Should I return to acting or enter the health field? After hiking down the canyon, I went on to get a master's degree in nutrition, followed by a chiropractic degree, along with numerous courses at naturopathic colleges.

Dr. Jonathan V. Wright, the doctor who has promoted alternative medicine in so many ways, had a cutting-edge program of medical rotations in integrative medicine, to which I applied eagerly. (Wright developed his methods at his Tahoma medical clinic, in Kent, Washington.) The year he picked me, Dr. Alan R. Gaby was also there, and the three of us became colleagues and friends. For the last two decades we have been scouring the scientific journals on a monthly basis, finding nutritional studies relevant to clinical practice and employing a full-time researcher to keep on top of this monumental task.

When I was in practice in one of the first multidisciplinary clinics in the country, I designed one of the earliest product lines of natural nutrients for menopause (as well as for other female problems), since there has always been a question about the safety of DES daughters taking synthetic hormones. Later I ran my own clinic in Mt. View, California, working with cardiologists, internists, body workers, and nutritionists in an integrative approach to health care. I specialized in women's health and nutrition and saw thousands of patients, while also working as a nutritional consultant to other physicians.

Yet time and again I'd hit another hormonal nightmare. I would read volumes of scientific literature, searching for answers. I eventually learned how to treat a wide variety of female problems through diet, nutrition, and herbs. I shared much of this information in my radio show in the Bay Area, through my fourteen years of lecturing to M.D.s, dentists, acupuncturists, chiropractors, and naturopathic physicians on nutrition in clinical practice, and as a professor of nutrition at several colleges. I was chosen Chiropractor of the Year for all of California, picked a second time as Chiropractor of the Year in Northern California, and was invited to be a member of several medical societies in which I was the only nonmedical doctor.

But it wasn't easy coming down with almost every condition to which DES daughters are prone. Spiritual leaders remind us to use our lives as curriculum, that if suffering can serve, the pain hurts less. I have tried to embrace this concept.

I left practice almost a decade ago. This has enabled me to dive more fully into researching the scientific literature, a luxury most doctors don't have. I have extensively investigated the role of nutrition and hormones, especially the female estrogens, in health. Over the last four years I have hung out on the phone, often late at night, with many women who were suffering with hormonal diseases like breast cancer, assisting them in getting second opinions and interpretations of pathology reports.

My DES-instigated fate inspired me to write *Hormone Deception* (Contemporary/McGraw-Hill, 2000), which is about substances in our environment similar to weaker forms of DES that can act like hormones. I interviewed sixty top scientists in this field. People in the know said I couldn't reach Dr. John McLachlan, one of the most visionary men in the field of environmental estrogens and a father of DES research. But when Dr. McLachlan heard my story, he gave me many hours of input on the phone over three consecutive nights. He asked me to lecture in New Orleans and invited me to work with him, which is how I arrived at my present position as consulting scholar at the Center for Bioenvironmental Research (CBR), Tulane and Xavier Universities. The CBR studies everything to do with estrogens, and I get to be a communications expert for this internationally respected research institution and think tank.

I give talks nationally, such as at Newcomb College Center for Research on Women, and have taught in "hormone salons" (sharing emerging data) at different universities, rape-crisis centers, etc. But women and doctors alike everywhere are still understandably confused about hormones. This has led to my writing this book in an attempt to expand women's present understanding of the role of hormones in female health.

This work is my mission. But it can be extremely stressful, with ringing phones, publishing deadlines, website details, debating controversial new data with leading researchers, and the trials and tribulations of having three books coming out one after another. While juggling these chainsaws, I check in to see how my cells are doing. Do they feel frantic? Am I at risk of losing my health while helping others to find theirs? When I feel off-center, I do breath exercises, try to remember soft belly (page 55), and do whatever it takes to get back to a comfortable center. I sip a glass of water and look through my lace curtains at the piñon-dotted hillside.

And I remind myself that laughter and passion, not vitamins B or C, are our most essential nutrients.

PART ONE

This section of the book covers basic information to help you fully understand and effectively use the information about specific conditions you'll find in Part Two. Read this information, then refer back to it after learning about the conditions of particular interest to you. When taking nutrients or medications, you must *first* read the interactions section to make sure you are taking them safely.

HOW TO PUT YOUR HEALTH TOGETHER

You Are Worth It

Many women fall into the trap of doing for everyone else—their kids, parents, mates, and friends. They think they are not being good women, good people, if they put their own needs first. Ironically, you can only share with someone else what you already have. If you don't have a mango in your bag, you can't give it away. If you don't have your own health, how can you help keep others healthy?

If you give, give, and give away your love, time, and energy to everyone else without adequately giving to yourself, you can become depleted, angry, fatigued, and stressed. Take time for yourself. Eat well, spend some money or time on good exercise, food, and fun. When you have a full reservoir, you can freely give to others. If you are frazzled and constantly tired, not taking care of or loving yourself, those around you will treat you the way you treat yourself—with no respect. But when others see you living sensibly, having boundaries, and generally taking good care of yourself, they will respect you and feel better about themselves as well. A vital aspect of health is being aware of the choices you make about managing your body, mind, emotions, and spirit.

As it turns out, martyrdom really only works for martyrs.

Think it costs too much to take care of yourself? Not all lifestyle and alternative medicine choices are expensive. Start by improving

31

Sometimes natural solutions to health problems don't work or aren't the best choice. Certain cases require antibiotics or other medications or surgery. These decisions must be made by you and your doctor according to your individual situation. This book adds to your choices. It's not necessarily an either/or situation. Natural therapies can decrease the side effects of traditional treatments and can be used after a course of treatment is finished to help eliminate the cause of the disease and prevent its recurrence.

the quality of most of your meals, taking the time to walk, to sit and contemplate your navel, to breathe deeply and look around at what is happening. You can be the master of your domain rather than a stressed-out victim hanging on by her fingertips. Try simple solutions first; if they don't bring the energy and health you want and deserve, then go on to more sophisticated and costly answers. You're worth it.

Choosing a Doctor

A doctor is supposed to be your ally, your cohort. For decades we pictured a doctor as someone sitting patiently by a sick person's bed, dispensing medical wisdom with care and compassion. But times have changed. It is ironic and tragic that while more and more valid information about alternative medicine is piling up, most doctors are encouraged by large health-care organizations to see patients in shorter and shorter visits. In fact, health maintenance organizations (HMOs) sometimes sue doctors or drop them from insurance if they tell patients about alternative therapies.

It's not an easy time to be a doctor.

There are doctors who are open to new information, but they are constantly pressured to move patients quickly through their offices. They know what they learned in medical school, which (in most cases) was seriously deficient in nutrition and alternative medicine, and, if they have the time, they can just manage to keep up with what is happening in their own fields. They are told not to go beyond what is "usual and customary"—and alternative/integrative medicine is not usual and customary. To use alternative medicine effectively takes precious time—to review your lifestyle, diet, nutrients, and family history so that a complete program can be customized for you. Also, what most doctors hear about alternative medicine is biased. Inaccurate articles get quoted for years, and inflammatory literature gets passed around continually and fraudulently.

Once again women will have to lead the way. We have done it before and we can do it again. We need to stretch our physician's perceptions so they can appreciate what nutrition can do. If a doctor belittles your concerns or ideas, find another doctor or practitioner who understands your issues and can explain his or her recommendations. We need to point out the link between our health concerns and our cycling hormones. We have to learn not to be intimidated by angry or arrogant responses from medical personnel who dismiss us as being too far "out there." We need to bring alternative medicine into public acceptance for ourselves and our mothers and daughters and granddaughters.

Don't be afraid to ask questions of your doctors. Come prepared with your queries, test results, and the information you have gathered from outside sources and internal observation. Surf the web. If you don't know how to use the Internet, someone at the library can show you how. Don't be intimidated or made to feel small. Demand that your doctor review your diet, your nutrients, your family history—and for that, a three- to five-minute consultation simply won't do. Talk over your responses to lifestyle changes and nutrients. Keep customizing and optimizing your program. When you stand up for yourself, you are standing up for all of us.

There are well-documented stories of cancer patients who were told by their doctors that there was no hope and all that was left was to go home and get their affairs in order. One woman who had been handed just such a death sentence read online that several months earlier a university hospital had discovered a complete cure for her cancer, but her doctor had never heard about it. Well, this is how it is for all health care. We need to take an active part in finding out the facts and news about our particular conditions rather than relying solely on our doctors. Also, most physicians are not aware of the effectiveness of alternative therapies, and you may get negative reactions until you find a physician who understands how to work with these protocols.

Our health journeys can be long and winding and are extremely individual. You can go to numerous doctors before finding the one who correctly diagnoses underactive thyroid as the cause of your headaches, while your best friend may have headaches due to a magnesium deficiency caused by chronic stress. This is the art of medicine, mixed in with the science. There are no simple answers.

Good caring doctors are out there. Look for doctors who will be inspired to work with you. Check out holistic physicians, naturopaths, chiropractors, nurse practitioners, and osteopaths. Pass their names on to other women. Start demanding that health insurance companies cover their services if they don't already do so. And keep working at your health, understanding that your doctors are advocates, but it is up to you to work hand in hand with them.

Nutrients

Most blood tests are notorious for not picking up nutrient deficiencies until late in the game when vital stores are extremely depleted and have been so for a long time. Our nutrients actually speak to us through body signals. Simple physical signs—along with general symptoms like energy levels, sleeping patterns, irritability or mood changes, vitality, digestion, and various other personal symptoms—are your best guide to what nutrients are optimal for your body.

Most women have an average need for most nutrients, which can be met by a multivitamin/mineral supplement, with greater requirements for one to three specific nutrients. All women should take a multivitamin/mineral supplement that does not contain iron unless blood tests clearly indicate they really require iron. Excess iron can promote heart disease and cancer. Look for multivitamins that contain mixed tocopherols (vitamin E).

Check the physical signs on the charts on pages 35–39 to see where you may have persistent signs, especially if they come up in several places, that suggest which particular nutrients you need to supplement in addition to your regular multivitamin/mineral. If you have several symptoms, take nutrients singly along with a backup multivitamin/mineral supplement for several months. After your

Whole Body Nutrient Diagnosis
Physical signs suggesting low levels of nutrients

Blood tests often don't pick up inadequacies until tissue levels are extremely low. Body "signals" often occur first and help you identify which nutrients you need to supplement as well as monitor your progress.

Inadequate levels of vitamin A
- Poor night vision and dark adaptation
- Dry eyes
- Tendency to recurrent infections and colds
- Tendency to food allergies
- Tendency to diarrhea
- Rough or "chicken skin" on arms and/or thighs
- Chronic acne
- Crohn's disease
- Peptic ulcers

Inadequate levels of magnesium
- Tendency to constipation
- Tendency to spasm/cramp/twitch
  (especially in neck, back, abdomen, calf)
- Chronic stress and/or nervousness/anxiety
- Noise sensitivity
- Irregular heartbeats
- Depression and/or sense of doom
- Tendency to irritable bowel syndrome
- PMS
- B$_6$ and/or essential fatty acid deficiencies
- Excess ear wax and/or dandruff
- Tendency to breast problems like cysts

Inadequate levels of zinc
- Poor sweet taste so overconsume sweets
- Slow wound healing
- Scars easily
- Feet smell poorly
- Tendency toward infections
- Tendency toward diarrhea
- Acne and/or rashes
- White spots on fingernails is suggestive
- Excess exposure to copper, iron, calcium, magnesium, and/or N-acetyl-cysteine without adequate supplementation of zinc
- History of Crohn's disease

Inadequate levels of digestive enzymes
- Chronic bloating, gas, intestinal discomfort, maldigestion
- Frequently feel cold in hands and/or feet
- Do not respond to improving lifestyle and/or taking nutrients
- Chronic skin, gallbladder, asthma, food allergy, digestive disorder, menstrual difficulties
- Dentures hurt, can't get them to fit well
- Tendency to tongue pain
- Chronic skin, hair, or nail problems
- Chronic nutrient deficiencies that do not respond to supplementation
- Unopposed estrogen problems that do not respond to treatment
- Any health problems, not just intestinal, that do not respond to treatment
- Feel worse after eating

Inadequate levels of calcium
- Muscle cramps and/or twitching
  (especially around eyes and in calves)
- Nervousness and/or anxiety
- Irregular heartbeats
- Tendency toward headaches
- Chronic stress, maldigestion, gallbladder problems
- Heavy caffeine/sugar/ protein consumption

Imbalance or deficiency of amino acids
- Attention deficit disorders (ADHD)
- Mood swings
- Learning disabilities
- Poor resistance to healing

Inadequate levels of B vitamins
- Chronic fatigue and/or moodiness, irritability
- Afternoon energy slump
- Poor digestion
- Frequently feel cold, or cold hands and feet
- Thin, splitting hair and nails suggests inadequate levels of biotin and/or stomach acid or essential fatty acids
- Tendency to tongue and mouth pain

Inadequate levels of vitamin C
- Bruises easily
- Puffy and/or red, bleeding gums
- Poor resistance to illness
- Injure joints and/or soft tissue easily

Inadequate levels of vitamin B$_6$
- Poor dream recall
- Excess ear wax and/or dandruff
- PMS
- Water retention especially in fingers and/or around eyes in morning
- Swollen and/or stiff fingers in morning
- Carpal tunnel syndrome
- Magnesium deficiency that doesn't respond to taking magnesium
- Essential fatty acid (EFA) deficiency that doesn't respond to taking EFAs
- Tendency to breast problems like cysts

Inadequate levels (or imbalance) of essential fatty acids
- Rough and/or chicken skin on upper arms and thighs
- Ridged, cracking, peeling nails
- Magnesium or B$_6$ deficiencies that do not respond to supplementation
- Excess ear wax and/or dandruff
- Tendency to inflamed soft tissue and/or joints
- Severe dry skin; cracks in heels, bad cuticles, red cuticles
- Tendency to breast problems like cysts
- Unopposed estrogen/ low progesterone problems
- Chronic respiratory problems
- Tendency to constipation
- Tendency to skin problems

Whole Body Nutrient Diagnosis (continued)

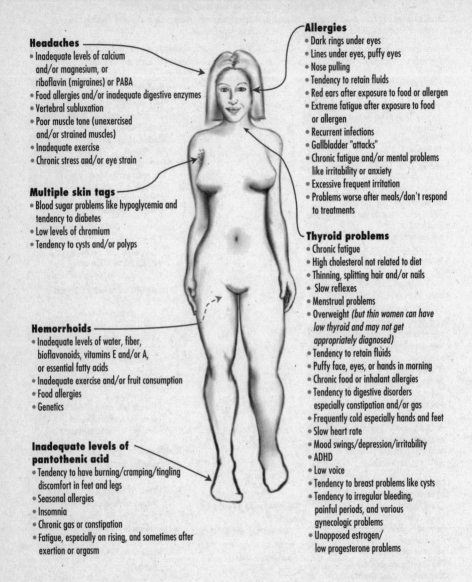

Headaches
- Inadequate levels of calcium and/or magnesium, or riboflavin (migraines) or PABA
- Food allergies and/or inadequate digestive enzymes
- Vertebral subluxation
- Poor muscle tone (unexercised and/or strained muscles)
- Inadequate exercise
- Chronic stress and/or eye strain

Multiple skin tags
- Blood sugar problems like hypoglycemia and tendency to diabetes
- Low levels of chromium
- Tendency to cysts and/or polyps

Hemorrhoids
- Inadequate levels of water, fiber, bioflavonoids, vitamins E and/or A, or essential fatty acids
- Inadequate exercise and/or fruit consumption
- Food allergies
- Genetics

Inadequate levels of pantothenic acid
- Tendency to have burning/cramping/tingling discomfort in feet and legs
- Seasonal allergies
- Insomnia
- Chronic gas or constipation
- Fatigue, especially on rising, and sometimes after exertion or orgasm

Allergies
- Dark rings under eyes
- Lines under eyes, puffy eyes
- Nose pulling
- Tendency to retain fluids
- Red ears after exposure to food or allergen
- Extreme fatigue after exposure to food or allergen
- Recurrent infections
- Gallbladder "attacks"
- Chronic fatigue and/or mental problems like irritability or anxiety
- Excessive frequent irritation
- Problems worse after meals/don't respond to treatments

Thyroid problems
- Chronic fatigue
- High cholesterol not related to diet
- Thinning, splitting hair and/or nails
- Slow reflexes
- Menstrual problems
- Overweight *(but thin women can have low thyroid and may not get appropriately diagnosed)*
- Tendency to retain fluids
- Puffy face, eyes, or hands in morning
- Chronic food or inhalant allergies
- Tendency to digestive disorders especially constipation and/or gas
- Frequently cold especially hands and feet
- Slow heart rate
- Mood swings/depression/irritability
- ADHD
- Low voice
- Tendency to breast problems like cysts
- Tendency to irregular bleeding, painful periods, and various gynecologic problems
- Unopposed estrogen/low progesterone problems

symptoms go away for several weeks, switch to taking only the multivitamin. When a long list of nutrients is recommended in Part Two for a specific condition, the information from these charts will help you decide which nutrients are the most important ones for you. The listed nutrients are options, and it is not meant for you to take all the ones on the list. Use your understanding of your body to pick the nutrients that are most important for you.

Nail Diagnosis

(These signs suggest these problems. Any unusual ongoing changes should be told to your doctor.)

Splitting cuticles
- Essential fatty acid imbalance or deficiency
- Overconsumption of processed oils
- Food allergies
- Inadequate levels of pancreatic enzymes and/or bile

Splitting, breaking nails
- Inadequate levels of biotin
- Inadequate levels of essential fatty acids
- Inadequate levels of vitamin B_6
- Inadequate levels of magnesium
- Low stomach acid

Excessive vertical ridges
- Inadequate levels of B vitamins, especially B_{12}
- Maldigestion
- Gallbladder problems
- A slight amount of ridging after forty years is okay, but more is suggestive of a problem

White Spots
- Inadequate levels of zinc

Moons
(half moon at base of nail)
- Large—suggest good constitutional reserve of energy. Should heal quickly
- Small—short on most nails, especially thumbs, suggests lower constitutional energy. May take longer to respond to natural programs.
- Large moons on little fingers, plus ear lobe creases and/or reddish tip of tongue suggest tendency to heart problems

Beau's lines
(deep horizontal ridge)
- Illness *(such as bronchitis)*
- Maldigestion
- Malnutrition in general
- Local trauma
- Nervous scratching
- Adrenal stress

Pitting
- Tendency to immune problems
- Inadequate levels of selenium
- Maldigestion

Pale or bluish nails
- Iron deficiency

Yellowish, bulging, bending, breaking nails
- Suggest fungal infection like candidiasis

Clubbing
(nails grow downward, end of finger noticeably enlarges, nails break in odd ways)
- Sign of poor oxygenation linked to various serious lung, liver, or kidney diseases. See doctor.

How to Take Nutrients

The recommended dosages for nutrients throughout this book are meant for adults. Children and lighter-weight or severely debilitated women or women with severe chemical sensitivities are usually treated with lower dosages, based on body weight and recommendations from the physicians who understand their particular needs. Women who are pregnant, about to undergo surgery, or have advanced kidney failure, liver insufficiency, or history of liver disease

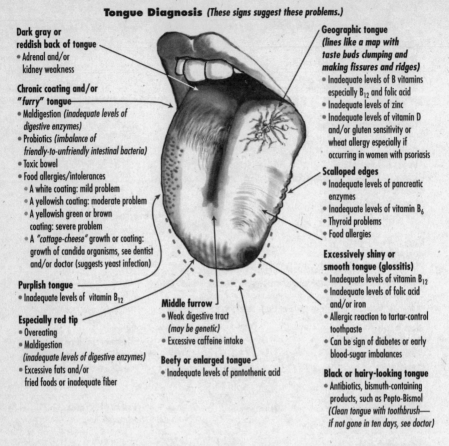

Tongue Diagnosis *(These signs suggest these problems.)*

Dark gray or reddish back of tongue
- Adrenal and/or kidney weakness

Chronic coating and/or "furry" tongue
- Maldigestion *(inadequate levels of digestive enzymes)*
- Probiotics *(imbalance of friendly-to-unfriendly intestinal bacteria)*
- Toxic bowel
- Food allergies/intolerances
  - A white coating: mild problem
  - A yellowish coating: moderate problem
  - A yellowish green or brown coating: severe problem
  - A *"cottage-cheese"* growth or coating: growth of candida organisms, see dentist and/or doctor (suggests yeast infection)

Purplish tongue
- Inadequate levels of vitamin B_{12}

Especially red tip
- Overeating
- Maldigestion *(inadequate levels of digestive enzymes)*
- Excessive fats and/or fried foods or inadequate fiber

Middle furrow
- Weak digestive tract *(may be genetic)*
- Excessive caffeine intake

Beefy or enlarged tongue
- Inadequate levels of pantothenic acid

Geographic tongue *(lines like a map with taste buds clumping and making fissures and ridges)*
- Inadequate levels of B vitamins especially B_{12} and folic acid
- Inadequate levels of zinc
- Inadequate levels of vitamin D and/or gluten sensitivity or wheat allergy especially if occurring in women with psoriasis

Scalloped edges
- Inadequate levels of pancreatic enzymes
- Inadequate levels of vitamin B_6
- Thyroid problems
- Food allergies

Excessively shiny or smooth tongue (glossitis)
- Inadequate levels of vitamin B_{12}
- Inadequate levels of folic acid and/or iron
- Allergic reaction to tartar-control toothpaste
- Can be sign of diabetes or early blood-sugar imbalances

Black or hairy-looking tongue
- Antibiotics, bismuth-containing products, such as Pepto-Bismol *(Clean tongue with toothbrush—if not gone in ten days, see doctor)*

may develop toxicity from nutrients even at low dosages. Supplementation should be done with supervision and extreme caution.

Most of the healing programs recommended in this book are meant to be taken for several weeks to several months. Once symptoms start to improve for ten days to one month, try cutting down dosages to see if you can maintain the improvement at lower levels. Most conditions do not require ongoing supplementation. Occasionally intravenous (IV) or intramuscular (IM) nutrients are suggested for those who may be very low in a nutrient or whose ability to absorb the nutrient in other forms may be hampered. IV and IM nutrients can kick-start the body, like priming the pump, and are short-term solutions. Work with your doctor. In some cases, good health may require ongoing low-dose maintenance nutrients. For example, eating a whole-foods diet only provides 15 IU of vitamin E per day, while the average woman does best with 100–300 IU per day.

Lip and Mouth Diagnosis
(These signs suggest these problems.)

Your mouth reflects daily changes in your intestinal tract. Monitoring ongoing signals of the mouth gives you information.

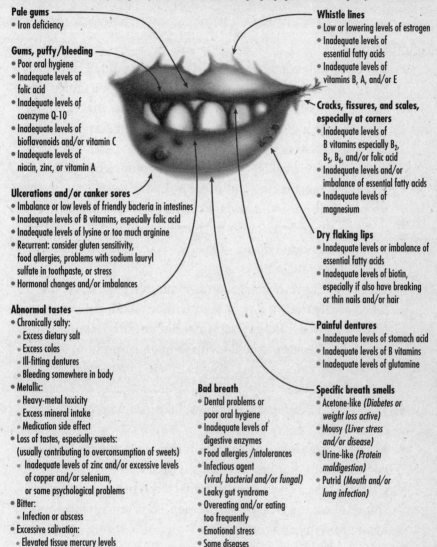

Pale gums
- Iron deficiency

Gums, puffy/bleeding
- Poor oral hygiene
- Inadequate levels of folic acid
- Inadequate levels of coenzyme Q-10
- Inadequate levels of bioflavonoids and/or vitamin C
- Inadequate levels of niacin, zinc, or vitamin A

Ulcerations and/or canker sores
- Imbalance or low levels of friendly bacteria in intestines
- Inadequate levels of B vitamins, especially folic acid
- Inadequate levels of lysine or too much arginine
- Recurrent: consider gluten sensitivity, food allergies, problems with sodium lauryl sulfate in toothpaste, or stress
- Hormonal changes and/or imbalances

Abnormal tastes
- Chronically salty:
  - Excess dietary salt
  - Excess colas
  - Ill-fitting dentures
  - Bleeding somewhere in body
- Metallic:
  - Heavy-metal toxicity
  - Excess mineral intake
  - Medication side effect
- Loss of tastes, especially sweets: (usually contributing to overconsumption of sweets)
  - Inadequate levels of zinc and/or excessive levels of copper and/or selenium, or some psychological problems
- Bitter:
  - Infection or abscess
- Excessive salivation:
  - Elevated tissue mercury levels

Bad breath
- Dental problems or poor oral hygiene
- Inadequate levels of digestive enzymes
- Food allergies /intolerances
- Infectious agent (viral, bacterial and/or fungal)
- Leaky gut syndrome
- Overeating and/or eating too frequently
- Emotional stress
- Some diseases

Whistle lines
- Low or lowering levels of estrogen
- Inadequate levels of essential fatty acids
- Inadequate levels of vitamins B, A, and/or E

Cracks, fissures, and scales, especially at corners
- Inadequate levels of B vitamins especially B_2, B_5, B_6, and/or folic acid
- Inadequate levels and/or imbalance of essential fatty acids
- Inadequate levels of magnesium

Dry flaking lips
- Inadequate levels or imbalance of essential fatty acids
- Inadequate levels of biotin, especially if also have breaking or thin nails and/or hair

Painful dentures
- Inadequate levels of stomach acid
- Inadequate levels of B vitamins
- Inadequate levels of glutamine

Specific breath smells
- Acetone-like *(Diabetes or weight loss active)*
- Mousy *(Liver stress and/or disease)*
- Urine-like *(Protein maldigestion)*
- Putrid *(Mouth and/or lung infection)*

When embarking on a healing program, add any new item at the rate of one per day, whether it be a nutrient, herb, exercise, or meditation technique. In this way your body acclimates to new things, and if one of them does not agree with you, it can easily be identified and eliminated. *Sometimes people don't get beneficial results from nutrients or herbs because they are either low in digestive enzymes or need detoxification or are starting too many things at once.* Sometimes taking digestive enzymes with nutrients for the first several weeks helps in acclimating to supplementation.

Helpful Notes

- Some sections contain a long list of recommended nutrients. Be aware that holistic physicians and health food stores often carry supplements that are inclusive formulas that combine all the recommended nutrients for that particular condition. You don't have to buy a long list of separate pills, making it easier on your pocketbook and on your stomach.
- When I suggest taking a nutrient in *divided doses*, that means to split up the amount and take it at different times during the day. For example, if it says to "take bromelain, 500–1,000 mg per day in divided doses," take 250–500 mg in the morning and 250–500 mg in the evening.
- Water-soluble nutrients, such as vitamins B and C, can be taken at any time of day with or without food. However, some sensitive folks get intestinal discomfort or nausea unless they take supplements with food or throughout a meal. And in rare cases, some women absorb even these nutrients better with food.
- When taking isolated B vitamins, take a backup vitamin B complex.
- When taking isolated vitamins or minerals, always take a backup multivitamin/mineral supplement.
- Calcium taken on an empty stomach can promote kidney stones in some predisposed women, so take with food and away from thyroid medication.
- Take most amino acids, herbs, and probiotics on an *empty stomach* (20 minutes before or one hour after eating).
- Essential fatty acids: Rotate whichever essential fatty acids you use, such as flaxseed oil, fish oil, and evening primrose oil, and take extra vitamin E for balance and oxidative protection. If you have trouble tolerating the oils, try enterically coated forms (tablets or capsules with a special coating that

prevents their release and absorption until they reach the intestines), or take with pancreatic enzymes (pages 468 and 469). Take with meals that contain fats.

- Fat-soluble nutrients, such as vitamin E, fat-soluble coenzyme Q-10, and essential oils are also best taken with meals that contain some fat.
- Fish oils can raise blood sugar, so work with a doctor when taking high doses of these nutrients. If this happens to you, try adding vitamin E, pectin, or garlic, which may stop these possible side effects. One tablespoon of cod liver oil equals many capsules, so consider the oral form, but avoid fish oils if you are on pharmaceutical blood thinners.
- Some supplements taken on an empty stomach can cause nausea, especially zinc, copper, iron, and 100 mg or more of niacinamide. *Bite tablets in half for the best effect.*
- Too much magnesium can cause loose stools and/or diarrhea, but this goes away when you reduce the dose.
- Bruising after beginning supplements suggests an allergic reaction to something in them.

Where to Purchase Nutrients

Most of the products mentioned in this book can be purchased from health food stores and vitamin discount houses (many of which have catalogs or can be found on the Internet). Holistic practitioners often sell these products as well. Many health food store products do not contain substances like binders, fillers, and colorings, but be sure to read all labels. Not everything sold in a health food store is healthy. A number of brand name products have one name when sold through a health-care practitioner and another in the health food stores. For example, doctors sell Allergy Research products, while health food stores sell a similar line called Ecological Formulas. Unfortunately, studies have demonstrated that just because a product has a brand name does not mean it's better for you, although I have found that the products sold through both practitioners and health food stores seem to be of the highest quality. Pharmacies tend to sell more inexpensive lines, which may not be as reliable.

Use only reputable brands of nutrients. Studies show that some less than reputable companies are putting in fewer nutrients than are listed on the labels. If you're not feeling better from your nutrients or herbs, you may not be getting the dose you think you're taking. This has been shown in various products such as St. John's wort or *Lactobacillus acidophilus*. Also, you can have a toxic reaction to any vitamin, mineral, essential oil, or herb, especially herbs. Some herbs have been found to be contaminated—another reason to use reputable brands and not to take anything without checking with appropriate health professionals. Report any reaction to your doctor. Most herbal treatments should be done for several weeks to one or two months at most, not for the long term! If you are already taking medication, work with your doctor to lower the dosage while adding nutrients. Stay monitored.

 Another reason you might not be benefiting from your nutrients/herbs is that you are not sufficiently digesting and absorbing them. See appendix F.

Lifestyle Factors

What? Me Exercise?

If I were up against a wall with a gun to my head, and my assailant was demanding to know which was more important, nutrition or exercise, I would have to admit that exercise is up there in a class all its own. And I say this even though I have been a nutritionist all my adult life. I know lots of regular exercisers who eat a poor diet yet still experience better health than fastidious eaters who are couch potatoes.

Regular exercise is a must!

Most of us have a thousand reasons why we don't have time to exercise, but it has to be like brushing your teeth, something you just do as a regular habit. Exercise has many benefits. One in particular is that exercise creates more *mitochondria*, the body's cellular energy machines. So while many women don't exercise because they are too tired, the irony is that exercising regularly eventually gives us more energy. It usually takes six to eight weeks to see the benefits begin rolling in, like better muscle tone and increased energy on rising and throughout the day. Those first weeks can be hell, and you may need to cajole and discipline yourself to do it, but keep remembering that soon you will be feeling more alive and more vital.

What kind of exercise is best? Any kind that you will do. But don't get stuck in an exercise rut. The body is clever and accommodates to our exercise regimes, so smart programs alter the exercises a little every few weeks to keep positive stresses and benefits coming from the sweat of our brows.

The best exercise programs for women combine cardiovascular workouts with resistance weight training of some kind. This protects our hearts and bones and keeps our metabolism up so we can enjoy more food, burn more calories, and maintain healthy muscles, bones, and organs.

Particular conditions may emphasize one over another form of exercise. For example, weight lifting is not good for treating high blood pressure, whereas it is optimal for preventing bone loss. I will discuss these issues under specific topics later in the book.

A body that is regularly exercised gets injured less, heals quicker, and feels better to live in. It's a proven fact that doctors who do not exercise or are overweight themselves often don't encourage someone with a moderate problem to work out or lose weight. You have to take care of yourself. There are many excellent books on exercise available, but I can't emphasize enough the power of motion. Need more encouragement? Studies show that moderate aerobic exercise, even without eating less, causes weight loss, particularly around your middle—no ifs, ands, or buts. Do it!

Are You Confused About Diet? Make It Simple

You eat at least twenty-one meals a week. Those who eat more frequent, smaller portions have even more. This means there are plenty of meals available for getting quality nutrition by having the majority of your meals contain sensible and healthy food choices. You don't

USE IT OR LOSE IT

Exercising three times a week only keeps the fitness you already have, so you need to exercise five to six times a week if you are on an improvement program. Vary your program to trick your incredibly clever body.

have to follow a rigid diet. *Perfect eating doesn't guarantee perfect health, and it's too stressful to worry about being perfect. That is not healthy.* Far more important is balance, moderation, and peace. Don't agonize over food. It is what you eat *most of the time* that adds up to health. If you occasionally want to eat out, consume junk food, or splurge on a great dessert, do it. Allow yourself that flexibility, knowing you have basic quality nutrition most of the week.

How to Begin, Live, and End Your Day

- *Start your day* with one to two glasses of filtered water, an antioxidant, B complex (25–50 mg), and 500–1,000 mg of vitamin C.
- *Eat colorfully*—Food colors come from different flavonoids, chlorophyll, carotenoids, and minerals. The more colors on your plate—luscious reds, greens, yellows, purples, oranges—the more beneficial nutrients in your body. If all your food is white—as in rice, potatoes, chicken, pasta, milk, cheese, etc.—you're not eating enough fruits and vegetables. Add tomato puree to foods several times a week for a big hit of carotenoids and lycopenes (health-promoting substances).
- *Vary fruits and veggies*—Try to eat at least three different vegetables and two different fruits a day. Fruits can be either half or whole portions of the fruit. Vary the color and type. This includes juicing your fruits and vegetables. Don't drink store-bought pasteurized and processed juices, which don't contain any fiber, or mix the juice with half or two-thirds water to reduce sugar exposure.
- *Keep it interesting*—The real secret of healthy eating is to consume different foods over the course of a week rather than eating the same basic ones each day. Each type of food has different amino acids, minerals, vitamins, etc., so variety is indeed the spice of a healthy life and prevents various adverse reactions to foods.
- *Watch portion size*—Most people overeat, which is a major cause of stress on the body. We have come to accept trough-sized portions as normal. An optimal serving of fish or meat (3–4 oz.) is about the size of a deck of cards.

A Balanced Dinner Plate

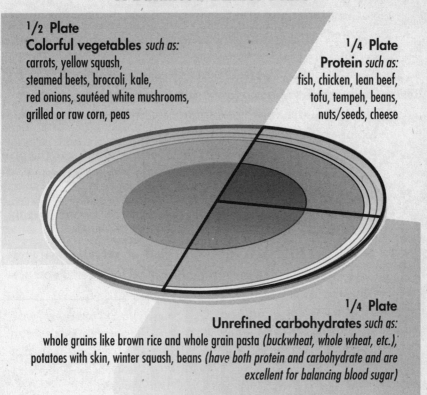

¹/₂ Plate
Colorful vegetables *such as:*
carrots, yellow squash,
steamed beets, broccoli, kale,
red onions, sautéed white mushrooms,
grilled or raw corn, peas

¹/₄ Plate
Protein *such as:*
fish, chicken, lean beef,
tofu, tempeh, beans,
nuts/seeds, cheese

¹/₄ Plate
Unrefined carbohydrates *such as:*
whole grains like brown rice and whole grain pasta *(buckwheat, whole wheat, etc.),*
potatoes with skin, winter squash, beans *(have both protein and carbohydrate and are
excellent for balancing blood sugar)*

- *Include whole grains*—Try to eat at least one whole grain a day.
  Try cooked whole grains, such as rolled oats, brown rice, millet, wheat or rye berries, or sprouted-grain breads, muffins,
  or whole-grain pastas. Food made from processed white
  flour is not a healthy choice. Processed wheat has some forty
  nutrients removed and only two to five put back in (and
  then it's called "enriched"!). Many psychological problems are made worse by inadequate B vitamins, yet we
  remove the Bs from whole grains, get depressed, then take
  medication.
- *Eat beans*—Eat some beans such as mung, azuki, garbanzo,
  lentils, fava, or red beans several times a week. If you have
  trouble digesting them, try cooking beans by soaking them
  first with ginger or adding seaweed to the water.

- *Nibble on seeds and nuts*—Snack on raw seeds and nuts (for flavor, mix different kinds together, and add in some roasted or flavored ones). Uncooked nuts retain their essential oils. Again, variety is the key; try walnuts, pumpkin seeds, almonds, sunflower seeds, pecans, cashews, hazelnuts, etc. Try mixing with various organic dried fruits like cranberries or raisins. Nuts should be *substituted* for other fats, not added on top of a high-fat diet!
- *Remember healthy proteins*—Try to consume one vegetable protein (like soy or beans) and one animal protein a day (such as yogurt or eggs or turkey).
- *End your day* with one to two glasses of filtered water and an antioxidant.
- *Eat this way for at least ten to fifteen meals a week*, and then you can be more flexible the rest of the time. However, if you are trying to use nutrition to heal a serious health condition, you may need to be more strict for the first several months.

> You have at least twenty-one meals in a week. Don't agonize over all your meals. It is what you eat *most of the time* that adds up to health.

Simple Food Facts

- *Overeating is worse than eating junk food.* Get this fact into your head. Most of us overeat while our cells starve. Overeating creates a tremendous stress on the intestinal tract and our overall health. Eat less, chew more, have faith your hunger will stop within ten minutes after finishing your first plateful and walking away from the table. There is no perfect diet. The closest diet to perfection is undereating (and exercise)!
- *Check your symptoms in relationship to food.* If you have depression, headaches, or fatigue when you miss a meal, this suggests low blood sugar. Feeling better avoiding food, or feeling worse right after or within hours of consuming food, suggests food allergies, hypersensitivities, or low digestive enzymes.
- *Women are more sensitive than men.* They have more adverse reactions to alcohol, caffeine, refined sugars, and tobacco than

men. (Life isn't fair.) Avoid daily excessive consumption of the first three, and don't smoke! Avoid passive smoke, too.

- *Don't eat while doing anything else*—driving, talking on the phone, standing up, tickling your beloved, or rushing. Stop, bite, and chew!

- *Eating organic is not a fad*—it's sensible. Pesticides and related substances are being actively studied and linked to widespread health problems. Try to buy as much organic food as possible, especially fatty ones like dairy, butter, and oils. Organic food not only has less bad stuff, it has better, higher quality nutrients. Recent data from the U.S. Department of Agriculture indicates that there are some drastic drops (in comparison to vegetables several decades ago) in the vitamin and mineral content of nonorganic vegetables, such as a 50 percent drop in calcium found in broccoli, an 88 percent drop of iron in watercress, and a 40 percent drop in the vitamin C content of cauliflower. The National Academy of Sciences issued an alert noting that it takes twice as many vegetables to get the daily requirements of vitamin A as previously thought. Support your local organic growers.

- *Eating sweets can throw everything off balance*—Sleep and workouts have many health benefits that can be blocked by eating sweet snacks or juices, including electrolyte drinks, before, during, or after workouts or thirty to sixty minutes before going to bed. Try to consume simple sugars (fruit juices, candy, power bars, etc.) before 1:00 to 3:00 P.M., especially if you are trying to lose weight or have insulin resistance. See *Insulin Resistance*.

- *Balance carbs with protein.* When most Americans started to consume diets lower in fat, they unfortunately added too many carbohydrates, which turned out to be a bad idea. Instead, consume a balanced ratio of protein to carbohydrates, making sure to avoid excessive consumption of white pasta, veggie chips, and many of the foods that look like health foods but aren't. Whole-grain pastas are available in health food stores. Especially avoid *processed* cereals and excess carbs first thing in the morning and later in the evening.

- *Include sprouted grains*—Sprouted-grain products cause fewer allergic reactions than whole-wheat flour products and are high in nutrients.
- *Cook smart*—Soak seeds in water overnight to give excellent flavor and enhanced nutrition. Eat whole or blend with water to make seed milks. Cut onions right before eating. Let garlic sit for ten minutes after removing skin for higher nutritional value. Blackened meat or fish (from grilling or broiling to the point where it turns black) contains unhealthy substances. Try healthy cooking methods, such as poaching meats and fish in vegetable broth, or water with a little wine, or part water to part chicken broth, or water with added olive oil and soy sauce. Save the water you steam veggies in and mix with olive oil, soy sauce, and garlic or other items like bouillon to make tasty and nutritious sauces. Use tomato paste and juice generously.

Simple Fat Facts
- *Academy Award–winning fats*—fish (not shellfish), olives, nuts, seeds (especially pumpkin and flaxseeds), and beans (like soy). Reduce saturated (mostly animal) fats and avoid and replace trans unsaturated fats (most margarines and shortenings) with oils like olive, walnut, flax, and fish.
- *Margarine myth*—Margarine and shortening both have trans fatty acids that actually elevate bad cholesterol and lower good cholesterol. The margarine advertising campaign (meant to maximize profits, of course) had encouraged the public to believe that margarine is better than butter. Trans fatty acids in the diet have been implicated in thirty thousand premature deaths per year. *We hated being manipulated by men, so we scrupulously avoid being manipulated by advertising.*
- *Extra-virgin* dark *green olive oil* protects arteries and heart more than yellowish or refined olive oils. Olive oil protects against various cancers and makes skin soft. Cook with olive oil.
- *Reduce oil in sautéing and frying* by mixing half oil with half water in the pan. To reduce splattering, lower heat or get a splatter screen to put around the burner.

- *Stir-frying is healthier than deep frying.* Use olive or peanut oil, which are more stable and create fewer toxic substances when heated than other oils.
- *Oxidized oils are bad for us.* Avoid high-temperature cooking with butter or lard. Poaching or baking creates less toxicity than broiling and scrambling. So when you eat eggs, poach or boil much of the time and enjoy omelets on Sunday morning. That's balance. Roasting nuts oxidizes some of their fats. Eat most nuts raw.
- *Fats store chemicals.* If you're looking to save money and only buy some organic foods, focus on organic oils, butter, olives, meats, and nuts. Cut fat off chicken and meat before cooking.
- *Fats to avoid in excess*—animal fats and palm kernel oil. Don't use polyunsaturated oils (corn, sunflower, safflower oil) too often: when heated in air, they produce toxic substances. Until more is known about the purity of canola oil, it's best to avoid it on a daily basis unless it's organic. When using soy and grain milks, avoid regular use of those with added oils and consume nonfat ones.
- *Refrigerate nuts, butter, and vegetable oils;* keeping them at room temperature creates oxidized fats.
- *Avoid dried egg products, powdered milk, nondairy creamers, and processed meats,* which all contain unhealthy fats.
- *Fish fats*—Eating two to three fish meals per week protects your heart and body. It reduces the risk of stroke by 50 percent. Fish is rich in omega-3 fatty acids which contain protective substances called EPA and DHA. See *Fats and Essential Fatty Acids* in Part Two. Shellfish (shrimp, crab, crawfish, and scallops) are high in cholesterol; eat them sparingly. Pregnant and nursing women, and children, should avoid predator fish (tuna, shark, and swordfish), which are more likely to contain toxic chemicals, such as mercury, in their fat. In general, avoid the fattier parts of fish.

> Eating higher-quality fat is a more effective way to prevent heart disease in women than reducing overall fat in the diet!

What to Drink or Not to Drink, That Is Our Question

Drink five to eight 8-oz. glasses of water a day depending on how many fruits and veggies you eat and how much tea or other beverages (nonalcoholic) you drink. More fruits and vegetables reduces water demands slightly. The Nationwide Food Consumption Survey suggests that a major portion of Americans may be chronically mildly dehydrated. Just 2 percent dehydration (2 percent loss of body weight daily) has been linked to a variety of problems: poorer physiologic performance; chronic headaches; kidney stones; various cancers, including breast; mitral valve prolapse; poor overall health in the elderly; and on and on. Drink water!

Start the day with one or two glasses and end the day with one.

Confused by all the different types of water? This should help.

Spring water flows naturally from an underground source to the surface. *Mineral water* comes from an underground source and contains minerals like sodium and calcium (a good source of calcium). *Drinking water* is tap water that has been filtered and disinfected. *Distilled water* is vaporized and then condensed back into pure water minus minerals and oxygen (which is not a good thing). Being void of these substances makes distilled water aggressive, meaning it leaches copper, lead, and even aluminum out of your pipes and cooking utensils into your water and foods. On the other hand, *reverse osmosis* (RO) duplicates the body's own filtering membrane system, leaves in some minerals, keeps in oxygen (which gives it freshness and great taste), and is less aggressive than distilled water. Carbon filters, distilling, and RO processing all remove radon from water. However, RO removes more radioactive particles and aluminum (often added at the water-treatment plant as part of the cleaning process). If you drink distilled or RO water, it is a good idea to take a multiple mineral supplement. *Sparkling water* is filtered tap or spring water that is naturally carbonated or has added carbonation, but not necessarily the harmful phosphoric acid added to many colas.

Bottled waters taste better than tap water because bottlers use ozone as a disinfectant rather than chlorine. Ozone is odorless and tasteless. It's rarely used in public water systems because its effectiveness wears off when it's exposed to air.

When buying bottled water, look for brands that contain calcium and magnesium and are low in sodium. Ideally, spring water should state the specific source of the spring. Try to purchase water in glass containers or hard plastic. Soft plastic containers are implicated in leaching potentially harmful substances into the water. Don't reuse plastic bottles.

Water in the Air?

Most of us are concerned with the purity of the water we drink, yet two-thirds of our exposure to the chemicals in water comes from what we inhale and what is absorbed by our skin through showers and baths, flushing toilets, and running dishwashers and washing machines. Home filtration systems located at the source of entry, where the water comes into your home, make good economic and health sense. Call my hometown water guru for customized home filtration systems: Craig Friedman at Good Water Company, 505-471-9036.

Mineral and sparkling waters (without phosphoric acid) do not dissolve bone like colas do. Commercial colas add phosphoric acid, and this acidity hastens bone loss. *Just one cola a day has been shown to promote bone loss*, and teenagers who consume daily colas may be at increased risk of bone fractures. Some natural sodas use fruit acids instead of phosphoric acid, which may not accelerate bone loss or may do so to a lesser degree.

Black tea has substances that protect our bones and heart with flavonoids. It also contains caffeine, though not as much as coffee. On one hand, caffeine has a better reputation these days. It improves cognition (how we think) and is being studied as a protective agent against cancer. On the other hand, caffeine continues to be implicated as a cause of lumpy, painful breasts, anxiety, insomnia, damage to chromosomes, irregular heartbeats, early fetal loss, etc.; and tea and coffee contain numerous acids that in *excess* are *not* a bone's best friend.

Milk is a good source of calcium but also has a troublesome side. Skim milk, fat-free dairy sources, and yogurt, as well as full-fat dairy products like butter and cheese, contain various substances that actually protect us against certain cancers (like colon cancer) and recurrences (as with bladder cancer). However, infants who drink cow's milk may increase their risk of juvenile diabetes (studies support both sides); milk is also implicated in heart disease in adults, and it may worsen certain female problems (from premenstrual syndrome [PMS] and cramps to fibroids and endometriosis). Milk, and especially yogurt are, however, much better sources of calcium than cottage cheese and most cheeses, which actually rob the body of calcium.

Some people are *lactose intolerant*, meaning that they lack the enzyme needed to digest milk sugar, or they are allergic to milk. Dairy allergies have been linked to numerous conditions such as recurrent ear infections, asthma, PMS, skin conditions, irritable bowel syndrome, recurrent tonsillitis, certain cases of ulcers, and even depression.

Don't overconsume milk and other dairy products. If you are allergic and can't eat dairy products, make sure to take calcium supplements (the most absorbable forms are calcium citrate and calcium lactate; see page 352), and take them with magnesium citrate, aspartate, or glycinate. Calcium-rich foods include dark green vegetables (except spinach), whole grains, and beans.

Most of the nutrition recommended in this book is in the form of foods and nutrient supplements. Every so often, special injections (IV nutrients) are recommended. See appendix G.

Stress-Reduction Techniques

An essential facet of healing is being able to relax: the antidote to modern-day, all-pervasive stress. There are numerous techniques that use the mind-body connection to help reduce stress. Mind-body tools have been shown to hasten healing, decrease drug requirements, decrease length of hospital stays, prevent recurrence, and make you feel more empowered and in control. This is more than a good thing when we are talking about taking your health to another level as well as healing disease. Try a number of options and find the ones that work best for you. Different ones may work at different times in your life.

STOP PASSING A DRUG CULTURE
ON TO OUR CHILDREN

It's more than alarming to see all the drug commercials on television teaching our children to reach for a quick drug fix rather than to wisely scrutinize their lives for true causes of their problems. Understand that science is now tainted by drug-company money. Nearly half the articles assessing drugs in the prestigious *New England Journal of Medicine* since 1997 were authored by scientists who received major research funds from these companies or were paid advisers to them. Using food, diet, and lifestyle as your first lines of therapeutic defense makes sense!

—*U.S. News & World Report*, March 6, 2000, p. 12

Self-Guided Relaxation

Put aside ten to fifteen minutes for you alone. Comfortably sit in a chair or lie on a bed or on the floor. Close your eyes and take three deep breaths. With each exhalation, let your muscles go soft over your bones. Take a moment to experience what it feels like to live inside your body. How does your abdomen feel, your heart, your feet? Feel inside. Learn to be aware of what you're feeling. Part of health is *awareness*, which comes through practice.

Now, go through your body, bottom to top, first tightening each part separately so it can then be more fully relaxed. Starting with both feet, stretch them out, tighten as hard as you can, and lift them into the air, holding them taut for a long inhalation. Then release, letting them gently return to the floor. Wiggle them, and then let them relax completely, as if sinking into the floor. Continue this technique up through your body, doing both legs, tightening your kneecaps and thighs, lifting, holding for an inhalation, tighter and tighter, and then, with an exhalation, letting them gently fall to the ground and relax. Continue with your buttocks and hips, back, chest, shoulders, arms and hands, then neck, face, and head. When you have tightened and then relaxed every part, feel yourself melt into the floor like a big slab of butter on a hot ear of corn.

Just lie there, enjoying the sensation of complete body relaxation. Let yourself just *be*. After a comfortable time, observe what it feels like inside, as you did at the beginning. How different do your abdomen, heart, face, and throat feel? Has your breathing changed? When you have explored the results of your relaxation, remember these feelings.

Every so often throughout your day, check in with your body and evaluate how it feels. Are you holding tension? What does the tension feel like and where is it? Remember your previous feeling of relaxation, and when you become aware of feeling tense, take a few breaths and try to re-create the body memory of relaxation. This exercise can eventually become a tool to bring more restful awareness and reduce stress at any time of day, in the midst of actually living your life.

The Breath

Yogis have known for many thousands of years that the mind follows the breath and the body follows the mind. So conscious breathing helps to restore the mindfulness and peace that can hasten healing in the physical body.

Simple Breathing Exercise: Comfortably sit in a chair or lie down. Close your eyes. Inhale in three parts, filling up the lower third of your abdomen, then the middle, and finally the upper part of your chest. Then exhale in reverse order. Be aware at the end of your exhalation to make your belly soft. Mindful breathing brings peace to our tissues and cells. Breathe in and out with the awareness of filling and emptying all three parts. An alternative way of doing this exercise is to simply "breathe" in and out of your belly as if your navel were a nose.

The Counting Breath: Comfortably sit in a chair or lie down. Inhale gently, using all parts of the abdomen, for a count of three on the inhalation and slower, for a count of six, on the exhalation. If this is too difficult for you, make do with a count of four on the exhalation. The exhalation is the relaxing breath, and we are lengthening the relaxation effect with this exercise. Breathe gently in this manner for five to ten minutes. If you get out of breath, relax and start again. Over time, try to increase the counts, but only to a comfortable number. For example, breathe in on the count of six and exhale for the count of ten to twelve, depending on your capacity. When you are done, sit quietly and enjoy the fruits of your efforts.

Soft Belly Exercise: Sit quietly. Take a moment to become aware of what you feel like. How do your face, shoulders, back, and chest feel? Place both palms on your belly and let it go soft under your hands. Don't worry about what your belly looks like or think about the scale. Take three long, deep breaths into your palms, feeling your belly enlarge as you breathe in and go soft when you breathe out. Sit and experience the benefits of a soft belly. How do your face, shoulders, back, and chest feel now? With just the awareness and softening of the belly, the whole body relaxes.

Remember soft belly. Throughout your hectic day—whenever you are feeling stressed, fearful, rushed, or angry—take three breaths and let your belly soften. It is hard to stay stressed with the awareness of soft belly. Use this simple technique, without anyone else needing to know, to bring more calm and health into your day.

Meditation

Meditation is a time to come into touch with that part of ourselves that is called the *witness* (or call it what you will—the soul, atman, spirit, or force). This is the part that is not our personality, body, mind, emotions, roles in life (mother, daughter, teacher, etc.), or ego. By practicing connection with the witness, we construct a place inside where we can view with dispassion all that is happening to us. This short-circuits our tendency to buy whole hog into our dramas, emotions, fears, illnesses, and symptoms. By being more aware of that which is not involved in all the details of daily life, we can live in peace, vitality, and freedom. This awareness paves the way for integrated health on all levels.

Meditation is one tool for becoming aware. It is only a tool, not an end in itself. Eventually, all such practices are meant to make us more mindful and healthy within all the moments of our lives, not just during the times of sitting or practicing. Expect that meditation will work for you. In other words, you will learn to *be* effectively, and your being and health will improve.

Simple Meditation: While sitting or lying down, tighten all your muscles as best you can for about thirty seconds and then let go and start to relax. Take long, gentle, deep breaths and consciously feel your muscles go soft and your entire body drain of tension.

There are many methods of meditation. A simple method used by the Harvard Mind/Body Institute is to use repetitive words, said silently in the mind. Focusing on these words helps to quiet the mind. It can be one word, like *thanks*, or *peace*, or *God*; a sentence, such as *I give thanks*; or a *mantra* (spiritual words or syllables in an ancient language) that you gently repeat over and over while keeping a relaxed state of being. Another method of meditation is to use the breathing techniques (see the breathing section, page 54) and focus on observing the in and out breath as it enters and exits your nose, or count your breaths.

The point is not to stop your thoughts. The mind is always thinking; that's its job. Your job is to focus your awareness on the object of your meditation practice—the words or breath—and let your thoughts simply drift downstream. When you become aware that your thoughts have captured your attention (which will certainly happen), gently return to repeating your words or watching your breath, with no guilt. The mind behaves like an unruly child (or as the Hindus say, like a drunken monkey stung by a scorpion), jumping from thought to thought. Just keep returning your attention to the focus of your practice.

Delicately and quietly sit with that part of yourself that is witnessing it all—you repeating your words, you watching your breath, the you that is sitting, the you that is struggling, the you that is obviously not all of you, since the witness is able to witness it.

After a comfortable period of time (start with five minutes and build up to twenty or more minutes), take a few deep breaths and gently stretch. Try to do your meditation practice at the same time each day.

Visualizations and Affirmations

Science has shown that *visualization* activates areas in the brain as though we were actually experiencing that which we are imagining. Thus, using visualizations on a regular basis can be a powerful healing tool. *Affirmations* are sentences that are repeated out loud to inform your cells and tissues of your intention and acceptance of healing. They are the reset buttons in the link between body and mind to get your mind to help heal your body.

At the end of the simple meditation given in the previous section, after you take a few deep breaths and relax, add visualizations and affirmations.

Visualize that you are well, and focus specifically on the part of your body that requires energy. See it as perfect, glowing with good health. Use either a metaphor that works for you (such as an army of enthusiastic soldiers cleaning up your liver, or a flower looking beautiful and perfect, or just the organ as you visualize it in your mind's eye, looking healthy and functioning optimally). Hold whichever vision works for you for at least five minutes. If your attention strays, gently bring it back to this vision.

Next, affirm out loud a sentence that feels appropriate to your healing. For example, you can say, "My estrogen levels are perfect and balanced; my intestinal tract is strong" or "My blood vessels are elastic and shiny."

Finish by giving thanks. Gratitude gets short shrift in our society, and being grateful has power. Affirm out loud: "I give thanks for the healing of ———."

Being Your Own Healer

Before you get out of bed in the morning, lie there and take three deep breaths. Smile. Smiling relaxes the entire physical body as well as the emotional body. Think of three things for which you are grateful. See them in your mind's eye, then let them into your heart.

Feel your gratitude for having these things. For example, "I give thanks for my healthy child, my best friend, and for having a roof over my head." Anything that keeps you smiling. Let the feeling of gratitude fill you. Gratitude heals. Let your healing begin before your feet hit the ground.

Prayer has been shown to help various diseases, such as rheumatoid arthritis and heart disease. If you are comfortable with this notion, pray, and have others pray for you. In twenty-three different studies, prayer, mental healing, spiritual healing, and therapeutic touch have been shown to have a positive healing effect almost 60 percent of the time.

Knowing Your Unknown

If you bring forth what is within you, what you bring forth will save you. If you do not bring forth what is within you, what you do not bring forth will destroy you. That which we do not know rules us because we aren't aware of it and either can't fix it or defend ourselves against it. So having emotional and physical blind spots or denying what ails our heads, hearts, and bodies leads to unwellness on all levels.

Don't be afraid to roll up your mental shirtsleeves and dig into what is at the core of your illness, unhappiness, fears, and despair. It is hard work. It may seem that others have it easier than you. Oh how green the grass is on our neighbor's lawn! But your unwellness is the grist for your personal mill, the shovel with which you can dig deep into who you really are. The wise woman chooses to use her life as a university. It is your curriculum to go inside and find out what isn't working and, by developing more awareness and information, to get it to work better.

This in no way means that everyone who gets sick does so to learn life lessons. The New Age-y concept that your thoughts create your illness only manages to make people feel guilty about being sick. Your illness is not necessarily your fault. It just helps to see whatever comes your way as another new opportunity, not simply as mindless pain. Use your life as a map to see where you are going and how you are getting there. Your condition has brought you to the point of reading this book, which encourages you to evaluate your diet, exercise, thoughts, and relaxation techniques. It is good for everyone to do this periodically. Through the use of mind-body tools and nutrients, you can take a bigger part in drawing a map of your world as you most want it to be.

PART TWO

Information contained in this book is based on numerous articles published in peer-reviewed scientific literature—which means studies deemed by a board of certified doctors to have merit in the eyes of the medical community—as well as thousands of hours of clinical observation by doctors at the top of their fields. Each condition lists a number of treatment possibilities. *Do not use all of them.* Work with your doctor to review your individual and family history and decide which treatments are best for you. The most important nutrients for each condition are starred (**). But these suggestions are not set recipes to be followed without pertinent clinical evaluation.

A

ABORTION

A medically induced termination of pregnancy.

Women in every age and every culture have always obtained abortions, despite legal, religious, and ethical obstacles. In the United States, an abortion is a private matter between a woman and her physician up to the twelfth week of pregnancy, after which state laws regulate the procedure. Approximately 50 percent of abortions are performed as a result of contraceptive failure. Early abortion is one of the safest procedures in medicine—about twenty times safer than childbirth—but the emotional stress involved may require consultation with a therapist or counselor.

A *therapeutic abortion* is done to save the life or health of the mother. Conditions that may worsen during pregnancy (and possibly become life-threatening) include severe heart disease, chronic kidney disease, and cancer (especially breast or cervical). Termination may be recommended if a woman contracts German measles (rubella) during the early stages of pregnancy because of possible damage to the fetus; for certain fetal conditions, such as severe developmental defects such as anencephaly, an absence of the brain; or for serious chromosomal abnormalities such as Down syndrome.

Early abortion (between the seventh and twelfth weeks of pregnancy) is done through safe vacuum suction techniques or through new hormonal treatments. Between thirteen and sixteen weeks, a D&E (dilatation and evacuation) procedure is performed. Late abortion (after sixteen weeks) is usually done by injecting a saline solution or a prostaglandin hormone into the uterus.

Complications are possible in a very small percentage of cases. These include bleeding, uterine damage, and anesthesia-related problems. The World Health Organization (WHO) reports that women who have two or more abortions risk a two to three times greater chance of miscarriage, premature delivery, or bearing a low birthweight infant in subsequent pregnancies.

Abortifacients are herbal drugs or home remedies that are claimed to cause abortion, such as large doses of castor oil, gin by the bottle, or very hot baths. None is effective.

Nutrients

Take for two to four weeks after abortion.

- PABA (para-aminobenzoic acid), 500 mg twice a day
- Zinc, 20 mg twice a day (balance with multivitamin/mineral supplement containing 2–4 mg copper)
- Vitamin C, 1,000 mg twice a day
- Vitamin B complex, 25–50 mg twice a day
- Protein/flaxseed Green Drink once a day (see page 465) for two weeks then two to four times a week for several more

ACNE (Acne Vulgaris)

A chronic skin disorder caused by inflammation of the hair follicles and the sebaceous glands, possibly involving bacterial infection of the skin. Largely the bane of adolescence (when it affects 75 percent of women), about 20 percent of all cases occur in adults. The skin can mirror our intake of essential fatty acids, the nutrients that help metabolize them, or the functioning of our digestive tracts. See *Fats and Essential Fatty Acids* and appendix F.

Symptoms: Blackheads (comedones, plugged hair follicles), whiteheads (small whitish bumps), papules (small pink bumps on the skin), pustules (pimples or yellowheads), nodules (solid swellings below the skin), and cysts (deep, inflamed, pus-filled lesions that can cause pain). Pustules and cysts form scar tissue during the healing process, leaving the pits sometimes seen on the face, neck, shoulders, or back of acne sufferers.

Causes: The main cause of acne is an imbalance in androgens—male hormones produced in small amounts by the ovaries and adrenal glands in women. During puberty, a temporary hormone imbalance increases the ratio of androgens to estrogens, causing acne. Genetic factors play a role. Some drugs may bring on or aggravate acne, such as corticosteroids, lithium, and barbiturates. Acne is *not* caused by eating rich or fatty foods (however, it can be secondary to maldigestion), lack of exercise, alcohol abuse, or masturbation. However, eating too much sugar can lead to acne because a rise in blood sugar is multiplied by five when it gets to the skin, and sugar-saturated skin is susceptible to acne. Excessive caffeine can also contribute to acne. Deficiencies in certain nutrients such as zinc and/or food allergies can cause acne.

Acne can be aggravated by environmental insults (such as pollution and high humidity), squeezing or picking at blemishes, hard scrubbing of the skin, and stress—especially when stress is severe or prolonged.

Uniquely Female: Women are more likely than men to have mild to moderate acne into their thirties and beyond. Changing hormone levels may cause an acne flare-up two to seven days before the menstrual period starts. Peri- and postmenopausal women and women with polycystic ovaries may have an excess of testosterone, which may cause acne, especially if the woman had acne during puberty. Women who do not ovulate regularly have increased androgen production in their ovaries, which can lead to acne. Hormonal changes related to pregnancy, starting or stopping birth control pills, or hormonal therapy (especially progestins, estrogens, and DHEA) can cause acne. Certain birth control pills can also aggravate the condition; ask your doctor to prescribe a different pill or another birth control method. Pregnant women or women planning pregnancy in the near future should not take the drug Accutane (a vitamin A derivative), which is sometimes used in severe cases; the drug can cause birth defects.

What to Do

- Check for food allergies (especially dairy) as well as allergies to facial creams, soaps, shampoos, and makeup.
- Read labels and avoid products that contain lanolin, isopropyl myristate, sodium lauryl sulfate, laureth-4, and D & C red dyes.
- Small doses of sunlight can be helpful, but stay out of the sun if using acne medications.

Topical Options

These preparations are available through your holistic practitioner:

- ** 4 percent niacinamide gel, applied twice a day to the affected areas for several months
- 20 percent azelaic acid cream applied once a day to the affected areas for one week and then twice a day for two to three months, or up to one year. For severe cystic acne, azelaic acid cream may be used in combination with 100 mg of oral minocycline (a tetracycline derivative). These topicals should be monitored by a doctor.
- Wipe affected areas morning and night with vitamin A-E emulsion, liquid chlorophyll, and aloe vera gel; stevia extract directly on skin; or use tea tree oil on sores three times a day.
- Wipe three times a day with tea made from alfalfa, burdock root, echinacea, with a teaspoon of apple cider vinegar and a dash of cayenne pepper. You can substitute 1 tsp. of brewer's yeast for the herbs.

Masks

- Apply white clay and let dry three times a day.
- Mix 1 Tbsp. brewer's yeast with 1 tsp. apple cider vinegar and ⅛ tsp. cayenne pepper. Spread on face and let dry completely. Wash off gently. This may be too strong for extremely sensitive skin, but it is a wonderful way to increase circulation and enhance healing.
- Try an enzyme face wash, available at health food stores.

The Makeup Connection

In adult women, oil-based makeup is a major cause of acne out-breaks. Avoid oils, greasy cleansing creams, and other cosmetics. Check to see that makeup is labeled "oil-free," "noncomedogenic," or "nonacnegenic." If you use Retin-A, ask for it in gel form. Wash your hands before applying makeup and remove all makeup when washing your face at night. Unused eye makeup should be thrown out after three or four months, and don't use anyone else's makeup.

Diet: Daily Green Drink with options (page 465). Eat a whole-food diet with an emphasis on green vegetables (four to five servings per day; try to eat raw half the time) and whole fruits (one to three servings per day). Increase fiber.

Avoid: Sugar and refined carbohydrates, such as processed foods like colas, candies, and frozen prepackaged foods, especially after 1:00 P.M. Too much iodine in the diet can be a problem for some people with acne, especially those who eat a lot of fast foods (which could be high in iodine). Limit seafood and other foods that contain iodine, such as wheat germ, kelp, cheese, citrus, asparagus, beef liver, and iodized salt. Avoid potential stressor foods such as caffeine, hydro-genated oils, and milk. Chocolate may aggravate some acne, even though studies don't always support this link.

Nutrients: Skin problems are some of the slowest conditions to respond to natural therapies (requiring six to twelve months and sometimes longer), but the response is often more complete than with drugs.

For Moderate Acne

** Vitamin A, 25,000 IU twice a day for two weeks, then reduce to once a day. In fourth week, reduce vitamin A to 10,000 IU daily. Fifth week, reduce to 5,000 IU daily. Work with doctor.

HOW TO TEST FOR OIL IN COSMETICS

Rub a streak of makeup onto a sheet of 25 percent cotton bond paper. Wait twenty-four hours, then check for an oil ring. The bigger the ring, the greasier the makeup.

** Vitamin E, 800 IU per day

** Zinc, 20 mg twice a day for two weeks (if you get nauseated, cut the dosage to once a day), and copper, 2–3 mg per day

- Niacinamide, topical 4 percent gel, apply twice a day to affected skin for several months

- Vitamin B complex, 50 mg twice a day

If that doesn't work, try the following:

** Essential fatty acids, 2–4 g per day for at least one year

** Chlorophyll (1 tsp. twice a day) if not doing Green Drink

** Proteolytic enzymes, 1–2 g twice a day on an empty stomach for three to five weeks

- Beta-carotene, 50,000 IU daily for one month, then reduce to 25,000 IU daily

- B complex, two to three times a day, with added vitamins B_6 and B_1

For Severe, Difficult-to-Treat Acne

** Vitamin A, 100,000 IU per day for two weeks, then reduce to 50,000 IU per day for several months. Take with vitamin E, 800–1,200 IU per day. (If you notice toxic symptoms, stop immediately: see appendix J.) Work with a doctor.

** Zinc picolinate or citrate, 30 mg two to three times a day for several months. Do not use zinc sulfate. After three months, reduce dosage to once a day. Balance with copper, 2–3 mg per day. Note: Too much zinc will make you nauseated. Lower the dose if this happens. *This combination of zinc, vitamin A, and copper has been found in some studies to be as effective as oral antibiotics in treating acne.*

** Vitamin B_6, 25 mg twice a day, and vitamin B complex, 25–50 mg per day

For Premenstrual or Midcycle Acne

** Vitamin B_6, 20 mg once a day for a month, then twice a day for several days before the time your face usually gets worse

- Magnesium, 200–300 mg per day

- Zinc, 15 mg per day

- Folic acid, 800 mcg per day, if gum problems coexist
- Vitamin B complex, 25 mg per day.
- Vitex (an herbal supplement), 40 drops of concentrated liquid in a glass of water in the morning for one to six months

For Blackheads
- Magnesium, 250 mg per day, and vitamin A, 10,000–25,000 IU per day

For Chronic, Numerous Whiteheads
- Vitamin B_1, 25 mg per day, or see remedies for maldigestion problems (pages 209, 468)

For Acne Scars
- Take bromelain, 500–1,000 mg per day in divided doses on an empty stomach for two to six months. Stop if there is no noticeable difference in two months.

For chronic cases that do not respond to any of the treatments, consider intestinal detoxification programs (read my book *Healthy Digestion the Natural Way,* John Wiley, 2000).

ADDICTION

Physiological and psychological dependence on and craving for a chemical substance. Almost half of all women between the ages of fifteen and forty-five have used some sort of recreational drug at least once in their lives. During the past year, more than 3.7 million women have taken prescription drugs such as tranquilizers, sedatives, and diet pills. And more than 70 percent of AIDS cases among women are drug-related.

Alcoholism

Alcohol dependence is a major addiction in women. It is habitual, compulsive, long-term heavy consumption of alcohol and the development of withdrawal symptoms when drinking stops. Genetic background and environment are factors, but anyone who drinks heavily for a prolonged period can become an alcoholic.

Uniquely Female: Women make up one third of the 15 million alcoholics in the United States. There are at least 2 to 3 million women alcoholics of reproductive age. Sixty-seven percent relate their drinking to their menstrual cycles, with drinking bouts often taking place during the premenstrual phase.

Women experience ill effects of alcohol earlier than men and at lower consumption levels because women have less water in their bodies so the alcohol is less diluted and has a greater impact. Also, women do not metabolize alcohol as efficiently as men, since our livers are smaller. Drink for drink, a woman will have a 30 percent higher blood alcohol level than a man of the same weight. Female drinkers have heavier, more painful periods as well as higher rates of stroke, osteoporosis, and infertility than do nondrinkers. Moderate to heavy alcohol consumption in women elevates blood levels of estrogen; has been associated with a number of unopposed estrogen illnesses (see *Estrogen Dominance*) such as breast cancer, as well as increased risk of vaginal infections; and can delay menopause by up to two years. Estrogenic and other possible adverse effects of hormone replacement therapy are increased with moderate to heavy alcohol consumption.

It is estimated that 19 percent of women consume alcohol during pregnancy, accounting for up to 5 percent of all birth defects. Alcohol easily crosses the placenta; the fetus receives as much alcohol as the mother but burns it up half as fast. Drinking more than five to seven drinks per week,* or even one drinking binge (four or more drinks over several hours), particularly in early pregnancy, increases the risk to 30 to 50 percent of having a child born with fetal alcohol syndrome or other serious fetal problems, including mental retardation. Healthy women should not consume more than five to six drinks per week. This means about one drink a day (not every day) and certainly not more than two in one day.

---

* One drink equals one 12-oz. bottle of beer (5 percent alcohol), 5-oz. glass of wine (12 percent alcohol), or 1.5 oz. liquor (40 percent alcohol).

What to Do

** Do a liver-cleansing program (page 311). No detox program
   will work unless the liver is functioning properly, and liver
   detoxification shortens withdrawal time significantly.

• Abuse of alcohol lowers B vitamins, which raises homocysteine levels (page 269), which in turn increases risk of heart
  disease and stroke. When women become menopausal and
  their risks of these illnesses increase, they should not overconsume alcohol and, when drinking, they should take
  vitamin B complex along with additional folic acid and
  vitamins B_6 and B_{12}. This will also help reduce symptoms
  of withdrawal from alcohol.

• Check for digestive enzymes (page 468)

Diet: When blood-sugar levels fall, alcoholics tend to develop
anxiety attacks and crave easily absorbed carbohydrates, such as alcohol and refined sugars like candy. Eat small, frequent meals to
counteract this tendency.

Avoid: Refined sugar and other refined carbohydrates (such as
white flour), caffeine, and chemical food additives.

Nutrients

** Chromium picolinate or aspartate, 500 mcg twice a day
** High-potency multivitamin/mineral (with selenium) daily
** Magnesium, 250–1,000 mg per day
** Niacin (vitamin B_3), 100 mg twice a day. Don't take higher
   dosages without medical supervision and regular blood tests.
** Essential fatty acids (EFAs), to correct deficiency of prosta-
   glandin levels. Use flaxseed oil, cod liver oil, or evening
   primrose oil, several grams per day. Alcohol abuse depletes
   docosahexaenoic acid, or DHA (found in fish oil), which contributes to the secondary depression of alcoholism. See *Fats
   and Essential Fatty Acids.*
** Vitamin E, 400 IU per day
• L-glutathione, 500 mg twice a day, or NAC (N-acetyl-
  cysteine), 250 mg one to three times a day. See doctor.

- High-potency vitamin B complex. Ask your doctor about vitamin B_{12} injections.
- Vitamin C with bioflavonoids, 2,000 to 3,000 mg per day, in divided doses
- Ask your doctor about L-tryptophan (by prescription), an amino acid that is a precursor to serotonin. Take 1,000–1,500 mg twice a day in between meals for depression and/or insomnia. Gamma-hydroxybutyrate (GHB), which is currently a Schedule I controlled drug, has been shown to promote abstinence but should be taken under strict medical supervision.

To Reduce Cravings

- ** L-glutamine, 500–1,000 mg two to three times a day, decreases alcohol craving for two to three months. Do not use glutamic acid.
- Free-form amino acids, 500 mg two to three times a day, taken away from mealtime and separately from glutamine. Some doctors can run blood and urine levels of your amino acids and then customize formulas for you based on your individual levels.
- ½ tsp. baking soda in water between meals, twice a day for two weeks
- Buffered vitamin C, 1,000 mg two to three times a day. Ask your doctor about intravenous (IV) nutrients, twice a week for six to eight weeks, then taper off.
- SAMe (S-adenosyl-methionine) is a food supplement that helps the brain receive neurotransmitter signals better. Some women can be helped by as little as 200 mg per day, finding that it elevates mood and decreases cravings.
- Those who suffer severe depression when not drinking may be helped by DHEA (dehydroepiandrosterone). Have your doctor test your levels of DHEA.
- Regular exercise, fifteen minutes twice a day, helps reduce cravings, stabilize blood sugar, and increase the energy you need to maintain your program.

Herbs: Milk thistle, 150–300 mg one to three times a day for one to two months, is especially useful in repairing the liver. For women, three cups daily of angelica and scullcap tea mixed together eases withdrawal and controls craving. Valerian, one to two 300–500 mg capsules of extract once or twice a day on an empty stomach, and B complex several times a day helps with anxiety attacks and mood swings. Kudzu, 30–100 mg two to three times a day, can be helpful.

Drug Dependence

Drug dependence is the compulsion to continue taking a drug, either to produce the desired "high" or to prevent the ill effects that occur when it is not taken.

Millions of Americans are dependent on nicotine and caffeine. Many others are dependent on mood- or behavior-altering drugs, such as tranquilizers or marijuana. Other commonly abused drugs include stimulants (amphetamines), depressants (alcohol and barbiturates), psychedelics (LSD), narcotics (cocaine and heroin), and anabolic steroids. Cocaine and heroin have been shown to cause angina, heart attack, coronary artery spasm, and life-threatening damage to the heart muscle. Prolonged dependence may cause lung and heart disease (tobacco dependence), liver disease, mental problems such as anxiety and depression, hepatitis or AIDS (IV drug use), and overdose. Narcotic analgesics, such as morphine, used briefly to relieve pain rarely lead to dependence.

Drug dependence is a signal that your life is out of balance, and often family-of-origin issues need to be uncovered and resolved. You must work with professionals for support and exploration of what is wrong and how to fix it. However, cleaning up your diet, exercising, and adding nutrients will make your healing time easier and shorter.

About marijuana: Today's marijuana has a 200 percent higher tetrahydrocannabinol (THC) content than what was grown twenty-five years ago. The effects of smoking marijuana last four hours; effects from ingestion last up to twelve hours. Marijuana affects blood sugar balance, muscle coordination, reaction time, short- and long-term memory, and possibly the immune system. The smoke contains the same carcinogens as tobacco smoke and can lead to lung damage. If you smoke, eat a lot of brown and Chinese red rice and broccoli (some raw); take antioxidants, vitamin B complex, and vitamin C with bioflavonoids, and do liver detoxification programs one to two times a year (page 311).

Symptoms of Dependence

Narcotics: Extreme drowsiness or confusion; loss of appetite; slow, shallow breathing; cold, clammy skin

Barbiturates, sleeping pills, tranquilizers: Slurred speech; staggering gait; disorientation; extreme drowsiness; slow, shallow breathing; cold, clammy skin

Stimulants (diet pills, cocaine): Agitation or extreme nervousness; excitation or irritability; hallucinations, dilated pupils

Diet: Moderation and consistency help stabilize blood sugar and moods, which helps reduce cravings. Healthy food helps stabilize the body. Do a Protein Green Drink daily (page 465), and follow instructions for a basic sensible diet (pages 43–49).

Avoid: Processed oils and refined sugars, alcohol, caffeine, and refined carbohydrates, because they aggravate cravings for drugs. Identify and avoid food allergies and intolerances. Avoid long periods of time between meals, and don't indulge in overeating binges.

Nutrients

To reduce cravings: See previous section on alcoholism.

<u>To Remedy Nutritional Deficiencies</u>
  - ** Vitamin B complex, 50 mg per day
  - ** Multivitamin/mineral complex, high potency, as prescribed on label
  - ** Sodium ascorbate (buffered vitamin C), 500 mg every three hours to detoxify your system and lessen cravings for one to two weeks. Intravenous (IV) C under a doctor's supervision.
  - ** Pantothenic acid (vitamin B_5), 500–1,000 mg three times a day, helps greatly with energy to maintain program and attitude.
  - ** Magnesium, 250 mg at bedtime (try aspartate ferm)
  - • Calcium, 500–1,000 mg with meals

- Niacinamide, 500 mg three times a day, and phosphatidylser-ine, 100 mg taken with fatty meals, to enhance brain function
- Alpha-lipoic acid, 100–250 mg once or twice a day, for free radical scavenging (take backup biotin, 2 mg per day).

Herbs: Siberian ginseng helps cocaine withdrawal; rosemary and valerian tea several times a day assist depression; oatstraw tea as an anti-addictive; chamomile for stress reduction; gotu kola for energy/nerve health; and scullcap to calm anxiety.

ADHESIONS

Adhesions are internal scar tissue. When women have abdominal surgery (either by cutting into the abdomen or through laparoscopy, which goes in through a small slit in the navel) there is always the risk of adhesions. Adhesions are formed from fibrous tissue by the irritation caused by blood and handling of tissues. Adhesions can make tissues stick together abnormally and can cause pulling, discomfort, and severe enough disability and pain to warrant further surgeries to remove the adhesions.

If you are about to have abdominal surgery (for almost anything other than hysterectomy), we highly recommend you consider the following surgical technique (see box, page 74). Dr. Myron Moorehead, a surgeon from Metairie, Louisiana, devised and has used the following procedure for eighteen years to minimize both blood loss and adhesion formation. If your surgeon has questions, have him call Myron E. Moorehead, M.D., at the Women's Laser Institute, 504-837-0010. Dr. Moorehead specializes in fibroid removal while saving the uterus and reducing adhesions and complications. Call for a consultation before undergoing a hysterectomy due to fibroids.

Note: Taking inositol, 500 mg twice a day for a week prior to abdominal surgery, significantly decreases painful gas after surgery.

DR. MOOREHEAD'S LOW-ADHESION SURGICAL TECHNIQUE

Adhesions were once thought to be a natural side effect of surgery, especially within the abdomen. In many of Dr. Moorehead's cases, patients have been able to go on to have babies, some of which were delivered by Cesarean section. This provided an opportunity to have a second look into the mothers' abdomens. The surgeons performing the C-sections said that in forty-two patients, they found no adhesions—not one. This is more than impressive.

For Your Doctor

This technique is appropriate for the removal of fibroids, endometriosis, and pelvic adhesions, but not for hysterectomies.

Dr. Moorehead's technique involves careful handling of all tissue intra-abdominally, followed by control of blood loss (accomplished by use of the laser for dissection and the injection of Pitressin into the uterus for vasoconstriction). Throughout the operative procedure, it is important to keep the tissue moist by frequent irrigation using a saline solution with heparin added. Following the surgery, the uterus is covered with an adhesive barrier, Interceed (TC7). Prior to complete closure of the abdomen, 100 cc of Hyskon is instilled into the pelvis, which functions to prevent the intestines and uterus from being in apposition for the first seventy-two hours. Postoperatively, the patients are placed on Danocrine, 200 mg three times a day, to suppress ovarian function and to put the patient in a hypoestrogenic state.

ADRENAL HORMONES, see *Hormones*

ADRENAL INSUFFICIENCY and ADRENAL FATIGUE

Outright adrenal insufficiency is called Addison's disease. However, many women suffer with *subclinical adrenal fatigue,* a real condition not yet recognized in conventional medical practice and that comes from continual low-level stress or periods of severe traumatic stress. This is the condition covered in this section.

Symptoms: Fatigue (especially on rising, after exercise, after orgasm, severe energy drops at various times in the day, such as late in the afternoon), dizziness upon standing up suddenly, low blood pressure, low blood sugar, weakness, nervousness, midafternoon headaches, nausea, and irritability. Joint and muscle pain is common. Sometimes darkening of areas of the skin may develop (hyperpigmentation). Other symptoms: feeling better if you sleep later in the morning, tendencies to inflammatory conditions in joints and skin, recurrent illness after exertion, multiple allergies, tendency to underweight, and frequent urination during night.

What to Do

Have your doctor

- Evaluate your thyroid.
- Run DHEA and DHEA-S levels.
- Run saliva or twenty-four-hour urine cortisol levels.

Diet: Eat small, frequent meals. Consume healthy complex carbohydrates and sufficient salt. Eat tomato-based foods.

Avoid: Too much protein and salt-free or low-carbohydrate diets. Avoid sugar, caffeine, and alcohol.

Nutrients

- ** Pantothenic acid, 1–3 g per day in divided doses, sometimes higher
- ** Magnesium aspartate, 100–300 mg per day
- ** Vitamin C, 1,000–2,000 mg per day in divided doses
- ** Vitamin B complex, 25 mg twice a day
- Vitamin A, 10,000 IU per day
- Raw adrenal and raw adrenal cortex glandular extract, 50–150 mg one to three times a day
- Chromium, 100 mcg twice a day
- Essential fatty acids, several grams per day
- Ask your doctor about oral hydrocortisone (5–10 mg three to four times a day for three to ten days; these are physiological doses of cortisol). Read Dr. William Jeffries's book *Safe Uses of Cortisol*, second edition (Charles C. Thomas Ltd., 1996).

- If your cortisol is elevated, take 100 mg of phosphatidylserine once a day with a fatty meal.
- DHEA improves well-being, energy, and sexuality.

Herbs: Licorice root extract, 200–500 mg two to three times per day for several weeks to months can be especially helpful. The glycyrrhiza in licorice taken in capsules, drops, or tea reduces the workload of adrenals. Siberian ginseng, 10 mg once or twice a day. Both should be avoided if you have high blood pressure (which is rare with adrenal fatigue). Holy basil, 400–1,000 mg, once or twice a day.

AGING

The physical and mental changes that occur in a person over time. Very few people live beyond one hundred years (although this group is increasing), and the average life span for women, in the absence of disease, is around eighty-five years. More American women than ever before in history live a third (or more) of their lives in the postmenopausal years. Growing old is inevitable, but feeling old is a state of mind. The aging process is often feared as bringing only frailty and increased vulnerability to disease and injury, but many societies value the wisdom and experience of their elders, and we must start doing this within our own families and communities.

All organs and tissues naturally undergo some loss in function due to aging. Aging is hastened by fatigue, low self-esteem, boredom, lack of interaction with community and friends, exposure to sun, smoking, excessive alcohol or drug consumption, air pollution, lack of exercise, a fatty or poor diet, overweight, and viral infections.

Vitality, self-esteem, gratitude, and service all contribute to a better relationship with aging. Of course, these attributes have their seeds in how we have been living our lives all along, just as our bone mass starts to bank its reserves in our youth. However, it is never too late to develop a good head on our shoulders and courage in our hearts. Start each day by reciting three things you have to be thankful for. Each day do one thing you love to do, help at least one other person, and do exercises for the body and the mind. You have the ability to cowrite the script of your life. Take risks and be creative. Read *Still Here* by Ram Dass (Riverhead, 2000).

Aging Starts in Youth

People younger than fifty can affect their old age positively. Early lifestyle habits of exercising regularly, combined with emphasis on coping skills of meditation, breathing, relaxation, and good eating habits, set the stage for a healthier senior life. According to a psychiatrist and one of the authors of a study demonstrating that healthy aging depends on past habits, Dr. George E. Valliant says: "A successful old age may lie not so much in our stars and genes as in ourselves." Yes, ladies, life is a balancing act between living smart, as though you would last forever, and living in the moment, as if this is all there is.

Age Spots

These blemishes appear on the skin with increasing age. They can be brown or yellow slightly raised spots that can occur at any site; freckles; keratoses (small, wart-like capillaries caused by overexposure to the sun); and De Morgan's spots (cherry spots), which are harmless red blemishes that become more numerous with age but do not increase in size. Keratoses may progress to skin cancer and are usually frozen off with liquid nitrogen or removed surgically. Some aging spots that particularly vex you or occur in very obvious places can be removed by simple plastic surgery techniques or various skin peels. If you hate looking at them, get rid of them!

Wrinkles

Furrows in the skin, a natural feature of aging caused by a reduction in collagen production and loss of skin elasticity. The likelihood of getting wrinkles is increased by heredity; exposure during adolescence and young adulthood to sun and sea wind; marked changes in weight; and cigarette smoking. Premature deep wrinkling is usually caused by overexposure to sunlight. Consuming good fats as well as using Retin-A and vitamin C cream also decrease wrinkles. See *Fats and Essential Fatty Acids*. Plastic surgeons now have many options to

THINNING SKIN AND INTESTINAL LINING

When we age, most things start to thin except for our waistline (bummer). As the lining of the intestinal tract thins, we make less digestive enzymes, which are necessary to break our food down into health-supporting nutrients. This is especially a problem for women in their late sixties and older. Get your stomach acid tested with a Heidelberg Capsule test performed by a holistic doctor (see page 468).

Low stomach acid is also a serious cause of low levels of vitamin B_{12} in the elderly, predisposing them to many problems like depression, fatigue, and heart disease. Low stomach acid also predisposes people to infections with a bug called *H. pylori* that can contribute to loss of appetite, ulcers, cancer, and heart disease. Many pharmaceuticals like H_2-receptor antagonists (antacids), sold over the counter or overprescribed or taken for too long, especially by the elderly, block normal secretions of stomach acid, which encourages vitamin B_{12} deficiency. Doctors should run a homocysteine test, which demonstrates, if the results are elevated, a need for more B vitamins and perhaps stomach acid, even if the B vitamin levels in the blood are normal.

—*Journal of Clinical Gastroenterology* 30 (1):4–6, 2000

offer, and these procedures may give some of us a needed emotional boost.

Sexuality

After menopause, a woman cannot reproduce, but she can continue to enjoy her sexuality into old age. Sexual desire, sexual arousal, and response to sexual stimulus can stay strong. Many women have greater sexual desire and pleasure after menopause because they are no longer afraid of getting pregnant; they know their bodies better and have higher self-esteem and less embarrassment. The reduction in available estrogen after menopause can lead to less clitoral enlargement and slower vaginal lubrication, and it may take longer to reach orgasm, but this varies from woman to woman. If intercourse becomes painful due to a thinning of the lining of the vagina (from a decrease in estrogen), there are treatment options (see section on vaginal atrophy under *Vaginal Problems*). More than 70 percent of couples have regular sexual intercourse in their late sixties, and 10 percent still enjoy intercourse in their eighties. (Let's stretch these numbers, ladies.) Usually, intercourse ceases because the male partner can no longer have or maintain an erection. If you're concerned about your sexual response, have your doctor test your levels of hormones (three major estrogens, testosterone and DHEA [dehydroepiandrosterone]), since low levels of hormones can decrease your sexual desire and enjoyment, whereas supplementation can improve them. PABA (para-aminobenzoic acid) helps, too.

Mortality

Being more active in leisure time is inversely related to all causes of death. Move it or lose it! Women who eat more whole grains and/or are optimistic in their world-life viewpoint are less likely to die from all causes, while eating refined grains (like white flour) increases risk in all areas. It's a proven fact that eating more whole grains, fruits, vegetables, fish, and eggs, and fewer refined foods increases longevity.

What to Do

These simple measures can reduce the physical and mental effects of aging:

- Mounting evidence suggests that oxidative stress and hyper-insulinism promote aging. Take antioxidants daily and avoid excess refined sugars, refined flours, and overeating.
- Have regular checkups by a doctor.
- Eat an optimal diet most of the time (pages 43–49), then eat out occasionally and have fun.
- Enjoy regular, moderate exercise, especially in the fresh air. Resistance exercises, even just once or twice a week, improve health and reduce the risk of falls and fractures. You don't have to be an athlete to get results.
- Minimize risk factors for heart disease (page 262).
- Learn to manage stress (pages 52–58) and meditate.
- Maintain good body and oral hygiene.
- Remain curious about life, passionate about causes.
- Keep your mind exercised. New research suggests that senior women can engage new and more brain areas as they grow older.

- Keep interacting with other people.
- Be an optimist. They live longer than pessimists.
- Get levels of digestive enzymes tested.

Diet: Science has long demonstrated two factors known to increase life span. The most important is healthy undereating—not starving or fasting, just eating quality food that sustains you without overeating, which strains you. (The second factor is lowered body temperature.) Eat less by eating smaller meals or "grazing" throughout the day. Consume whole foods. Eat more at the beginning and middle of the day and less at night. Foods associated with increased longevity and decreased chronic degenerative illness are natural foods high in fiber, especially if taken with green tea; unrefined dark green olive oil and rice bran oil; garlic; fermented foods such as yogurt, kefir, and sauerkraut; goat's milk products rather than cow's; and grains such as millet, buckwheat, quinoa, and amaranth.

Drink lots of pure water to keep body and brain from getting dehydrated. Chlorine may accelerate the aging process by inducing free-radical damage to cells. Chlorinated water may also increase the risk of heart disease and some types of cancer, especially bladder cancer. Fluoride in water can lead to hip fractures. Drink pure water—bottled spring or filtered water. If you do drink chlorinated water, take antioxidants. Or you can boil the water and the chlorine will evaporate. *Moderate* alcohol intake in the elderly is linked to better long-term survival.

Avoid: Overeating; processed foods; and excessive consumption of stressor foods such as alcohol, caffeinated beverages, deep-fried food, refined sugars, processed oils, excessive salt, and smoked foods.

Nutrients
   ** Start and end each day with one to two glasses of filtered water and an antioxidant.
   ** A mega-multivitamin supplement with trace chelated minerals, including at least 50 mg of B vitamins and selenium, 200 mcg per day, decreases risk of a number of chronic diseases
   ** Calcium aspartate or chelate, 800–1,000 mg per day

** Magnesium, 250–500 mg per day

** Essential oils: evening primrose oil; fish oil, 2–6 g per day in divided doses; and/or 1 Tbsp. flaxseed oil or ⅛ tsp. ground flaxseeds

** Vitamin E: start with 200 IU per day and slowly increase over several weeks to 800 IU per day.

- Vitamin D, 400–600 mg per day (avoid if you have a history of kidney stones or heart disease)

- Glutamine, 500 mg twice a day, to increase digestive capabilities. Also consider digestive enzymes (page 468).

- Coenzyme Q-10, 25–100 mg per day

- Free-form amino acids, twice a day taken on an empty stomach (it's best to get your amino acid levels tested and have a formula customized for you)

- Probiotics as directed

- Raw thymus glandular, 500 mg per day, to stimulate your immune system

- Consider SAMe (S-adenosyl-methionine), a food supplement that helps the brain receive better signals and is also associated with improving the symptoms of aging, as well as helping joint and liver function. Try 200 mg daily and see if it makes you feel more vital; if not, try a higher dose, such as 600, 800, or 1,000 mg per day. SAMe's effects are often seen immediately, but can be delayed up to two weeks after starting (page 496).

- Phosphatidylserine, 100 mg per day with a fatty meal, helps memory and cognition, as proven in many studies.

Herbs: For longevity take ginseng; ginkgo biloba; and ashwaganda, an Ayurvedic (East Indian approach to healing) herb.

"Do not try to live forever. You will not succeed."

—*George Bernard Shaw*

ALLERGIES

Your body is its own universe set inside the outer universe. When some of the outside world gains entry into your body and you can't process the foreign substances appropriately (breaking them down into benign pieces), various inflammatory responses cause a collection of symptoms we call allergies. You can be exposed to these foreign particles through skin contact (such as with a metal like nickel, which is found in various kinds of jewelry); by breathing in dust, pollen, or environmental pollutants; or by eating various foods. Allergies are an often undiagnosed cause or exacerbator of many health conditions; in fact, undiagnosed allergies are a potential hidden contributor to osteoporosis from a woman's teen years on.

Simplistically speaking, there are two basic kinds of allergic responses:

1. Immediate—instantaneous and obvious reactions
2. Delayed/cumulative (and thus hidden)—reactions that occur too far after exposure to let you make an obvious connection, or occur intermittently with repeated and cumulative exposure.

About half of all allergies take the form of hidden reactions, which makes them difficult to identify. Skin testing picks up immediate reactions, such as a histamine reaction to a particular substance (juniper, mold, etc.) that causes an identifiable swelling on the arm. Allergies that are not caused by this mechanism are harder to identify and thus create confusion and the controversial "politics" of allergies.

Uniquely Female: Hormones play a large role in immune function.

- At puberty, especially at younger ages, girls menstruate but often do not ovulate. Thus, they produce estrogen but not progesterone (ovulation produces progesterone). This *unopposed estrogen* environment can cause liver stress, which may contribute to allergies. Girls who develop allergies at puberty should be treated by having them avoid the identified aller-

---

ALLERGIC THRESHOLD

The allergic threshold is an imaginary line dividing overt allergy symptoms from no symptoms.

No Symptoms

ALLERGIC THRESHOLD _____

Symptoms

Certain conditions lower the threshold and cause and/or increase the severity of various allergic symptoms. Hormone fluctuations and imbalances, such as during premenstrual and peri- and postmenopausal times, can significantly lower the threshold and worsen or create new allergic symptoms. Other conditions that lower the threshold include maldigestion; physical trauma; underlying disorders, such as undiagnosed thyroid problems; environmental chemical exposure; and chronic use of certain medications that may tax the body's ability to deal with foreign substances, e.g., long-term use of acetaminophen, non-steroidal anti-inflammatory drugs (NSAIDs), such as Ibuprofen, and non-enterically-coated adult aspirin.

---

gens and by taking milk thistle, B vitamins, pantothenic acid, essential fatty acids, and a multivitamin/mineral supplement. Evaluate the need for digestive enzymes if there are maldigestive symptoms (pages 208, 468).

- During the reproductive years, women with cyclical allergy symptoms or worsening of allergy symptoms anywhere from midcycle to several days into the menses may have a possible hormonal imbalance. Have your doctor run your hormone levels, and consider taking vitamin B_6, 25–50 mg per day; B complex, 25 mg per day; magnesium, 250–400 mg per day; essential fatty acids, 2–6 g per day; and herbs like vitex. Rule out progesterone deficiency.

- Some premenopausal women, on the other hand, can be allergic to their own progesterone. This allergy can manifest as endometriosis or as severe premenstrual syndrome (PMS) that does not respond to any therapy, including progesterone. See *Premenstrual Syndrome*. In rare cases, some women need to be "desensitized" to their own progesterone by an allergist, nutritional doctor, or an environmental medicine practitioner.

- Any time during peri- or postmenopause, the changing hormonal milieu can either suddenly cause allergies in a woman who never had them, worsen an already allergic condition, or suddenly improve or stop old allergies from occurring. Ask your doctor to run full hormone tests, including DHEA (dehydroepiandrosterone), cortisol, and testosterone. Supplement low hormones, adding vitamin B_6, B complex, and magnesium (see doses on page 83), as well as free-form amino acids (take as directed on label), and PABA (para-aminobenzoic acid), 300 mg one to three times a day, and avoid allergens.
- During menopause, declining hormonal levels can result in greater reactivity to allergens and chemicals. In women who develop allergies at menopause, the digestive tract and immune system need boosting. Evaluate for digestive enzymes (page 468). Supplement with glutamine (several hundred milligrams, in divided dosages), B vitamins (25–50 mg a day), and PABA (several hundred milligrams a day). Hormone potentiators or replacement therapy often decrease allergic reactions, so consider trying these before treating allergies. See *Immune Enhancement.*
- Allergic reactions can cause the adrenal glands to secrete stress hormones, which promote bone loss and impede the body's ability to use testosterone to build bone.
- Women who go through puberty early and women who eat a diet high in total fat and/or saturated fat may have children predisposed to allergies.

Food Allergies

Food allergies are not the same as *food intolerance,* in which certain enzymes needed for digestion are lacking (such as in lactose intolerance, which is the inability to digest dairy foods). Some latex-sensitive individuals will also react to certain foods like bananas, avocados, and chestnuts.

Symptoms: Extreme fatigue immediately after eating or up to one hour later; indigestion, such as burping, gas, and intestinal discomfort; recurrent diarrhea; recurrent infections, such as middle ear infections, bronchitis, and vaginitis; ears getting red within an hour of eating; nose itching, or nose and ear pulling; dark circles under the eyes, called "allergic shiners"; lines and/or puffiness under the eyes; headaches; depression or mood swings; mental problems or learning problems; behavioral problems, such as hyperactivity; poor resistance to numerous health problems, such as flu; and rashes and hives. Even chronic fatigue and fibromyalgia are worsened by food allergies. Many of these symptoms overlap with other illnesses, and it is necessary to figure out if your health problems are caused or exacerbated by food allergies.

Some diseases particularly linked to food allergies are severe premenstrual syndrome; chronic diarrhea and/or constipation, irritable bowel syndrome, Crohn's disease, ulcerative colitis; cyclical headaches or migraines; palpitations; and various types of chronic joint problems. But food allergies can cause *any* kind of health problem. They may show up in women as unexplained and poorly responsive bone loss; recurring infections, such as bladder, respiratory, or yeast infections; frequent urination; digestive disorders; migraines; arthritis; asthma; fatigue; depression; and nasal congestion.

Cyclic vomiting syndrome, on the rise in high school girls, has been linked to food allergies in some children.

Causes: Eating the same foods over and over again; inadequate digestive enzymes (page 468); nutrient deficiencies and junk food diets; eating chemically altered, sprayed, or processed foods; inherited food sensitivities; food additives; stress; intestinal and/or chronic infections; and emotional trauma. Food allergies make stress worse, and stress makes food allergies worse.

What to Do

Testing for food allergies is not easy. Skin testing for hidden (delayed) allergies is unreliable. We recommend the following testing methods, none of which is *totally* foolproof.

- *Elimination-challenge test* (two weeks): This method is difficult, but it teaches you to become aware of symptoms caused by allergy-provoking foods. It is the most complete of the home tests, while being the most difficult to do.

  Eliminate all common food allergens for ten days to two

weeks. You should continue the test only if your symptoms improve or go away during this time. Once you are symptom free for at least several days, add foods back one at a time to figure out which provoke symptoms. If you are very ill, elimination diets can make the body more sensitive and reactions can be severe, so work with a doctor. Read my book *Healthy Digestion the Natural Way* (John Wiley, 2000) for details.

The most common allergens to be removed include foods you crave, foods you know you react to, foods you eat more than three times a week, and all processed foods and oils. Also eliminate dairy products, cereals (especially wheat), corn, eggs, soy products, shellfish, beef, citrus fruits, strawberries, tomatoes, peanuts, coffee, tea, alcohol, refined foods, tap water, and certain food dyes (such as yellow #5). Other additives known to cause reactions are vanillin, benzyldehyde, eucalyptol, monosodium glutamate (MSG), BHT-BHA, benzoates, sulfites, and annatto.

What's left to eat? Try whole grains such as millet, amaranth, or others you don't normally eat (not whole wheat), vegetables, beans (if you can digest them), nuts (not peanuts), seeds, fish (not shellfish), unprocessed cold-pressed oils. Eat simple meals of foods you don't usually eat and vary them throughout the week. After identifying and eliminating food allergens, rebuilding digestion, and improving diet, some foods can be retested after three months and again at six months to see if they are now safe to eat. Some foods may be reactive forever. Eating a variety of different foods every day is the best way to reduce reactions.

- *Elimination-challenge for four days.* Remove a food completely for four days. On the fifth eat *only* that food in large amounts first thing in the morning and see how you feel over the course of the day and the next. (From lunchtime on, you can eat some foods you already have been eating.)
- *Eliminate one food for six weeks to three months* and see if you feel better.
- *The Food Antibody Assessment IgE and IgG blood tests* provide information on immediate-onset allergies and delayed aller-

gic responses. Your doctor can order testing kits from labs listed in appendix A. Although not perfect, these tests are helpful and are used by many holistic practitioners.

- *Provocative neutralization* is a treatment for food allergies that desensitizes the body to foods. It is used by some allergists and environmental doctors to help your body overcome sensitivities.
- *Chiropractic kinesiology* is a hands-on method of allergy diagnosis using "muscle testing." It is surprisingly effective for some women.
- *Pulse test:* Sit down, relax, and take your pulse (at the wrist). Count the number of beats in a sixty-second period (normal count is 52–70 per minute). Eat the food you are testing. Wait fifteen to twenty minutes and take your pulse again. If the rate has increased more than 10 beats per minute, eliminate this food for one month, then retest. This test is not conclusive, but a significant rise in your pulse suggests a problem.
- *Hormone test:* Thyroid and adrenal problems can cause or aggravate food allergies, so test hormone levels.

Note: The Food and Drug Administration requires safety testing but *not* labeling of genetically engineered foods that may contain genes from the most common allergenic foods. There is concern that lesser-known antigens can be transferred to these modified foods. If you are a very sensitive individual, it may behoove you to avoid genetically altered foods as much as possible.

Nutrients

- ** Consider digestive enzymes (page 468).
- ** Pantothenic acid, up to several hundred milligrams three times a day
- ** *L. acidophilus* and *Bifidobacterium bifidum* (probiotics help reduce allergic inflammatory reactions)
- ** Vitamin C with bioflavonoids, 500–1,000 mg one to several times a day. It is such a powerful antihistamine that if you are planning to have allergy testing done, discontinue taking

vitamin C for three weeks beforehand in order to get accurate results.
** Vitamin B complex, 50–100 mg per day
• Zinc, 20 mg per day
• Multimineral with manganese

Inhalant Allergies

Sensitivity to airborne allergens.

Symptoms: Runny, itchy nose and watery eyes; sneezing and coughing attacks; sore throat; chronic lung, bronchial, and sinus infections; itchy skin; rashes; asthma; shortness of breath; frontal headaches; insomnia; menstrual disorders; hypoglycemia; learning disabilities.

Causes: Common immediate reactions are often caused by flowers, grasses, tree pollens, mold, animal dander, house dust, dust mites, and yeasts. Exposure to heavy traffic may worsen hay fever. House dust mites, or mattress mites, can cause problems for years without being diagnosed, and they often cause chronic problems like skin rashes. Get diagnosed and try special mattress covers.

If you suffer from inhalant allergies, use locally produced honey (from as close to your geographical area as possible; it improves the immune system response to allergens from local plants and flowers) throughout the year as your sweetener. Take pantothenic acid, 1–5 g per day, and avoid wheat and dairy products for two months before the allergy season starts. During allergy season, rub one third of a 5,000 IU vitamin A capsule on the inside of your nostrils once a day.

Chemical Sensitivity

Chemical sensitivity can affect any organ system in the body, especially the nervous system. See *Multiple Chemical Sensitivities*. Women who spend hours in front of computers may be more prone to skin rashes or other symptoms from flame-retardant chemicals that outgas from the heated plastic.

A critical link in the present-day rise of allergies is our omnipresent exposure to environmental chemicals that overload our system, junk food diets, and stressful lifestyles, which lead to nutrient deficiencies and maldigestion. Hormonal imbalances such as in severe PMS or in peri- or postmenopause can cause any kind of allergies.

Other types of allergic reactions are responsible for a lung disease (allergic alveolitis), skin swellings after booster vaccinations, or contact dermatitis (a rash caused by contact with substances such as nickel, detergents, and cosmetics). See the section on dermatitis under *Skin*.

Five to 10 percent of women who wear latex gloves at work may develop multiple allergic symptoms, including dermatitis, nasal congestion, asthma, multiple food allergies (to foods handled by workers wearing latex gloves), vaginal itching, low blood pressure, and even infertility. A latex allergy may take years to develop and will thus be difficult to identify.

ANEMIA, IRON DEFICIENCY

The most common form of anemia—inadequate oxygenation of blood—develops when the amount of iron in the blood is insufficient to make hemoglobin, the substance in red blood cells that carries oxygen from the lungs to the rest of the body. Iron is essential for the formation of hemoglobin. Iron-deficiency anemia is seen most frequently in women, children, and older adults. Vitamin B_{12} deficiency, or pernicious anemia, causes anemia with symptoms of weakness, light-headedness, vertigo, ringing in the ears, palpitations, angina, and symptoms that can mimic congestive heart failure.

Symptoms: During the early stages of anemia, there may be no symptoms; when symptoms do appear, they may be vague, confusing, and mimic other conditions. Typical symptoms are fatigue, headache, inability to think clearly, irritability, loss of appetite, pale blue whites of the eyes, pale skin, rapid heartbeat, shortness of breath during exercise, poor endurance, abdominal pain, coldness, dizziness, fainting, weakness, sore mouth or tongue, brittle nails and/or hair, and, in severe cases, breathlessness and pain in the center of the chest. Specific signs of iron deficiency in chronic and severe cases include a strong desire to eat ice, paint, or dirt; smooth tongue; and spoon-shaped nails.

Causes: Excessive menstruation; loss of iron from abnormally heavy or persistent gastrointestinal bleeding; recurring infections and chronic illness; pregnancy; autoimmune conditions; parasites. Other causes are poor absorption of iron due to stomach surgery or digestive disorders, malfunctioning kidneys, or a diet that does not provide enough iron. People with milk allergies or lactose intolerance can lose blood in their stools after eating dairy products, but this may go unnoticed, because the stools are not always black and tarry as in the case of internal bleeding. Inadequate stomach acid (especially in peri- and postmenopausal women), junk food diets, diuretics, and the drugs omeprazole (Prilosec) and lansoprazole (Prevacid) may inhibit iron absorption.

Uniquely Female: Women of childbearing age tend to have low, or no, built-up stores of iron because of menstrual bleeding, and thus they can become anemic more quickly than others. Particularly heavy periods from conditions such as fibroids or unopposed estrogen syndrome; some diseases (gastritis, peptic ulcer, inflammatory conditions of the intestinal tract, and stomach cancer); and prolonged treatment with aspirin and other NSAIDs (nonsteroidal anti-inflammatory drugs) can cause iron-deficiency anemia from bleeding that usually goes undetected until the problem is advanced. This commonly causes fatigue in women. Anemia affects over half of all pregnancies and is more common in women who have had more than one baby, especially if the children were closely spaced. Pregnancy stops the loss of menstrual blood, but the growing baby places an even greater drain on the mother's iron stores. In postmenopausal women, severe anemia is usually caused by stomach ulcers, inadequate stomach acid (hydrochloric acid), or an intestinal tumor. Women who use intrauterine devices (IUDs) are prone to heavy periods, which can contribute to anemia through excessive loss of blood.

What to Do
   ** Evaluate your need for stomach acid (page 469).
   • Excess iron has been linked to several health problems, such as aggravating cancer, so iron supplements should be taken only if needed.

- Check for thyroid deficiency, heavy-metal toxicity, and food allergies (wheat and milk).
- Rule out *H. pylori* infection (a bug that can infect the stomach and lower production of stomach acid. It usually causes stomach burning, pain, ulcers, and loss of appetite, especially in the elderly).

Diet: The body absorbs only a small amount of the iron in food. Red meat is the best source, especially liver and organ meats (animals raised organically are the safest source of organ meats). Other iron-rich foods include beans (lima, kidney, chickpeas, lentils); blackstrap molasses; dried fruits (figs, prunes, raisins, apricots); nuts; whole grains, particularly brown rice; yams; seafood; eggs and poultry; leafy green vegetables; cherries or cherry juice; and parsley. Cooking in iron skillets adds iron to the food.

Avoid: Uncooked foods high in oxalic acid (almonds, asparagus, beets, kale, rhubarb, colas, spinach, Swiss chard), which interferes with iron absorption, as do some food additives, excessive tea and coffee (tannins in black tea, polyphenols in coffee), and lead and cadmium (in tobacco smoke [even passive exposure] and car exhaust).

Nutrients
- ** Iron supplements: Ferrous sulfate irritates the gut wall and often causes constipation as well as damaging blood fats (it promotes the oxidation of lipoproteins). Ferrous peptonate is gentle and easily absorbed. The next-best-tolerated forms are ferrous chelates and gluconates. Supplement only if blood iron or serum ferritin levels are low or below normal.
- ** Vitamin C enhances absorption of iron and should be taken with iron supplements.
- Multivitamin/mineral with vitamin A (several hundred IUs), which helps you digest iron
- Vitamin B_6 (pyridoxine), 25 mg per day
- Vitamin E, 200 IU per day
- Zinc supplementation (15–60 mg per day, with backup copper, 2–4 mg per day) can help overcome anemia in endurance

runners, disabled women, and premature infants. A mild deficiency of zinc in pregnant women may worsen iron-deficiency anemia. When zinc is combined with iron, it increases hemoglobin levels significantly in pregnant women.

- Check for folic acid deficiency, as folic acid works with vitamin B$_{12}$ to prevent *pernicious anemia.* Birth control pills and epileptic medications can create folic acid deficiency.

ANGINA PECTORIS

Discomfort or pain in the chest (a dull ache in the middle of the chest or a feeling of pressure that may spread to the neck or down the arms), usually brought on by emotional stress, exposure to cold or exertion, or toxic chemical fumes, and relieved by rest. See *Heart Disease.*

Diet: Very low fat diet (make sure to include essential fatty acids). Limit animal foods. Consume whole foods. Do not overeat. Read about the Pritikin and Dean Ornish diets.

Avoid: Refined foods and sugar, alcohol. Limit caffeine (five cups or more of coffee per day increases your risk of angina).

What to Do

Take one aspirin immediately if you think your angina is serious enough for you to go to the hospital. Identify and avoid food allergies and low blood sugar problems. Reduce stress (see pages 52–58).

Nutrients

** Magnesium, 300–600 mg per day; ask your doctor about intravenous (IV) injections once or twice a week for six weeks. Alan R. Gaby, M.D., recommends various kinds of IV formulas at specific doses and rates. For information on training tapes about IV uses and procedures, refer to (www.dralangaby.com).

** Vitamin E, 400–800 IU per day

** L-arginine, 500 mg three times a day

** Coenzyme Q-10, 60–100 mg one to three times a day

ANGINA AS A WARNING SIGN OF A HEART ATTACK

If you have recurring, sudden, intense chest pains, lasting thirty seconds to one minute, with a viselike grip of pressure across the chest, this is *not* indigestion—call 911. Call your doctor if angina is more painful each time you have it

 or it occurs more often, lasts longer than ten to fifteen minutes even after rest, wakes you from sleep, or occurs during exercise and doesn't go away with rest.

** Omega-3 flax or fish oil, 2–6 g per day in divided doses
** High-potency multivitamin/mineral supplement
- L-carnitine, 500 mg three times a day
- Extra vitamin C decreases angina in drinkers.
- Some people need to consider chelation and/or hormonal therapy with testosterone or estrogen.
- Ask your doctor to evaluate your thyroid function. If it's abnormal, remember that great care must be taken with thyroid supplementation, as excessive doses (higher than you need) can stress the heart.
- Ask your doctor about IV or oral N-acetyl-cysteine (NAC) and IV glutathione (600 mg) along with nitrogylcerin to reduce the threat of heart attack with unstable angina.

Herbs: Hawthorn berry, 80–300 mg two to three times a day, is very helpful. Ginger, 1–4 g one to three times a day, plus cayenne; infusion of sage and lime flowers (two pinches each per cup of water), two or three cups a day.

ANXIETY

An unpleasant emotional state ranging from mild unease to intense fear, with a sense of impending doom although there is no obvious threat. Anxiety becomes a disorder when it disrupts normal daily activities. More than 25 million Americans have had debilitating anxiety at some time in their lives. Anxiety can be linked to high blood pressure, heart spasms, and fatal heart disease.

Symptoms: Difficulty breathing, nameless terror, fear for the future, trembling, "butterflies" in the stomach, heart palpitations, fatigue, headaches, chest pain, muscular weakness, dizziness, nausea, muscular tightness, changes in appetite, a tendency to sigh or hyperventilate, an inability to relax, and a feeling of unreality. Uncommon symptoms include diarrhea, "pins and needles," visual disturbances, phobias, or a sense of impending death. Other symptoms include sweating, blushing, pallor, or a constant need to urinate or defecate. There often is a feeling of being cut off from oneself or from the world.

Causes: Lack of regular exercise; imbalanced diet and nutrient deficiencies; unresolved conflict issues; chronic or severe stress; currently being in a situation that is not optimal for well-being; hormonal imbalance (usually a progesterone deficiency, estrogen excess, or thyroid hormone excess); underlying undiagnosed illness that is stressing the immune system; chemical sensitivities; allergies or intolerances; hypoglycemia; excess caffeinated beverages or foods; and possibly habitual patterns of negative thinking. Hidden celiac disease (see page 174) has now been found to cause anxiety.

Uniquely Female:

- For midcycle or premenstrual syndrome–associated anxiety, take 20 mg of pyridoxal-5'-phosphate once or twice a day, L-tyrosine, 500 mg morning and evening on an empty stomach, along with vitamin A emulsion, 10,000 IU per day for three months.
- During puberty, add zinc, 20 mg daily.
- Around perimenopause, consider low-dose progesterone supplementation.
- At menopause, get all of your hormones tested and supplement wherever appropriate, especially DHEA (dehydroepiandrosterone). Consider hormone potentiators such as PABA (para-aminobenzoic acid).
- Anxiety during pregnancy may be related to problems handling elevated levels of estrogen, so consider two capsules of

milk thistle with breakfast for two weeks, avoid caffeinated beverages and refined sugars, and add vitamin B complex, 25 mg, even if you are already on a multivitamin/mineral formula (make sure you do not exceed 25 mg of vitamin B_6 per day, as it can lower milk production).

What to Do

- Identify and eliminate food allergens.
- Avoid toxic chemical exposures.
- Learn stress-reduction techniques (page 52).
- Get an antigliadin antibody test to rule out celiac disease. If you test positive, avoid gluten and see how you fare.
- Adapton is a naturally occurring extract of a deep-sea fish that is used widely in Europe for anxiety, stress, and depression. It decreases sensations of anxiety and improves mood, feelings of well-being, and sleep. It appears to have no side effects. Take 4 capsules on an empty stomach in the morning for fifteen days and then reduce to 2 capsules until improved. To order, call 800-544-4440.
- Try Rescue Remedy (one of the Bach flower essence remedies), ten drops under your tongue every fifteen minutes until you feel improved, then take twice a day for several days.
- Exercise: Put your legs on a bed, buttocks on the floor, cover your face with your arms, and breathe deeply. Inhale through your mouth and exhale through your nose, then reverse. Repeat slowly for five minutes. Then exhale, saying "AHHHH" out loud. Keep repeating for as long as it's comfortable.

Diet: Have a Protein Green Drink (page 465) once a day; the magnesium in this drink acts as a natural sedative. Consume yogurt and dark green leafy vegetables. Foods rich in B vitamins (such as whole grains, beans, nuts, and nutritional yeast) support energy, digestion, and the adrenal glands.

Avoid: All stressor foods, such as caffeine (including chocolate and colas), refined sugars, alcohol, and food allergens. Avoid aspartame and low-calorie sweeteners.

Nutrients

- ** Magnesium, 250–600 mg several times a day (too much can cause loose stools)
- ** Vitamin B complex, 25–50 mg once or twice a day with meals
- • Calcium, 600–1,200 mg per day
- • Vitamin B_{12} injections, 1,000 mcg intramuscularly as needed
- • L-tryptophan (by prescription), 1,000 mg twice a day on an empty stomach
- • Inositol, 500 mg twice a day up to 12 g per day for panic attacks and agoraphobia

Herbs

- • Tea made with chamomile and ½ dropper of valerian or kava-kava. Kava, in a standardized extract of 45–250 mg of two to three times a day (contraindicated if you're taking benzodiazepine drugs)
- • For palpitations: Hawthorn berries
- • For shakiness: Take adrenal glandulars (1–2 capsules, two to three times a day), vitamin C (1 g twice a day), and pantothenic acid (500–1,000 mg several times a day).
- • For fear: Kava, valerian root, or scullcap
- • For hopelessness: St. John's wort

Panic Attacks

Panic attacks are a type of anxiety disorder marked by overwhelming feelings of fear, especially fear of dying or losing one's mind, that last anywhere from a few minutes to an hour or two.

Panic attacks must include at least four of the following symptoms: palpitations, pounding heart, or accelerated heart rate; sweating; trembling or shaking; shortness of breath or a sensation of smothering; feeling of choking; chest pain or discomfort; nausea or abdominal distress; feeling dizzy, unsteady, light-headed, or faint; feelings of unreality or being detached from oneself; fear of losing control or of going crazy; fear of dying; numbness or tingling sensations; chills or hot flashes.

Causes: Illness, stress, certain medicines, and chemicals may trigger the first attack. Past injuries and dangers may also be a factor. Fear of additional attacks can actually set them off. Adrenaline, the body's hormonal response to danger (real or imagined), causes many of the body changes typically felt during a panic attack.

Uniquely Female: Peri- and postmenopause, or any other time of fluctuating hormones (such as the week before the onset of menses), can result in disorientation, anxiety, and panic attacks.

What to Do
- Check for underlying physical disorders.
- Certain tranquilizers and antidepressant medications can relieve the attacks. Take any medications exactly as prescribed. If you feel the medicine is not helping, let your doctor know, but don't stop taking it on your own. Don't take tranquilizers for more than a few days at a time.
- Counseling may help. It is important to stick with a regular program of therapy.
- Learn stress-reduction techniques (pages 52–58) and meditation.
- Try to spend time outdoors.
- Get plenty of rest.
- Try to identify what triggers your attacks.
- Aerobic exercise (such as walking) can help you relax.

Avoid: Don't smoke, use drugs, drink alcohol, or consume high-caffeine foods and beverages, such as coffee, tea, soda, and chocolate. They can either cause anxiety or make your symptoms worse. Those who have repeated panic attacks may be ultrasensitive to caffeine.

Nutrients
- GABA (Gamma-aminobutyric Acid), 500–1,000 mg, once or twice a day.
- See herbs for anxiety (page 96); ask your doctor about propranolol, 10 mg per day.
- Tests show that cortisol levels elevate during panic attacks. Keep vitamin C lozenges on hand and suck at the first sign of panic to lower cortisol levels.
- If peri- or postmenopause is part of the problem, refer to those sections.

ARRHYTHMIAS
(Premature Ventricular Contractions, PVCs)

Healthy people can be suddenly aware of their heart beating out of sequence, racing, or "fluttering" (*palpitations*), which can cause considerable anxiety. EKGs (electrocardiograms) show the heart rhythm only over a short period of time, and arrhythmias are often intermittent. The heartbeats can be fast or slow, regular or irregular, brief or prolonged, and can happen at rest or only during activity. Pacemakers are used to treat severely slow heart rates. When a person with arrhythmias also has light-headedness, dizziness, and fainting, it means the heart's ability to pump blood is endangered and needs prompt medical attention.

Causes: When your heart "skips a beat" or beats too loudly (called *ventricular ectopic beats*) you may be in love, but it's probably from too much stress or taking over-the-counter remedies for colds or too much cappuccino. Risk factors include smoking, stress, high blood pressure, obesity, lack of exercise, diabetes, and poor diet with too much refined sugar, caffeine, alcohol, and saturated fat.

Uniquely Female: Harmless arrhythmias are common, especially in women in their thirties, and are usually triggered by too much alcohol, caffeine, smoking, stress, or exercise. Premature ventricular contractions (PVCs) can be worse right before the onset of menses and may improve with extra magnesium (250–400 mg per day) and vitamin B_6 (25 mg per day taken with B complex, 25–50 mg per day) the last two weeks of the menstrual cycle.

What to Do
- Plunge your face into cold water to stop palpitations.
- Avoid sodas. The phosphoric acid binds magnesium and makes it unavailable for regulating the heart.
- Identify and avoid allergic foods.
- Have your DHEA (dehydroepiandrosterone) level checked.

Diet: Eat a lot of fish and a diet low in hydrogenated and saturated fats and reduce salt.

HOW TO TAKE YOUR PULSE

Place your fingertips across the wrist of the opposite hand on the thumb side to feel the heartbeat. Count the number of beats during one minute (or count for fifteen seconds and multiply by four). If the rhythm is irregular or the rate is over 100 after resting for five minutes, call your doctor.

Avoid: Coffee, tea, alcohol, and nicotine if you are prone to arrhythmias.

Nutrients

Arrhythmias sometimes respond to nutrition, whereas atrial fibrillation usually only responds to intravenous (IV) magnesium. See *Heart Disease*.

- ** Magnesium, 250–500 mg per day, and potassium, 99 mg per day as aspartates; ask your doctor about IVs.
- ** Multivitamin/mineral supplement containing trace minerals like selenium, copper, and manganese
- ** Fish oil, 2–6 g per day, or 1 Tbsp. cod liver oil (balance with vitamin E, 800 IU per day)
- ** Taurine, 1,000 mg twice a day on an empty stomach
- ** Coenzyme Q-10, 30–100 mg per day
- • Vitamin D, 400–800 IU per day

Herbs: Hawthorn berry, 80–300 mg two to three times a day, is especially helpful, or ginger, 1–3 g two to three times a day.

ARTHRITIS

Inflammation of a joint that can produce pain, swelling, stiffness, and redness. May involve one joint or many and varies from a mild ache and stiffness to severe pain and deformity. Arthritis is probably the oldest known ailment on earth; even dinosaurs had it. Nowadays almost 40 million Americans have arthritis.

Osteoarthritis

Osteoarthritis (OA), or degenerative arthritis, is the most common form of arthritis and usually results from gradual wear and tear and thinning of the joint, the synovial membrane surrounding the joint, and/or thickening and spurring of the adjacent bones. Over time, the cartilage that normally cushions the joint becomes inflamed, swells, and is then eroded by movement. Most common in the fingers, feet, knees, hips, and the back and neck regions of the spine. It occurs in 80 percent of people over the age of fifty and in almost all people over the age of sixty, although not all have symptoms. Earlier in life, injury to a joint may bring on osteoarthritis.

Symptoms: Pain, swelling, creaking, and stiffness (especially in the morning and at the end of the day) of one or more joints. Cold and damp weather may make the aching worse. An osteoarthritic joint can make popping, clicking, and banging noises. May interfere with activities such as walking or dressing and may disrupt sleep. The affected joints can become enlarged and distorted, causing various levels of disability and the gnarled appearance of arthritic hands. Bone "spurs" (pointed growths) can cause swelling and redness around the tissue.

Causes: Old traumas; repeated mechanical joint stress due to poor posture, lack of exercise, joint malalignment, and poor muscle health; obesity; and aging. Genetic factors may hasten disease at younger ages. Elevated levels of inflammatory and degenerative agents may be due to genetics, allergies, or imbalances of nutrients such as essential fatty acids.

Uniquely Female: Osteoarthritis affects three times as many women because hormonal imbalances may make joints more vulnerable to injury. Cyclical joint problems and finger swelling that occur before menstruation or during menopause may be helped by taking vitamin B_6, 25–50 mg once or twice a day, or pyridoxal-5'-phosphate (P-5-P), 20 mg once or twice a day, for several months and then reduce to several times a week. During pregnancy, joint problems may be helped by taking 5 mg of P-5-P daily along with a multivitamin/mineral supplement with adequate folic acid. Magnesium and fatty acids may help, too.

What to Do

- Slant board: Gravity compresses our joints throughout the day. Lie on a slant board for fifteen to twenty minutes at the end of the day to gently stretch out your joints and relieve pressure.
- Acupuncture and hands-on therapy by physical therapists and chiropractors helps OA of the knee and can delay or prevent the need for surgery. Manipulative treatment two to five days after surgery has been shown to shorten healing time. Five to ten minutes of quadriceps exercise twice a day can reduce pain and increase function of knees.
- Millions of people are driven to overconsumption of anti-inflammatory and pain medications, all of which have adverse side effects, such as chronic irritation of the intestinal lining, increased risk of upper gastrointestinal bleeding, and even bone loss! Enteric coating does not reduce risk. These drugs are only palliative and don't stop the disease progression. In the long haul, they may actually hasten it. Nutritional alternatives are worth a trial before resorting to drugs; in scientific studies, they are successful at least 75 percent of the time and are free of the side effects of conventional drugs.

<u>Avoid:</u> Identified food allergens, which are commonly dairy and beef (page 84). Eliminate plants from the nightshade family—tomato, bell pepper, eggplant, white potato, and tobacco—if nothing else helps and see what happens.

Nutrients

Nutrient therapy will work best if your case is mild to moderate, with some cartilage remaining in the joints. Joints with *no* cartilage do not respond.

- ** Glucosamine sulfate, 500 mg two to three times a day. Results take four to six weeks. Some people benefit just with this. If it doesn't help, add chondroitin sulfate, 400 mg two to three times a day, to enhance glucosamine's action. Give it a three-month trial. If no benefit, try the other substances listed below. These agents do not disrupt blood sugar (*Journal of Family Practice* 50 (5):2001).

** Niacinamide, 1,000 mg sustained-release twice a day, reduces joint pain and improves motion. Take for three months. If nauseated, stop and restart at a lower dose. You may need your doctor to monitor your liver function.

** Essential fatty acids (eicosapentaenoic acid [EPA] and docosahexaenoic acid [DHA]) in divided daily doses, either fish-oil concentrate, 5–10 g per day, or cod-liver oil, 1–2 Tbsp. per day; and ⅛ tsp. ground flaxseeds every other day or 1 Tbsp. flaxseed oil every other day. Start low and work up to the dose you can tolerate up to 1 Tbsp. a day. These oils decrease joint tenderness and enhance the effectiveness of anti-inflammatory medications, often lowering the dose needed for therapeutic benefit. Some people do better with enterically coated capsules.

- SAMe (S-adenosyl-methionine), 200–400 mg one to three times a day
- Vitamin C, 500–1,000 mg two to three times a day
- GLA (gamma-linolenic acid, found in evening primrose oil, borage oil, and black currant seed oil) has been shown to be effective. Try various oils at various dosages; 540 mg per day plus 10 g per day of fish oil reduces symptoms and can reduce doses of nonsteroidal anti-inflammatory drugs (NSAIDs) significantly.
- Vitamin D, 400–800 IU per day. Low levels of vitamin D increase the enzymes that destroy cartilage, especially in hips and knees.
- Vitamin E, 400–800 IU per day, has an anti-inflammatory effect.
- Boron, 1–3 mg twice a day (check with your doctor first if you had breast cancer)
- ASU (avocado/soybean unsaponifiables), 300 mg per day for six months, has been shown to help, but it may be hard to find in the United States.

Herbs: Nettle leaves, 500–800 mg twice a day.

Rheumatoid Arthritis

This chronic autoimmune disorder differs from osteoarthritis in that there can be more inflammation and joint deformity caused by the thickening synovial sac that surrounds the joints. Rheumatoid Arthritis (RA) can affect tissues other than joints (such as the temporal artery to the eye). Many joints become extremely painful, stiff, and deformed, although the joints of the hands, feet, and knees are most commonly affected. The disease is usually progressive but controllable, and early treatment may prevent deformities.

Symptoms: At the onset, there can be fatigue, loss of appetite, mild fever, and generalized aches and pains. Later, affected joints can become swollen, red, warm, painful, and stiff. Structures around the joint may become inflamed, resulting in weakened ligaments, tendons, and muscles, which result in loss of movement and eventual destruction of joints. Swelling of the wrist and carpal tunnel syndrome are common, as is Raynaud's phenomenon. Anemia usually accompanies the disease. Small nodules appear beneath the skin over the joint in about 20 percent of female sufferers. Joint stiffness is usually worst in the morning and subsides during the day.

Causes: Food allergies often play a role, especially in women between the ages of twenty-five and forty, as do infectious microbes, genetics, leaky gut syndrome, and possible deficiencies or problems with the metabolism of certain nutrients such as essential fatty acids. The RA that responds best to avoiding allergic foods is the type with hot, inflamed red joints and no deformities. Drinking four or more cups of coffee a day is linked to a higher risk of RA.

Uniquely Female: This disease affects more than 6 million Americans, most of them women. This may be due to the fact that many autoimmune disorders are estrogen driven (occur more in the presence of estrogen). See *Estrogen Dominance.*

What to Do

** Check for parasitic, bacterial, and yeast infections (unidentified parasitic infection can manifest as chronic joint problems). Use labs that require purge methods. Rule out Lyme disease, and/or mercury toxicity.

- Identify food allergens.
- Avoid toxic chemical exposures.
- Ask your physician about anti-amoebic treatment with metronidazole. Refer your doctor to *Medical Hypotheses* 5:1237–49, 1979.
- Check for thyroid imbalances and digestive enzyme deficiencies.
- Caution: An increasing number of cases of lymphoma are being seen in RA patients who are treated with methotrexate. It makes sense to try natural therapeutics!
- Try aloe vera creams on arthritic joints to lessen pain and improve range of motion, as well as drinking 1–2 oz. of liquid aloe vera each day.
- Cut down on coffee.
- Avoid smoking, even secondhand smoke.

Diet: Olive oil consumption is inversely related to incidence of RA. Eat a fish-enriched diet (several fish meals weekly) and consume raw food, Green Drinks (page 465), and fresh vegetable juices. A diet rich in fresh vegetables and fruits is high in natural antioxidants. Consume vegetable broth. Eat cherries, blueberries, or hawthorn berries or take their extract. Try ½ Tbsp. cod liver oil mixed in 2 Tbsp. fresh juice one half hour or more before breakfast for six months. Eat oat or rice bran daily. Consume eggs, onions, garlic, asparagus, green leafy vegetables, nonacidic fresh fruits, whole grains, oatmeal, brown and Chinese red rice.

Avoid: Food allergens, and too much cooked or lifeless food. Excess vitamin D can increase soreness in joints in some people. Also try eliminating red meat for several months and see if that helps. Limit refined foods and citrus fruits. Some people are helped by a more vegetarian diet. Do not take iron or a multivitamin that contains iron unless you have proven iron deficiency.

Nutrients

- ** Copper (in the form of sebacate), 2–4 mg per day
- ** Borage oil, 720–1,440 mg per day, and fish-oil concentrate, 5–12 g per day in divided doses, for six to twelve months.

Start at a low dosage and work up to a dose you can tolerate. Reduce as symptoms improve. These oils decrease joint tenderness and enhance effectiveness of medications. If you don't respond to these oils, try others, such as evening primrose oil.

- Zinc (picolinate or citrate), 30 mg two to three times a day. Reduce to once or twice a day after two months. Works best for aggressive form of RA with deformities. Take with meals.
- Vitamin E, 400–800 IU per day, reduces joint pain.
- Selenium, 200 mcg per day
- Bromelain, 300 mg two to three times a day on an empty stomach for several weeks
- MSM (methylsulfonylmethane), 3–5 g per day
- Vitamin D_3, 400–800 IU per day, taken under a doctor's supervision helps maintain your calcium levels if you're taking long-term corticosteroids. Ask your doctor about alphacalcidol, a form of vitamin D.
- Antioxidant formula daily
- Vitamin C, 500 mg twice a day
- Pantothenic acid, 500–1,000 mg once or twice a day
- D, L-phenylalanine, 75–1,500 mg per day, may help with pain
- Avoid melatonin, which may worsen RA.

Herbs: Ginger root powder, 2–5 g two or three times a day. Certain natural formulas contain salicylic derivatives from wintergreen and purple willow, but don't take these if you're allergic to aspirin. Devil's claw, 2 g twice a day. Ginger and turmeric are herbal anti-inflammatories, as are cayenne/ginger compresses. Raw lemon rubs and hot castor oil packs are beneficial. Boswellia is an Ayurvedic (East Indian medicinal) NSAID, 400–800 mg three times a day.

What to Do for Both Types of Arthritis
- If overweight, lose weight. The more weight you carry, the more stress and pressure on your joints, which increases stress on the cartilage, which, in turn, interferes with the bone and increases inflammation, swelling, and pain.

Long-term use of high-dose aspirin and NSAIDs is the conventional treatment for arthritis. However, high dosages of aspirin can cause gastrointestinal (GI) irritation and bleeding, decrease digestion of other nutrients, and cause ringing in the ears *(tinnitus)*. NSAIDs can also irritate the GI tract and have been shown in some studies to inhibit cartilage repair and hasten its degeneration. More than seven hundred patients a year die from NSAIDs, and toxicity from drug treatments are said to contribute to 60 percent of the cost of treating RA patients in the United States.

If you do take aspirin or NSAIDs, consider chewing DGL (deglycyrrhizinated licorice, hormone-free licorice) on an empty stomach twenty minutes prior to taking medications to reduce gastric irritation. Fish oil concentrates hasten positive benefits of NSAIDs and may reduce gastric irritation as well as the dosages of NSAIDs you'll require for relief.

- Apply heat. Put a warm heating pad or warm, moist towels on the painful joint, or soak it in a hot tub or whirlpool bath for ten to twenty minutes every waking hour for forty-eight hours.
- If your back is affected: Sleep on a firm mattress or place a piece of ¾-inch plywood between your mattress and the box springs. Waterbeds help some people.
- Regular exercise that doesn't traumatize the joints—especially walking, bicycling, or swimming—strengthens muscles and reduces symptoms. All experts agree that exercising in water significantly reduces pain. Yoga is good for movement with proper joint alignment.
- Apply a muscle ointment such as aloe vera cream at night before bed to reduce morning stiffness.
- Endorphins (natural brain opiates) help reduce pain. They're produced by your body when you enjoy things that make you joyful and passionate, such as art, music, sports, or sex.

Menopausal Arthritis

This disorder starts around menopause and includes pain, swelling, numbness, and tingling of fingers and hands; reduced gripping strength; and shoulder and knee pain and stiffness. Vitamin B_6, 50 mg two to three times a day, plus backup vitamin B complex usually helps within one to three weeks.

Gout

Gout is a form of arthritis in which uric acid crystals accumulate in joints (usually just one joint at a time), causing inflammation and pain.

Symptoms: An acute attack most commonly affects the foot or the joint at the base of the big toe, making it red, swollen, and extremely painful. Shoulder, elbow, knee, hand, ankle, or arm joints can also be affected, becoming hot, swollen, and very tender; the skin over the joint may look shiny and red. Joint pain may be accompanied by fever and chills.

Uniquely Female: In women, gout usually occurs after menopause or chemotherapy. High blood pressure and excess weight increase risk.

What to Do

- Avoid aspirin, which can raise uric acid levels. Acetaminophen can't fight inflammation; use ibuprofen for pain.
- Reduce high blood pressure.
- Fasting and rapid weight loss diets may aggravate gout attacks.
- Check for lead toxicity as certain gouts are caused by a buildup of lead in the body.
- Ginger compresses can help soothe the inflamed area. Or try rubbing fresh mint leaves on the joint to relieve pain.

Diet: Uric acid is a natural product of the breakdown of purine, a component of certain foods. Drink eight to ten large glasses of water and four glasses of black cherry juice a day to help your body get rid of uric acid. Eat foods high in potassium (fresh cherries, bananas, celery, broccoli, potatoes, and greens). Strawberries also neutralize uric acid.

During an Attack: Throughout the day, drink cherry juice or eat ½ pound of cherries and drink plenty of water (this may loosen stools a bit). If you can't get cherries, try strawberries or blueberries. Eat a raw-foods diet of vegetables and fruits, seeds, nuts, and some whole grains for two weeks, with plenty of fresh vegetable juices and *L. acidophilus* and other beneficial bacteria. Consume vegetable and potato soups or broth at least several times a week. Use ginger freely.

<u>Avoid:</u> High-purine foods most likely to induce gout—red meat, organ meats, poultry, shellfish, sardines, anchovies, and legumes. Limit fish, meat, and poultry to one 3-oz. serving five days a week for one to three months depending on the severity of the gout. Avoid refined sugar (especially sucrose and fructose) and alcohol (especially beer), as they increase production of uric acid. Limiting alcohol to one drink a day (if you regularly consume more) can reduce the number of attacks.

Nutrients

- ** Vitamin C, 1,000–2,000 mg two to three times a day. Start at 500 mg twice a day and build up to higher dosages. A high dose is contraindicated if kidney disease is present and/or gouty crystals occur within the kidneys. Work with doctor.
- ** Folic acid, 25 mg two to three times a day, along with 500 mg vitamin C
- ** Quercetin, 150–250 mg two to three times a day between meals
- ** High-potency multivitamin/mineral with zinc and copper
- • Low-dose lithium (orotate), 3–5 mg two to three times a day, which should be taken with flaxseed oil and vitamin E to avoid toxicity. Work with doctor.
- • B complex, 50 mg, with extra vitamin B_6, 250 mg, and folic acid, 800 mcg, one to three times a day
- • Don't take vitamin A and niacin during attacks as they may aggravate the gout.
- • Ask your doctor about intravenous colchicine.

<u>Herbs:</u> Bilberry, 80 mg three times a day.

ASTHMA, BRONCHIAL

Recurring attacks of breathlessness, usually accompanied by wheezing or mild coughing, caused by spasms in the muscles that surround the bronchi in the lungs. Although asthma frequently begins before the age of five, it can develop at any age. More than 10 million Americans have asthma. It is difficult to cure, but can be controlled by avoiding allergenic foods, various substances and chemicals, and taking nutritional supplements. Repeat attacks are common.

Symptoms: Trouble breathing, a tight feeling in the chest, coughing, and wheezing. Colds are accompanied by ear or bronchial infections. If you are sweating and have real difficulty breathing, your lips and nail beds turn a pale or blue color, or if your heart beats faster and you become very anxious, get help immediately. Symptoms vary widely from woman to woman.

Causes: Triggers (substances causing asthma attacks) may include allergies to something inhaled, such as pollens, house dust, animal fur or dander (interestingly, dark-colored cats are four times more likely to cause allergic reactions than light-colored ones), or an attack may follow a respiratory infection; exercise; exposure to tobacco smoke, chemical fumes, or other air pollutants; or from allergies to a particular food or drug (commonly aspirin). Stress or anxiety may precipitate attacks. Most common allergens include cow's milk products, shellfish, tomatoes, chocolate, nuts, fish, yeast, nightshade foods, foods high in salicylates, food colorings (especially yellow dye #5), and monosodium glutamate (MSG). Other causes include adrenal exhaustion, inadequate stomach acidity, hypoglycemia, poor circulation, chemical toxicity, emotional stress, very cold air, and low thyroid function. Asthma can also be a reaction to the hepatitis B vaccine.

Uniquely Female: Estrogen dominance is implicated in asthma; studies have found that women on hormone replacement therapy have a higher incidence of asthma and heavier women have more asthma (heavier women usually manufacture more estrogen). Oral contraceptives, hormone replacement therapy, and fertility drugs can trigger asthma.

What to Do

- Prolonged use of inhalers (corticosteroids) causes bone loss, so natural alternatives for asthma should be tried first.
- *To open up air passages*—4 oz. horseradish, 2 oz. lemon juice, 1 tsp. garlic juice, and 1 Tbsp. honey. Take 1 tsp. four times a day.
- *To stop an attack:* Mash raw cranberries through a strainer and add warm water; drink a cup every half hour for one hour.
- *For acute attacks:* Ask your doctor about an intravenous (IV) injection of magnesium, vitamin B_6, and other nutrients to stop an attack.
- *Topical treatment:* Try castor oil packs on the back around the kidneys and lungs.
- Identify and avoid food sensitivities (especially dairy) and stomach acid deficiency (especially in children).
- Avoid toxic chemicals (new carpets, paints, glues, pesticides, perfumes).
- Avoid living or working near heavily trafficked areas.
- Keep the amount of dust in your home to a minimum. Have guests wipe their feet twice on a mat or remove their shoes. Hire a company to clean out the air ducts and vents every year.
- Replace pillows or mattress with materials that don't cause allergies. Look for bedding that is made of urethane or foam rubber and is labeled "nonallergenic."
- Quit smoking and avoid passive smoke.
- Exercise daily to make your heart stronger, lower blood pressure, and keep you healthy.
- Lose excess weight so that your heart and lungs don't have to work as hard.
- Eliminate and desensitize inhalant allergens.
- Antibiotic use in infancy may be linked with increased risk of developing asthma later in life. Be judicious with antibiotic use and try to feed your growing children organic meat to avoid antibiotics fed to animals.
- Test for allergies to female hormones and desensitize if necessary.

> # IN A PINCH
>
> If you don't have your inhaler and you feel an attack coming on, drink several cups of strong coffee, black tea, caffeinated soda, cocoa, or eat a chocolate bar. Caffeine is similar to many asthma medications.

- Get a negative ion generator, especially for use in your bedroom.
- Acid reflux and heartburn can cause coughing in asthmatics. Control heartburn to take care of cough (see my book *Healthy Digestion the Natural Way*, John Wiley, 2000).

Diet: Drink eight to ten 12-oz. glasses of water each day. This (as well as bromelain, 500–1,000 mg once or twice a day) helps thin the sputum so it can be coughed up more easily. Keep blood sugar steady by eating smaller, more frequent meals and consuming potassium-rich foods like bananas, whole grains, avocados, and carrot juices and soups. Eat fish and fresh fruit, especially pears. Season foods with garlic, ginger, and cayenne. Bronchodilator foods include chili peppers, garlic, onions, mustard, and horseradish. Focus on fresh fruits and veggies, nuts and seeds, oatmeal, brown rice, and whole grains. Consume Protein Green Drink daily (page 465).

Avoid: Some asthmatics react to the following: aspirin or aspirin-like substances (salicylates) in foods (see box, page 112), yellow dye #5 (tartrazine), sulfite preservatives, BHA and BHT additives, and MSG. Explore avoiding furry animals; ask your vet or pet store about washes and rubdowns for your pet. Avoid refined carbohydrates and sugars. Consume fewer animal products (red meat can promote bronchial spasms in some people) and eat more raw foods such as salads with grated raw vegetables. Women with exercise-induced asthma may be helped by cutting down on salt.

Nutrients
** Regular use of high-potency multivitamin/mineral supplement reduces the number and severity of asthma attacks.

SALICYLATES (ASPIRIN-LIKE COMPOUNDS) IN FOODS

High: Most fruits, especially berries, apricots, and dried fruit like raisins and prunes; processed tomatoes (canned, soup, paste, and sauce); herbs like curry powder, paprika, licorice, thyme, dill powder, turmeric, oregano, tea (black and peppermint), mint, cloves, oil of wintergreen; coffee; and vegetables like bell peppers, cucumbers, and pickles. Peanuts and almonds with skins have moderate amounts.

Low: Whole grains, veggies, legumes, and fresh tomatoes.

Find one containing small amounts of molybdenum, which helps detoxify sulfites.

** Vitamin B_6, 25–50 mg one to two times a day, can decrease the number and severity of asthma attacks.

** Magnesium, 250–600 mg per day. Ask your doctor about IV magnesium.

** Cod liver oil, 1–2 Tbsp. per day, or fish oil, 3–6 g per day in divided doses, and ⅛ tsp. ground flaxseeds every other day.

** Check stomach acid (studies suggest low stomach acid occurs in up to 80 percent of child asthmatics) and supply sufficient grains (5–50) of hydrochloric acid with pepsin per meal.

• N-acetyl-cysteine, 100 mg twice a day, along with zinc, 20 mg, and copper, 2 mg, daily (ask your doctor about higher dosages, and do not take if you have a history of liver disease)

• Vitamin C, 500–1,000 mg one to three times a day (take the last dose before bed, which seems to decrease or lessen severity of attacks at 4:00 A.M.)

• Discuss short-term use of potassium iodide to mobilize secretions in the lungs, and have your DHEA (dehydroepiandrosterone) levels checked, especially if you are on oral or inhaled glucocorticoids.

• Folic acid together with L-tyrosine (an amino acid) reduces bronchial constriction by activating certain adrenal hormones.

• Beta-carotene daily and sublingual dimethylglycine (DMG) taken one-half hour before a workout may reduce exercise-induced asthma.

- According to Dr. Alan Gaby, Myer's cocktail (see appendix G) usually clears up an attack in a few minutes in a doctor's office.
- Ask doctor about nebulizing (inhaling) glutathrone (100–200 mg/cc) to immediately stop asthma attacks, and use periodically to prevent them. Can help get you off steroids.

Herbs: Lobelia extract may be helpful during an asthma attack, 1 ml one to three times a day, or use lobelia ointment applied liberally on the chest two to three times a day. Try ginkgo biloba, 40 mg three times a day for six weeks.

AUTOIMMUNE DISORDERS

In these disorders, a person's immune system (which is meant to attack invading bacteria or viruses) produces antibodies that attack the body's own cells and tissues.

Examples of autoimmune disorders are systemic lupus erythematosus, insulin-dependent diabetes, rheumatoid arthritis, and various thyroid and adrenal diseases (refer to each separately). Autoimmunity and problems with the immune system (immune dysfunction) are often tightly linked. People with immune systems that aren't regulated properly can develop autoimmunities. Approximately 8.5 million people in the United States suffer with autoimmune diseases, and 1.2 million new cases occur every five years. These numbers may be underestimated because autoimmune diseases are often misdiagnosed and have not been thoroughly studied.

Like allergies, autoimmune disorders produce hypersensitivity reactions, which are inappropriate responses of the immune system. Organs and tissues frequently affected include the endocrine glands (thyroid, pancreas, adrenals), parts of the blood (such as red blood cells), and connective tissues, including skin, muscles, and joints. In non-organ-specific disorders, autoimmune activity is spread throughout the body. Hormonal deficiencies and imbalances, such as a lack of thyroid hormone or insulin, or unopposed estrogen, may play a large part in certain autoimmune disorders.

Uniquely Female: Autoimmune illnesses occur more in women, appearing to be estrogen driven. Exposure in the womb to estrogenic environmental pollutants (hormone disruptors) may be contributing to today's increased incidence of autoimmune disorders. Daughters exposed in utero to DES (diethylstilbestrol), the first synthetic estrogen, are known to have a higher incidence of autoimmune disorders. With earlier puberty, fewer births, less time lactating, more obesity, more cycles of menstruation, junk food diets, and rapidly proliferating toxic chemicals in the environment all contributing to increased estrogen exposure, we can probably expect the number of autoimmune disorders to continue to increase. See *Estrogen Dominance.*

What to Do

** Deficiency or imbalance of hormones can worsen illness so have all hormone levels tested, including DHEA (dehydroepiandrosterone), and work with your doctor to supplement and balance hormones as well as take supportive nutrients.

** Allergies and chronic intestinal yeast infections are often associated with autoimmune disorders (see page 491). Identify and eliminate food and inhalant allergies and toxic chemical exposures.

** Check digestive enzymes (page 468).

** See *Immune Enhancement.*

B

BAD BREATH (Halitosis)

Foul-smelling breath.

Symptoms: Pull some floss between your teeth and then sniff it. If it smells bad to you, it probably does to others, too. Sometimes even if the floss doesn't smell, you could have bad breath that others detect. Ask an honest friend.

Causes: Usually a result of gum disease or tooth decay; smoking; drinking too much alcohol; poor digestion; food allergens; eating garlic or onions; poor oral and dental hygiene; or nose, throat, or sinus infections. A metallic smell may indicate diabetes or an active metabolism undergoing rapid weight loss (ketosis) or heavy-metal toxicity; sour smells may indicate stomach problems or tumors. Bad breath may come from intestinal problems such as parasites, deficiency of digestive enzymes, food allergies or intolerances, or overeating on a regular basis. Other causes include tuberculosis, syphilis, dehydration, and zinc deficiency. Certain drugs, such as penicillamine and lithium, can cause bad breath.

Uniquely Female: Girls at puberty or women during peri- and postmenopause may be particularly affected.

What to Do

** Floss and brush regularly. Remember to brush your tongue. Use a new toothbrush every two months. Try ultrasonic toothbrushes, which, I think, are the best.

** Test for food allergies, and/or have your doctor order a comprehensive stool analysis (page 492).

Diet: Go on a five-day program, eating at least 50 percent raw foods. Chew food well before swallowing. Try eating smaller more frequent meals. Increase consumption of cultured products such as yogurt, kefir, buttermilk, and sauerkraut.

Avoid: Overeating; drinking excessive fluids or iced drinks with meals; alcohol or coffee; highly spiced foods; garlic, hot peppers, and onions; strong cheeses (Camembert, Roquefort, blue); strong-smelling/tasting fish (such as anchovies); fried foods; heavy sweets.

Nutrients
   ** Probiotics, as directed on label
   ** Evaluate for digestive enzymes (page 468).
   ** Magnesium, 250 mg once or twice a day
   ** Vitamin B complex, 25 mg per day
   ** Rinse with folic acid or tea tree oil mouthwash. First floss
      well, then rinse for thirty to sixty seconds.
   ** Chlorophyll (alfalfa liquid or wheat grass or barley juice),
      1 Tbsp. in juice twice a day
   • Vitamin C, 1,000–2,000 mg per day

BALDNESS (Alopecia)

Baldness occurs more frequently in women than realized, often severely impairing self-esteem and even keeping women housebound because of depression and feelings of unattractiveness. Your doctor may need to take a biopsy from your scalp to determine what is causing your hair loss. There is no guaranteed cure, but there are viable alternatives that can improve your quality of life.

Female pattern baldness occurs when hair thins out all over the head and gets coarser and duller over time. It does not have a known cause, although genes, aging, and levels of male sex hormones (androgens) are often blamed. Exposure in the womb to environmental hormone disruptors may be contributing to an increased incidence of female baldness. This type of balding usually begins either at puberty or in the thirties and becomes more noticeable as time goes on.

Male patterned hair loss can occur in women and starts at the temples and top of the head. It may be caused by the immune system attacking hair follicles stimulated by an excess of male hormones. Get your hormones checked. This type of hair loss early in life may signal insulin resistance or celiac disease (see page 174).

Temporary hair loss can be caused by shedding, hair breakage caused by styling and perms, oral medications, certain skin diseases like fungal infections of the scalp, nutrient deficiency of biotin and/or iron, stomach acid deficiency, and immune disorders that cause *alopecia areata* (shedding in patches). At puberty and menopause, some women may experience accelerated hair loss, which may be caused by unopposed estrogen and/or the nutrient biotin, or inadequate levels of stomach acid. Women taking oral contraceptives can develop vitamin B_6 deficiencies, which may cause hair to fall out. Ask your doctor about testing all your hormones (especially thyroid). Consider therapeutic trials with various anti-androgen substances such as topical and oral progesterone as well as antioxidant creams (see Dr. Proctor's products on page 118).

Toxic baldness may be caused by a number of therapies, including chemotherapy, certain drugs, and mercury toxicity. Any time you start to lose hair, you should check the side effects of medications you are taking in the *Physician's Desk Reference* or ask your pharmacist. Some drugs that can cause hair loss are epilepsy medication, beta blocker drugs for high blood pressure, too high a dose of thyroid medication, cholesterol-lowering drugs, blood thinners, Parkinson's medication, anabolic steroids, antidepressants, antithyroid medications, drugs made from vitamin A. Toxic exposure in the environment, such as to pesticides, can also cause baldness. Severe stressful events can also be toxic to the hair follicles.

What to Do
- Learn stress-reduction techniques (page 52).
- Hair-replacement alternatives such as hair transplants, hairpieces, or hair extensions can improve self-image and are widely available.

- Some baldness may be caused by unopposed estrogen and progesterone deficiency (pages 226 and 286). Some women respond to treatment with progesterone, and others to pregnendone, by growing hair. Ask your doctor.
- Scalp reduction is a surgical technique that can eliminate patches of baldness. See a scalp surgeon.
- Use coloring creams that hide noticeable thinning. Call Derm-Match: 800-826-2824 (www.dermmatch.com).
- Ask your doctor about compounds such as the oral finasteride called Proscar, which is effective for treating male-pattern baldness.
- Potent hair-growth stimulators are topical antioxidant agents that may help, but the underlying immune dysfunction needs to be addressed. Hair-growth agents like Rogaine (minoxidil) can stimulate growth in some people, but we do not know how daily use affects women, and these agents should be avoided especially by pregnant women.
- Dr. Peter Proctor is a hair-treatment physician who has developed patented hair formulas that address all the causes of baldness and may be more effective than even minoxidil. He has written thirty scientific articles on this subject. He offers prescription and nonprescription products for mild to severe hair loss problems. Call 800-544-4400 or go online to www.lef.org. Discuss with your doctor.
- Exercises like the yoga plow and even merely sitting for several minutes with your head bent down toward your knees increase circulation to your scalp as does daily scalp massage, but these methods only seem to help a few women.

Nutrients
** Evaluate digestive enzymes, especially stomach acid (page 468).
** Biotin, 2–5 mg once a day
** Have your blood iron, ferritin, and thyroid tested to rule out iron deficiency and thyroid problems.
** Zinc, 30 mg twice a day, balanced with copper, 2–4 mg per day (most helpful with patchy alopecia areata)

** Multivitamin/mineral supplement daily
** Flaxseed oil, 1 Tbsp. once or twice a day, or ⅛ tsp. ground flaxseeds four to five times a week; balance with vitamin E, 400 IU per day
• Vitamin B$_6$, 25 mg twice a day, with low-dose vitamin B complex (25 mg per day)
• Ask your doctor about progesterone and other anti-androgens
• PABA (para-aminobenzoic acid), 300 mg to 2–6 g a day for alopecia areata and alopecia totalis
• If on oral contraceptives, take vitamin B$_6$, 50 mg per day and B complex

Herbs: Silicon by capsule or drops as directed on label has proven helpful.

BLADDER INFECTIONS, see *Urinary Problems*

BLOATING (Edema)

An abnormal accumulation of fluid in the body tissues that may be visible as a swelling. It can be local, as after an injury, or general, as in heart, liver, or kidney failure.

Symptoms: If you press your finger into the skin (usually over the shinbone) and are able to make an indentation that slowly flattens out, you have edema. Some women over the age of thirty find that they occasionally wake up with puffy hands and face. Over the course of the day, the belly can become distended and, by evening, ankles are swollen and retained fluid has caused a gain in weight. Along with the bloating may come irritability and depression and a tendency to suffer from constipation. The attack may last for one or more days, after which the symptoms may disappear. In heart disease, right-sided disease leads to swelling in the feet, ankles, legs, liver, and abdomen; left-sided disease leads to a build-up of fluid in the lungs *(pulmonary edema)*, which causes extreme shortness of breath and is a medical emergency.

Causes: Edema involving the hands and face may indicate extreme hypertension, especially when accompanied by headaches, blurred vision, or dizziness. It can also be caused by heart, liver, or kidney failure. Abdominal swelling without fluid retention elsewhere in the body is usually due to a digestive problem like gas, indigestion, hidden food allergies, or swallowing air. But abdominal swelling with chronic indigestion and vague intestinal pains may also be a sign of ovarian cancer. Puffy hands and face can be caused by low thyroid, food allergies, chemical sensitivities, or deficiencies of vitamin B_6, magnesium, or essential fatty acids.

Uniquely Female: By far the most common cause of bloating in women is premenstrual fluid retention (two to ten days before menstruation), especially for women in their thirties and forties. Estrogen can partially block salt and water excretion by the kidneys, so the body retains fluid. The more estrogen's actions are heightened by progesterone deficiency and/or DHEA (dehydroepiandrosterone) deficiency, the more fluid shifts and retention may occur. See the section on edema under *Pregnancy*. Puffy hands and face can worsen before the menses or at menopause.

What to Do
- ** Have a physical exam immediately to rule out disease, chronic venous insufficiency, or trauma.
- ** Check for food allergies, environmental sensitivities, and hypothyroidism.
- Don't overuse diuretics. Chronic use results in loss of potassium and magnesium, which causes weakness and muscle cramps.
- Learn stress-reduction techniques (pages 52–58).
- Exercise daily, at least twenty minutes of aerobic and light weights.
- Take hot baths or saunas twice a week.
- Stop smoking.

For Bloating from Hormonal Causes
- Restrict salt during the week before your period.
- See *Premenstrual Syndrome;* and if you don't respond to the natural therapies listed there, ask your doctor about low-dose estrogen birth control pills or mini-pills for several months.
- Some women experience congestion around the vulva when they are bloated. Sexual activity relieves vascular congestion.

Diet: Increase protein foods such as eggs and lean meats. When eating meals, take a bite of protein food first. Consume more raw fruits, veggies, and seeds and have more whole grains like rice or oats. Drink as much filtered water and herbal tea throughout the day as possible. Grate some foods from the cabbage family into raw salads several times a week.

Avoid: excess sugars and simple carbohydrates (if you do consume them, try to do so in the first half of the day), excess salt and caffeine, fried foods, soy sauce, pickles, olives, dairy products, dried shellfish, gravies, chocolate, alcohol, and tobacco.

Nutrients
- ** If it's hard to bend your fingers in the morning or if you have bloating midcycle or during the last weeks of your cycle, add vitamin B_6, 25 mg one to three times a day; a B complex, 25 mg once a day; and magnesium, 250 mg once a day.
- DIM (diindolylmethane) is the active ingredient in the cabbage and broccoli family and in indole 3-carbinol; 20 mg twice a day improves metabolism of estrogen and decreases water retention, and so theoretically it may help.
- If the above do not help, consider adding several grams per day of evening primrose oil and vary over the weeks with other essential fatty acids.
- Supplement proteins with protein drinks and/or free-form amino acid blends.
- Take potassium and magnesium with any diuretics (pharmaceutical or herbal).
- Ask your doctor about progesterone.

Herbs: Drink a strong tea of corn silk and watermelon seeds on rising and before bed for two weeks. If bloating is hormonally related, consider vitex, 40 drops of concentrated extract in a glass of water in the morning for one to three months.

BLOOD PRESSURE

The pressure of the blood in the main arteries rises and falls based on the activity of the heart and muscles during exercise, stress, and sleep. In a blood pressure reading, the first number is the *systolic*—the rising pressure created when the heart muscle is pumping. The second number is the *diastolic*—the falling pressure when the heart relaxes between beats. A healthy young adult has a blood pressure reading of about 110/75, which often rises to about 130/90 around age sixty. Less than 20 percent of people treated for high blood pressure achieve normal ranges. You must work with and be monitored by a doctor.

High Blood Pressure (Hypertension)

Hypertension is the most common chronic disease in older women and is a high risk factor for stroke, congestive heart disease, and kidney disease. It affects 60 million Americans. Blood pressure is considered high if *repeated* measurements show either the systolic number is 140 or more or the diastolic number is 90 or higher. *Mild hypertension*—a diastolic pressure between 90 and 105—usually responds to nondrug therapy, especially lifestyle changes. You must be monitored by a doctor to see if what you're doing is working. Controlling hypertension reduces the risk of heart disease and stroke. If you cannot control your blood pressure with lifestyle, you *must* take drugs. Abnormally high blood pressure, even at rest, usually occurs in later life, although it is being increasingly diagnosed in women between the ages of twenty-five and fifty-five.

Symptoms: Hypertension is sometimes called the "silent killer" because most people feel no ill effects in the early stages. Warning signs of more advanced high blood pressure include headaches, sweating, rapid pulse, dizziness, shortness of breath, and visual disturbances. There can also be irritability, ringing in the ears, flushed complexion, fatigue and sleeplessness, edema, depression, heart arrhythmia, or chronic respiratory problems.

Causes: No underlying cause is found in 85 or more percent of women with high blood pressure, a situation known as *primary* or *essential hypertension,* which is associated with hardening and narrowing of the walls of the blood vessels. It may be linked to insulin resistance (page 300). The other 15 percent have *secondary hypertension,* where high blood pressure is the result of other health conditions such as pregnancy, kidney or adrenal disease, the use of certain drugs (including diet pills or oral contraceptives), or chemical exposures (like lead, even in nonoccupationally exposed women). Other causes include calcium/fiber deficiency; poor sugar metabolism or excess refined sugars in the diet; salt sensitivity, magnesium deficiency, and food allergies; hyperthyroidism; excessive alcohol consumption or a high-fat diet; and lack of exercise. Risk factors include age (over fifty), tobacco smoking, obesity, diabetes, elevated blood cholesterol, genetic history, and psychological stress.

Uniquely Female: Men are more at risk of hypertension than women until women go through menopause. By age fifty, hypertension is more common in women than in men, especially in black women. Hypertension is the most common disorder of pregnancy, affecting as many as 5 to 10 percent of women. It is first treated by bed rest and increasing protein, but, if it becomes severe, labor may be induced early. It is a leading cause of maternal and newborn death and illness. It sometimes develops in women who are taking the birth control pill, which is a clear sign you should go off it. "White coat hypertension"—blood pressure that elevates when taken in the doctor's office—occurs in 20–40 percent of mild to moderate sufferers and is related to anxiety.

What to Do
- Women with a history of asthma, heart failure, liver or kidney disease, or diabetes should not take beta blockers, as they can cause a wide range of side effects.
- It is especially important for women with hypertension to maintain optimum weight, reduce salt intake, and stop taking

any synthetic hormones such as birth control pills, fertility drugs, or hormone replacement therapy.

- Ask your doctor about intravenous (IV) calcium/magnesium.
- There is an ongoing debate about whether calcium-channel blockers cause cancer. Ask your doctor.
- It takes four to twelve weeks for a nutritional and lifestyle program to work. You must be monitored by a doctor while making changes and may need drugs in the beginning. Be sure to tell your doctor everything you are taking, including herbs, nutrients, and over-the-counter medications.
- As many as 50 percent of those with high blood pressure may have Syndrome X (high blood pressure, blood fats, overweight, family history, and insulin resistance). For those with glucose intolerance and hyperinsulinemia, eat a diet lower in carbohydrates and read *The Zone* by Dr. Barry Sears (Regan Books, 1995) and *Protein Power* by Michael R. Eades, M.D., and Mary Ann Eades, M.D. (Bantam Books, 1996). See *Insulin Resistance.*
- If you have very high blood pressure, you may need to continue the use of medication in addition to natural approaches, but you may be able to lower your doses of medicine.
- Monitor your blood pressure regularly at home, especially if you get tense as soon as you walk into a doctor's office. If you are a heavy snorer, or have sleep apnea, also check your blood pressure regularly.
- Quit smoking. The chemicals in tobacco smoke elevate blood pressure.
- Lose excess weight (losing only two pounds drops one to two points of diastolic blood pressure). Fat around the waist especially contributes to high blood pressure.
- Women's hearts seem to be more vulnerable to stress than men's. Reduce stress (pages 52–58), including at work. Try massage, biofeedback, deep breathing, yoga, muscle relaxation, hypnosis, and meditation, which have all been shown to lower blood pressure.
- Do aerobic exercise (swimming, walking, bike riding). Moderate exercise (three times a week) decreases blood pressure

TO ELIMINATE SALT FROM YOUR DIET

Check labels for soda, sodium, or the symbol Na. Avoid monosodium glutamate (MSG); baking soda; canned vegetables; commercially prepared foods; over-the-counter medications that contain ibuprofen (Advil, Nuprin); diet soft drinks; foods with mold inhibitors, preservatives, and most sugar substitutes; meat tenderizers; softened water; and soy sauce.

by several points, and strenuous exercise (five to six times a week) can lower it even more. T'ai chi and even light exercise has been shown to help. Exercise helps even if you have been a couch potato all your life.

- Don't do isometrics, such as weight lifting, which may cause blood pressure to skyrocket, and don't overexert yourself in hot or humid weather.
- Get a pet. Pet owners are more likely than nonowners to still be alive a year after leaving a coronary care unit.
- Dry brush the skin all over your body to stimulate circulation.
- Check for food allergies, especially if you have migraines or nasal congestion. Have your hair lead levels tested; increased lead levels are a risk factor for hypertension in women.
- Avoid antihistamines.

Diet: Ask your doctor about the DASH diet. DASH is a fruit and vegetable diet with low-fat dairy products and is low in saturated and total fats. This reduces blood pressure in those with the disease and those at high risk.

Eat more raw vegetables. Increase potassium-rich foods: fruits (avocado, bananas, melons, citrus fruit, dried fruit); vegetables (asparagus, broccoli, cabbage, cauliflower, eggplant, green peas, potatoes, sweet potatoes, squash). Consume garlic and onions (right after cutting), ginger, kelp, shiitake and reishi mushrooms, brown rice, and whole oats. To avoid potassium loss in cooking, steam rather than boil your vegetables. Eat calcium-rich foods such as dairy products, leafy green vegetables, and nuts. Colorful fruits and vegetables, such as berries or red peppers, are high in flavonoids, which may help lower blood pressure as well as minimize damage to organs secondary to high blood pressure.

Consume fish and dark green virgin cold-processed olive oil generously. A slight reduction in saturated fat, along with the use of extra-virgin olive oil, has been shown to reduce the daily drug requirements needed to lower blood pressure. Consume vitamin K–rich foods (dark green leafy vegetables such as watercress and kale, green tea), as K deficiencies increase the harmful effects of salt. Foods high in L-arginine are also good, such as roasted soybeans, light turkey and chicken meat, pumpkin seeds, salmon, chickpeas, tofu, hummus, and black beans.

Avoid: Bacon, corned beef, pork, sausage, smoked or processed meats, aged cheeses, anchovies, chicken liver, chocolate, fava beans, pickled herring, sour cream, and full-fat dairy products. Avoid the amino acids phenylalanine (found in NutraSweet) and L-tyrosine. Try to consume less salt, animal products, and caffeinated beverages and foods. Daily coffee drinking raises blood pressure in hypertensives. Tea (green and black) elevates pressure while sitting, but not standing. Overconsumption even of green tea is not a grand idea. Don't drink grapefruit juice while taking antihypertensive drugs.

Nutrients
* ** Magnesium, 300–400 mg per day
* ** Calcium, 800–1,000 mg per day (helps only salt-sensitive types)

THE ALCOHOL-HEART CONNECTION

Heavy regular use of alcohol (three to four drinks per day) damages the heart muscle and is related to high blood pressure, strokes, and arrhythmia. On the other hand, a glass of red wine at night can actually lower stress and hypertension. However, this data is still controversial. You may get similar benefits from drinking red grape juice or eating the grapes (though in larger quantities), and we are reluctant to encourage drinking alcohol.

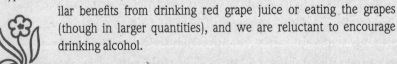

** Vitamin E, 100 IU per day for one week, then increase to 200 IU per day

** Fish oil, 3–9 g per day. Look for a formula high in DHA (docosahexaenoic acid), the main fish oil responsible for lowering blood pressure.

** L-arginine, 1,000–1,500 mg twice a day for salt-sensitive types

** Avoid melatonin. It may impair the effect of calcium-channel blockers in lowering blood pressure.

- Potassium, as directed by your doctor
- Coenzyme Q-10, 30–60 mg twice a day
- Chromium, 200 mcg per day to combat insulin resistance
- Vitamin C, 1,000 mg twice a day with bioflavonoids and rutin
- Quercetin, 500 mg twice a day
- Check your thyroid (including tests for subclinical hypo-thyroidism).
- Check for heavy-metal toxicity (cadmium and lead), especially if you suffer with high blood pressure but don't have other risk factors.
- Check blood insulin levels.

Herbs: Hawthorn berries, 100–300 mg two to three times a day.

Low Blood Pressure (Hypotension)

This condition most commonly occurs after standing or sitting up too quickly.

Symptoms: Light-headedness, fainting, fatigue and easy loss of energy, headaches, susceptibility to allergies and infections.

Causes: May be caused by antidepressant drugs or drugs used to treat high blood pressure. Other causes include poor diet, kidney and/or adrenal malfunction, and anemia.

Uniquely Female: Mostly women suffer from low blood pressure.

What to Do

- Stand up slowly. When first getting out of bed in the morning, dangle your feet over the edge before standing up.
- Before standing up, squeeze an isometric hand grip to raise your blood pressure momentarily. Or do some complex men-

tal arithmetic (like counting backward from one hundred by sevens), which works even better than physical activity.
- Sleep with the head of your bed elevated eight to twelve inches higher than the foot.
- Alternating hot and cold water therapy increases circulation.
- Deep breathing exercises bring more oxygen to the system.
- Eat smaller, more frequent meals. Don't restrict salt and fluid intake.
- Get professional assistance in developing an exercise program.
- Get tested for diabetes, anemia, and thyroid and adrenal function.
- Get tested for food allergies.
- Avoid toxic fumes.

Diet: Add generous portions of orange and yellow vegetables like cooked carrots and yams as well as garlic. Eat plenty of green vegetables. Do *not* restrict salt, as it is necessary to raise your blood pressure.

Nutrients
- ** L-tyrosine, 500 mg on an empty stomach in the morning
- ** Pantothenic acid, 500 mg per day, or up to several grams per day
- ** Licorice root extract, 250–500 mg two or three times a day for six to eight weeks only
- ** B complex, 50–100 mg per day
- Calcium, 500–800 mg per day, and magnesium, 250–400 mg per day
- Vitamin E, work up to 800 IU per day
- Bioflavonoids, 1,000 mg once a day

BLOOD SUGAR PROBLEMS (not Diabetes)

Glucose is the body's chief source of energy for cell metabolism. Your blood sugar level is normally kept within narrow limits by several hormones.

Hyperglycemia

A condition of abnormally high blood sugar; see *Diabetes Mellitus.*

Glucose intolerance (also called borderline diabetes, impaired glucose tolerance, and impaired fasting glucose) is a condition in which a person's blood sugar level is higher than normal but not high enough to be diagnosed as diabetic. If your fasting glucose level consistently tests between 100–126 mg/dl (diabetes is diagnosed as concentrations greater than 126 mg/dl), or you have an abnormal response on a six-hour glucose-tolerance test (even with normal blood glucose fasting levels), you have glucose intolerance and are at increased risk of developing diabetes in the future. Glucose intolerance (and insulin resistance, see page 300) can start early in life. If you or your child tends to put on weight easily, especially around the waist, have skin tags (little bits of skin on stalks under armpits and on neck and chest), low blood sugar, low good cholesterol, high triglycerides, high blood pressure, and a family history of diabetes, order a glucose-tolerance test, which is a better predictor of risk for blood sugar problems than the fasting blood glucose test. Catching dysfunctional carbohydrate metabolism years, even decades, early can prevent diabetes. The good news: glucose tolerance can improve within a single day (*European Journal of Clinical Nutrition* 54:24–8, 2000) by improving your diet, exercising, taking supplements, and losing weight.

What to Do
- Get a glucose-tolerance test.
- Test your insulin levels.
- Get tested for celiac disease, a permanent problem digesting wheat and usually all gluten-containing grains, such as rye, and barley. Gluten intolerance may aggravate blood glucose problems.
- Eat a healthy diet, lose weight, and exercise.
- Learn which foods are high on the *glycemic index* (GI), a measure of the effect of carbohydrate foods on blood sugar, and avoid overconsuming them. Fats and proteins don't affect blood sugar the way carbohydrates do. In general, high-GI foods are highly processed and rapidly digested carbohy-

drates, such as white rice, corn flakes, candy, white bread, colas, pizza, and popcorn, but the list also includes such foods as carrots, bananas, and baked potatoes. The glycemic index greatly affects cholesterol; eating foods lower on the index can raise your good cholesterol (high-density lipoprotein, or HDL).

- Certain herbs, like American ginseng, improve glucose tolerance in nondiabetic individuals (take 3–6 g per day for several months while improving diet).

Hypoglycemia

Hypoglycemia is an abnormally low level of sugar in the blood caused by oversecretion of insulin by the pancreas; pituitary or adrenal abnormalities; or a problem with the liver producing glucose or storing carbohydrates. *Reactive hypoglycemia* may occur at various times of the day, usually after consuming refined sugars, refined flours, or allergic foods, which make the body oversecrete insulin, which several hours later causes low blood sugar. Most common occurrences are midmorning or midafternoon symptoms that follow, for example, a breakfast of doughnuts or sugary cereals, or a lunch with colas and desserts.

Symptoms: Weakness, faintness, shaking, nervousness, fast heartbeat, cold sweat, dizziness, irritability, and headache if meals are missed. Craving for sweets; constant hunger. Other possible symptoms include mood swings, such as inappropriate anger; swollen feet or weakness in the legs; tight chest; excess weight; pain in the eyes; and insomnia. Neurologic symptoms can be caused by low blood sugar, especially in the elderly, and are often misdiagnosed as symptoms of cerebrovascular disease. These symptoms may include seizures, loss of speech, loss of sensation, muscular weakness on one side of the body, etc. These symptoms in diabetics should alert you to the possibility of hypoglycemia.

Causes: Poor eating habits: overconsumption of foods high in sugars (even natural ones) and insufficient quality essential fatty acids; not enough high-quality protein foods; skipping meals and then bingeing and overexercising; a complication of diabetes; inhalant or food allergies, chemical sensitivities; and from intestinal yeast overgrowth. Hypoglycemia is also associated with stomach surgery, certain medicines, liver disease, high fever, and a family history of diabetes. Almost 50 percent of those over the age of fifty with hypoglycemia have hypothyroidism. Two to four cups of coffee can aggravate hypoglycemia in Type 1 diabetics.

Uniquely Female: The "drama" of teenagehood may be caused or worsened by hypoglycemia. Hypoglycemia often afflicts women with premenstrual syndrome. Sweets can precipitate hypoglycemia, especially during the week before your period. There is a tendency to get hypoglycemic in early pregnancy as a result of frequent nausea and vomiting. Some oral contraceptives can cause glucose intolerance and poor sugar metabolism. A history of dieting and yo-yoing weight can cause or worsen the problem.

What to Do
- *Acute attack:* Drink fruit juice.
- Establish good eating habits. Eat six or seven small meals a day at regular intervals. Between meals, eat protein snacks such as eggs, chicken, nuts, cheese, or skim milk. Don't skip meals, especially breakfast. Avoid morning caffeine beverages and consume whole grains at least once a day.
- Identify and avoid food and inhalant allergens.
- Check for nutrient malabsorption. Evaluate digestive enzymes and rule out adrenal or thyroid problems.
- Avoid toxic chemicals.

Diet: Proper diet is the key factor for maintaining adequate levels of blood sugar. Eat sparingly foods high in carbohydrates (refined starches and sugar). Instead, eat foods high in protein and beneficial fats. Carry around raw seeds and nuts mixed with small amounts of dried fruits or roasted nuts for flavor and munch.

Avoid: Refined and processed foods, white flour, white rice, corn, soft drinks, and salt. Avoid sweet fruits and juices, such as grape and prune, or add them to a solution of three-fourths water to reduce the sugar. Caffeine, alcohol, and cigarette smoking induce major swings in blood sugar. Alcoholic beverages can trigger hypoglycemia, particularly when taken on an empty stomach.

Nutrients
- ** Chromium, 100 mcg three times a day
- ** Pyridoxal-5'-phosphate, 20 mg two to three times a day
- ** Vitamin B complex, 25 mg once or twice a day
- ** Pantothenic acid, 500 mg three times a day
- ** Vitamin C, 1,000 mg twice a day
- ** Magnesium, 250–400 mg daily (prevents bouts of severe loss of energy), especially in aspartate form
- ** Multivitamin/mineral supplement daily, including at least 20 mg zinc
- • Check for enzyme deficiencies and food allergies (page 84)
- • L-cysteine, 500 mg once a day; after two weeks increase to twice a day
- • Ask your doctor about injections of B complex plus pyridoxine and liver, twice a week for three months, then once a week for two months. They help hypoglycemics tolerate foods that produce low blood sugar reactions and help the elderly with malabsorption problems.

Syndrome X, see *Insulin Resistance*

BODY ODOR

Symptoms: Body odor is most noticeable in the armpits, under the breasts, and around the genital area because these areas are favorable to the growth of bacteria. Feet, which are in a warm, airless condition for hours on end, are also a perfect environment for bacteria.

Causes: The smell is caused by the by-products of bacterial activity from sweat on the surface of the skin. It may be particularly strong after eating garlic, curry, or other spicy foods. Stress can cause sweating on the palms and face.

Uniquely Female: Women may be most prone to body odor during puberty, especially if they start to menstruate early (ten years or younger). May occur during menopause from malabsorption of minerals (especially zinc) and other nutrients, as well as overgrowth of parasites, bacteria, and yeast. As hormones wane, the intestinal lining thins, which may contribute to deficiencies of various digestive enzymes.

What to Do
- ** Check digestive enzymes (page 468).
- ** Identify food allergies (page 84).
- Have a comprehensive stool analysis.
- Soap and water wash away both perspiration and bacteria.
- Deodorants remove bad-smelling odors using antiseptics (to destroy bacteria), perfumes (to mask odors), and antiperspirants (to reduce the production of sweat), but many contain toxic chemicals such as aluminum. Natural deodorants include dabbing underarms and feet with vinegar, or applying aloe vera gel or baking soda mixed in water under the arms. Some commercial products, such as Tom's of Maine, use natural ingredients.
- Keep your clothes washed.
- Wear natural fabrics. Cotton and other natural fabrics absorb perspiration and allow it to evaporate. Wear sandals when possible.
- Stay calm. Anxiety, nervousness, and sexual excitement can increase perspiration. See body-mind destressing exercises (pages 52–58).
- Pine soap or old-fashioned glycerin soap mask odors.
- If all else fails, use the old skunk remedy. Put a couple of cups of tomato (or lime) juice in your bathwater and soak for fifteen minutes.

Diet: Some foods and spices impart an odor hours after eating them, especially fish, cumin, curry, and garlic. Try eating fewer animal products and more cultured products.

Nutrients

- ** Vitamin B$_6$, 10–25 mg per day, and vitamin B complex, 25 mg per day
- ** Zinc, 15–50 mg per day, with backup copper, 2–4 mg per day
- ** Probiotics, two to three times a day
- ** Magnesium, 250 mg once or twice a day, is a natural bowel "sweetener" that can improve body odor.
- ** Multivitamin/mineral supplement
- • Liquid chlorophyll, 1 tsp. in a glass of water one to three times a day
- • Bromelain, 500–1,000 mg once or twice a day between meals

Herbs: Body-freshening teas: peppermint; fenugreek/sage; rosemary; alfalfa/mint. Detox baths: Combine some of these herbs in cheesecloth and place over tub faucet. Let the hot water run through. Add any of the following to your bath: ½ cup of baking soda; ½ cup of vinegar; 1 cup of Epsom salts. Fill the tub as high as possible and submerge as much of your body as you can. Repeat this bath three to four nights in a row for two to three weeks, and then once a week for several more weeks depending on response.

BOILS (Furuncles)

Inflamed, pus-filled areas of skin. A boil can appear suddenly and become very painful within twenty-four hours. If boils are very large, a doctor should drain them. A carbuncle occurs when the infection spreads and forms other boils.

Symptoms: Starts as a red, painful lump and swells as it fills with pus, becoming rounded with a yellowish head. Itching, mild pain, and localized swelling. Common sites include the back of the neck, face, breasts, buttocks, and moist areas such as the armpits and groin.

Causes: Boils are caused by bacteria, toxicity, infected hair follicle, blocked oil gland, low resistance after an infection, thyroid disorders, and rarely by poor hygiene. May be recurrent or occur in clusters in those with diabetes mellitus or other conditions in which general body immunity is impaired.

Uniquely Female: Anecdotally, a number of breast cancer patients report chronic infections such as boils and parasites in their early health history. If a girl experiences chronic boils, it is worth adding immune enhancers to her daily nutrient regime and monitoring her for unopposed estrogen signs and immune dysfunctions as she matures.

What to Do

- In general, do not squeeze a boil. If a small boil has come to a full head, sterilize a needle and make a small nick in the head, then squeeze. It may take five to seven days until the boil breaks on its own.
- Use warm wet compresses three times a day to bring the boil to a head. Continue compresses for three days after the boil opens to drain out all the pus. Keep the skin around a boil clean while it is draining. Hot compresses every several hours relieve discomfort and hasten drainage. Some effective choices:

  Hot Epsom salts pack (put 2 Tbsp. in 1 cup water and then soak a cloth with the solution)

  Castor oil poultice

  Tea tree oil drops in water (may irritate skin)

  Mixture of one part sesame oil and one part lime juice

  A wet black tea bag

- Or apply a mixture of honey, oil from vitamin E and A capsules, and some zinc oxide several times a day up to once an hour.
- Apply iodine drops to boils two times a day and rub gently into the surface, then wash hands.
- Wash hands well before preparing food.

Diet: Eat yogurt, kefir, and acidophilus. Drink six to eight glasses of pure water daily and some aloe vera juice each morning. Consume iodine-rich foods like fish.

Avoid: Hydrogenated and partially hydrogenated oils.

Nutrients
- ** Vitamin A, 100,000 IU for three days. Reduce to 50,000 IU for three days, then to 10,000 IU. *Do not use if pregnant.* Ask doctor.
- ** Proteolytic enzymes, 1–2 g two to three times a day on an empty stomach between meals
- ** Zinc, 20 mg once a day
- • B vitamin complex, 50 mg once a day
- • Liquid chlorophyll, 1 tsp. two to four times a day
- • Colloidal silver, internally or applied locally as directed on the package
- • If boils are recurrent, consider thymus glandular, 500 mg two or three times a day immediately before meals or thymic polyproteins, 4 mcg one to three times a day; fish or flaxseed oils, several grams per day; and detoxification programs.

<u>Herbs:</u> Oil of oregano, one or two 140 mg capsules after breakfast and dinner; echinacea, 300 mg two to three times a day (in homeopathic form it helps with recurrent boils); goldenseal, 250–400 mg capsules two to three times a day (do not take longer than three weeks); or combinations of these.

BREAST PROBLEMS (Benign)

The breast consists mainly of fatty tissue in which are embedded fifteen to twenty lobes of milk-secreting glands, which end in the nipple. Breast size and shape vary at different times in a woman's life—during the menstrual cycle, pregnancy and lactation, and after menopause. Around 70 percent of American women suffer from benign but uncomfortable breast changes at some point in their lives.

Breast cells are exquisitely sensitive to hormones such as estrogen, progesterone, prolactin, and thyroid as well as to chemicals in the environment that mimic hormones. The more "immature" breast cells are, the more sensitive they are, in a continuum from fetal breast cells (the most sensitive), through infants and young girls. It is not until late in the first pregnancy that breast cells become mature (turned into milk machines) and become less sensitive and vulnerable. Thus, exposure in the womb or during early childhood and teenage years to hormone disruptors such as pesticides and plastics (and other pollutants like cigarette smoke) may be setting the scene for breast problems later in life.

Fibrocystic Disease (Cystic Mastitis, Mammary Dysplasia)

Lumpy and/or tender breasts, mainly in women between the ages of thirty and fifty, often related to estrogen dominance (see page 226). One woman in five will detect a lump or a lumpy area at some time during her life, although 80 percent of lumps are benign.

In the two weeks before menstruation, breasts can become bigger and develop tender areas of knobby lumps, usually in the upper and outer part of each breast. Once menstruation starts, the tenderness goes away and the lumps disappear. This condition is part of premenstrual syndrome (PMS). Some women over the age of thirty develop another form of breast lumpiness that may persist throughout the menstrual cycle, possibly due to excessive sensitivity to the sex hormones, especially estrogen. Most commonly, these two conditions overlap and are called *benign fibrocystic breast disease.*

Most women with fibrocystic breasts are not at increased risk for breast cancer. However, having several breast biopsies during her lifetime, even if the lumps prove to be benign, does seem to increase a woman's risk of breast cancer. Any biopsy demonstrating hyperplasia or atypical cells indicates an increased risk. Also, if a woman develops fibrocystic breasts when she starts hormone replacement therapy (HRT), she is at increased risk of cancerous change and should probably go off HRT.

Symptoms

Symptoms of fibrocystic disease can be grouped in the following categories:

Cyclical Pain and Swelling—Painful or sensitive breasts, sometimes with a feeling of fullness. Relatively common just before menstruation, during midcycle, in early pregnancy, or while breast-feeding.

Pain may affect one or both breasts, may radiate dull ache to armpit or arm, affecting premenopausal women sensitive to *excess* hormones of estrogen, prolactin, and rarely progesterone or *deficien-*

cies of thyroid and/or progesterone. Chart pain to know if it's cyclical. Most breast pain is *not* cancerous.

Noncyclic Pain—not related to cycle or hormones. Usually affects one breast, often after age thirty, and linked to: fluid-filled cysts, fibroadenomas, duct problems, mastitis, injury, breast abscesses, a pinched nerve, inflamed cartilage between ribs, or inflamed veins. Noncyclic pain requires a doctor's care. Notify doctor of *any* recurring pain.

Breast Lumpiness—Lumps may be either cyclic or noncyclic and may or may not be painful. Cysts are round, either firm or soft, may be small or large, and move freely. (Most cancers do not move freely and are referred to as feeling "fixed.") Lumps that are not painful and not cyclical are more worrisome and must be checked by imaging techniques. Thickening and lumpiness most frequently occur in both breasts, but may also appear in just one.

Fibroadenomas are smooth, fibrous, benign tumors that are common in young women aged fifteen to thirty. The tumors seldom enlarge and shrink with the menstrual cycle, but they are still thought to be linked to unopposed estrogen. Once removed, they often recur.

Lumps that occur in only one breast are either nondominant masses (the lump merges in one or more places with the surrounding breast tissue) or dominant masses (a mass that is clearly distinct from surrounding lumps), which usually are fibroadenomas. Other lumps, especially hard, painless lumps, may turn out to be cancerous, which is why *all lumps should be checked by a doctor.*

Note: Breast cancer is occurring in younger and younger women these days. Often doctors will want to "watch" lumps in young women rather than testing immediately. Get a second opinion, as young women who lose time from an inaccurate diagnosis are at greater risk for breast cancer than are postmenopausal women. Consider your options in light of your personal and family health history. Read risk factors and preventative steps in the breast cancer section under *Cancer.*

Breast calcifications (calcium deposits) are common, and most are benign. They show up on mammograms and are not detected by manual exam. The deposits may be due to secretions from cells, cellular debris, inflammation, trauma, radiation, or foreign bodies. They

MAMMOGRAMS

There is conflicting data about whether or not to perform routine mammography, and how often, in women under fifty, with more agreement for women over fifty. Numerous studies have shown that screening lowers death from breast cancer by 29 percent in women between fifty and sixty-nine years of age. However, a recent study (*Lancet* 355:129, 2000) reanalyzed data and concluded that for every one thousand women screened every two years over twelve years, one breast cancer death is avoided, while the total number of deaths is increased by six. There are no easy answers, but we still do recommend mammograms every two years for women in their forties, and yearly for women fifty and older.

 What's a woman to do? Talk with your doctor, take your personal and family history into account, do regular breast self-exams, and make decisions based on your own risks.

are not related to calcium supplements. Sometimes they suggest cancerous changes.

Causes: Most fibrocystic breasts are thought to be caused by hormonal changes, especially increased levels of estrogen (and sometimes prolactin) and inadequate levels of progesterone, causing the breast cells to retain excess fluid. Iodine deficiency and an underactive thyroid make breasts more sensitive to estrogen. The birth control pill can cause breast tenderness in some women, while low-dose oral contraceptives may reduce it. Hormone replacement therapies can both help *or* worsen pain.

What to Do

- Do breast self-exams each month (see page 154). Get to know your own breasts. Rub your breasts with soap and water in the shower to detect lumps not often found by other palpation techniques. Report any lump that is not part of your normal cystic condition.
- Reduce or eliminate caffeine, including chocolate, tea, coffee, and cola. There is also caffeine in a number of over-the-counter drugs, such as NoDoz, Excedrin, Midol, Anacin, Empirin, and Dexatrim.

- Lose excess weight. In women, fat produces and stores estrogen. Breast tissue is very responsive to excess estrogen.
- Do a liver cleanse (see page 311). The liver is the main site for estrogen clearance and metabolism. An unhealthy liver can cause estrogen dominance, a state that contributes to changes in the breast tissue (page 226).
- Have regular, daily bowel movements. To have regularity, a higher-fiber diet is recommended over taking laxatives. Women who have fewer than three bowel movements a week have a four to five times greater risk of fibrocystic breasts than those who have at least one movement per day.
- Breast tissue responds to both thyroid hormone and iodine. With inadequate iodine, breast tissue is more sensitive to estrogen. Your doctor should evaluate and treat actual or subclinical hypothyroidism.
- Avoid tight-fitting bras that may obstruct the flow of lymph drainage.

For Breast Tenderness
- Use a heating pad (moderate heat) or hot water bottle or take hot baths or showers to relieve the pain. Try alternating heat and cold.
- Find a good support bra (without underwires).
- Gentle self-massage can help move extra breast fluids back into the lymph passageways. Soap up your breasts, then rotate the fingers along the surface in small circles. Use your hands to press the breasts in, then up and toward your armpits for enhanced lymphatic drainage. Or if you are squeamish about touching your own breasts, use a gentle massaging tool that you can purchase at a drugstore.
- A castor oil compress to relieve inflammation: Fold a wool flannel cloth into four layers and saturate it with castor oil. Put the cloth on the breast and cover with plastic. Apply a heating pad turned up to moderate, then hot. Leave on for an hour. Repeat for three to seven days.
- Test your progesterone levels, and supplement if low.
- Ask your doctor for SSKI, prescriptive iodine.

- Try vitamin B_6, 50 mg per day; magnesium, 250 mg per day; and evening primrose oil, several grams per day.
- If you're taking hormone replacement or oral contraceptives, consider lowering the dose or changing or stopping the medication.
- Try adding ⅛–¼ tsp. ground flaxseeds to yogurt, soup, etc., or take 1 Tbsp. flaxseed oil each day.

Diet: Low fat and high fiber. Eat raw cruciferous veggies like broccoli and grated cabbage in salads several times a week, and organic as much as possible. Eat brussels sprouts, nuts, fruit, whole grains, and beans. Consume seafood and seaweed.

Avoid: Hydrogenated and animal fats, alcohol; avoid all caffeinated beverages, food and drugs for one month and see if your pain and breast fluid retention decrease or go away. Avoid pesticides, and also avoid the kinds of chemicals found in many commercial perfumes and cosmetics.

Nutrients
- ** Vitamin B complex, 50–100 mg once a day, and 100–300 mg per day of vitamin B_2
- ** Magnesium, 250 mg once or twice a day
- ** Vitamin E, 400–800 IU per day
- ** Evening primrose oil, 1,500 mg twice a day, plus 1 Tbsp. flaxseed oil
- Methionine, 500 mg twice a day
- Choline, 500 mg twice a day
- *L. acidophilus,* 1 tsp. three times a day
- Indole-3-carbinol or its metabolite (diindolylmethane) reduces irritating metabolites of estrogen and *theoretically* may help. Your doctor can order a urinary estrogen metabolite test to see if it might help you.
- Ask your doctor about progesterone cream applied twice a day from midcycle to menses; *not on breasts.*
- If nothing else works, ask your doctor about prescription iodine, 3–6 mg per day.

- For severe breast pain, ask your doctor about painting your vagina with Lugol's iodine, or take diatomic-elemental iodine, eight drops per day. Ask your doctor about a slow (five- to fifteen-minute) intravenous (IV) injection of magnesium sulfate or magnesium chloride, taken one to two times each week for two to six weeks.
- If nothing else works, ask about low-dose oral contraceptives.

Herbs: Yarrow leaf capsules, 2–6 per day, or yarrow leaf liquid tincture or extract, ¼–1 tsp. per day; phytolacca oil—apply to the affected breast at night for two weeks, then three times a week, then once a week for another month; or vitex, 40 drops of concentrated extract to glass of water in the morning for four to eight weeks.

Breast discharges are common and often are not related to disease. Possible causes are hormonal imbalance, medications, or tumors (either benign or cancerous). *Normal discharge is cloudy white to milky*, often comes from both breasts, and can be caused by natural hormones before the period, during and after breast-feeding, or from sexual stimulation, excessive breast squeezing, trauma, or surgery. Early pregnancy may cause clear straw-colored discharge.

Galactorrhea is a milky discharge from both breasts, not related to breast-feeding or the menses, and may occur in the absence of menstrual periods. It is caused by high levels of prolactin due to medications, over the counter and prescribed; an underactive thyroid; or a tumor in the pituitary gland. Drugs can treat high prolactin levels. If it's due to a medication, change medicines.

Suspicious Discharges—Must See a Doctor
- Persistent throughout the whole month
- Any discharge coming from *one* breast
- Bloody, greenish gray, or clear and sticky—like egg white (Infections and benign and cancerous tumors can all cause bloody discharge.)
- Pus suggests an abscess

What to Do

There are a number of tests that are used to diagnose discharges. See your doctor, especially if the discharge is bloody or associated with cracking, scaling, or irritation around the nipples. During pregnancy, a milky discharge is very common. Simply wash away any dried milk with warm, soapy water so your nipples won't get sore.

BREAST-FEEDING (Lactation)

The natural method of infant feeding from birth to weaning. Human milk contains the ideal balance of nutrients and, ideally, breast milk should be the *only* food for the baby during the first four to six months of life. This is especially important for premature or low-birthweight infants. The production of milk depends on a number of hormones, especially prolactin. The "letdown" of milk is initiated by suckling (which sends a message to the brain via the hormone oxytocin).

Colostrum is the thick, yellowish fluid produced by the breasts during late pregnancy and in the first few days after childbirth. It has a high content of lymphocytes (a type of white blood cell) and immunoglobulins (antibodies), which help protect the baby from infection.

Breast-feeding also is good for the mother, because it helps the uterus to contract to its pre-pregnant size, thus reducing the chance of hemorrhage from the placental site, and it can be a bonding and nurturing experience for both mother and child. Breast-feeding correlates to more optimal thymus size in late infancy. Breast milk is high in DHA (docosahexaenoic acid), an essential fatty acid vital for your child's brain. Most commercial formulas over the last fifty years lacked DHA. DHA deficiencies are linked to attention deficit hyperactivity disorder, aggressive hostility, types of depression, and other disorders. Maternal alcoholism creates DHA deficiencies in utero that contribute to fetal alcohol syndrome. Early introduction of formula feeding (under three months) is associated with increased risk of type 1 diabetes in children.

Breast milk does have a shadow side. Breast milk is at the very top of the food chain and contains concentrated environmental pollutants. Approximately 40–60 percent of pollutants stored in the mother's body (coming from everyday background exposures) get transferred to the first suckling infant. Since breast-feeding passes so many beneficial nutrients to the infant, along with fostering important emotional bonding, breast milk is still considered the ideal food for all infants. However, this is becoming a controversial issue. If you have not yet had children, consider getting blood tests to detect common environmental pollutants. If you have higher than normal levels of these toxins in your body, there are methods for substantial detoxification before you decide to get pregnant. (Read my book *Hormone Deception,* Contemporary/McGraw-Hill, 2000.) Even the government suggests maternal blood and/or breast milk testing if you live in a polluted area. (Subcommittee on Nutrition During Lactation, Food and Nutrition Board, Institute of Medicine, National Academy of Sciences, 1991.)

What to Do
- Wear a good supportive nursing bra.
- Increase fluid intake to two or three quarts per day.
- Position the baby correctly (contact La Leche League for breast-feeding advice). Make sure the baby takes the full nipple and areola into his or her mouth. Moving the baby into different positions helps protect the nipple.
- During each feeding, nurse from both breasts. Remember, breast-fed babies nurse more often than those on a bottle.
- Relax. Breast-feeding is natural. Don't let your mind get in the way.

Nutrients
- ** If you have difficulty making adequate milk, take 1 tsp. brewer's yeast sprinkled on salad or mixed in juice, along with B vitamin complex, 15–25 mg per day.
- ** To maintain quality milk, take B complex with at least 500 mcg of folic acid; a daily multivitamin/mineral supplement with Vitamin A, 5,000 IU; and Vitamin K, 65 mcg.

BEWARE OF OVER-THE-COUNTER MEDICATIONS
WHILE BREAST-FEEDING

- Avoid aspirin, magnesium salicylate, and salicylamide; combination cough, cold, and allergy products; long-acting or high-dose antihistamines.
- Don't consume caffeine while taking products that contain theophylline. Asthma medications also accumulate in breast milk, so use products with the lowest amount of theophylline possible.
- In general, try to avoid medications that are maximum or extra strength, long-acting, and those with a variety of active ingredients. Take medications immediately after nursing or before the baby's longest sleep period.
- Be sure to ask your doctor about possible side effects any medication may produce in the baby. Ask about trying nonpharmaceutical therapies first.
- The American Academy of Pediatrics regards acetaminophen, ibuprofen, and naproxen to be safe to take while breast-feeding, with ibuprofen having the best documented safety record. Decongestants appear to be safe but may decrease milk production, so drink extra fluids.

- Do not take more than 25 mg of vitamin B_6 per day if you plan to nurse or are nursing, as high levels reduce milk production by reducing prolactin levels.

Herbs: Red raspberry leaf tea is the classic support for breast-feeding. Avoid black walnut, sage, yarrow, and large amounts of parsley, which all can decrease milk supply.

- Note for diabetics: While breast-feeding, your dose of insulin should be 25 percent less than the pre-pregnancy dose. Check with your doctor.

An *inverted nipple* is a structural defect that can be corrected before breast-feeding by using a breast shell for fifteen to twenty minutes a day, starting in the sixth or seventh month of pregnancy. If a previously normal nipple becomes inverted, have it checked out at once by a doctor; it may be due to breast cancer. *Cracked or sore nipples* are common during the last months of pregnancy and during breast-feeding. Cracks may lead to a breast infection called *mastitis*.

Especially during the first weeks of nursing, mothers can have problems with their nipples.

What to Do

- *To prevent sore nipples:* Keep nipples dry, letting them dry naturally in air after each feeding. Learn to break the baby's suction so you can comfortably change positions and rotate the pressure of the baby's mouth on the breast.
- Nurse on the least sore side first. If both breasts are sore, hand-express until letdown occurs and milk is readily available to the baby.
- After nursing, apply a very small amount of vitamin E (nonsynthetic D-tocopherol) or aloe vera to any crack.
- Calendula cream applied three times a day softens and soothes the nipple area.

Engorged Breasts

When the milk replaces colostrum in the first two to five days after childbirth, it is common for the breasts to become very swollen and tender. Sometimes the breasts will feel full, hard, and tight, and the skin will be hot, shiny, and distended.

What to Do

- *To prevent engorgement:* Allow the baby to empty each breast completely (about seven minutes on each side) at each feeding. Nurse the baby with short, frequent feedings (every 1½ to 2 hours).
- Use a breast pump or hand-express milk to empty breasts and relieve pressure.
- Apply moist heat half an hour before nursing and massage the breast during feedings to get the milk flowing.
- Application of hot towels or standing under a hot shower may help.

Mastitis (Caked Breasts)

Mastitis is an inflammation of the breast tissue often caused by bacterial infection, especially during the first month of breast-feeding when nipple cracks or plugged milk ducts most commonly occur. About 2 percent of breast-feeding mothers are affected. Remember, the infection is in the breast tissue and not in your milk. Breast abscesses occur in about 7 percent of women who have mastitis. After treatment with antibiotics, the abscess will have to be incised.

Symptoms: A tender area in the breast with a patch of reddened skin. One or both breasts may be involved. There can be pain, swelling, and hardness in the breast. You may also have fever, chills, flu-like pain, nausea, and vomiting. The breast could feel hot to the touch.

What to Do

- Ask your doctor if you need antibiotics, especially if you have a fever.
- Prevention includes emptying the breast regularly by feeding the baby frequently or by expressing the remaining milk by hand after each feeding.
- Do not stop nursing. The ducts can become overfull and can worsen the problem.
- Drink at least eight glasses of water and/or juice daily.
- Try to get plenty of rest (yeah, right).
- Use a hot water bottle, hot compresses, or heating pad on the affected area.
- Apply moist warm heat to the breast fifteen minutes before nursing.

Nutrients

- Green Drink daily, minus parlsey, one week (page 465)
- Lactobacillus and bifidobacteria, several caps of each per day, or a supplement that contains a combination of probiotics
- Vitamin C, 100 mg twice a day

Herbs: Blessed thistle, dandelion, nettle leaf, and raspberry.

BURSITIS

Inflammation of a bursa, one of the fluid-filled sacs that act as shock absorbers between the tendons and bones. The joints most likely to be affected are the shoulders, knees, hips, and elbows. There are eight bursae around each shoulder, eleven around each knee, and as many as seventy-eight on each side of the body.

Symptoms: Mild to severe debilitating pain, swelling, tenderness, and loss of movement in the affected joint, sometimes accompanied by fever. Pain can be particularly bad in the morning and in damp weather.

Causes: Usually the result of pressure, friction, or injury to the membrane, or overuse of the joint. The problem can also stem from nutrient imbalances, infection, arthritis or rheumatism, or be secondary to nerve pressure in the spine, gout, calcium deposits, food allergies, or periods of extreme stress.

Uniquely Female: Some women can get flare-ups of bursitis before the start of their menstrual period or during transitional hormonal times such as peri- and postmenopause. Take vitamin B_6, 25–50 mg per day; magnesium, 250–400 mg per day; and essential fatty acids, several grams per day, along with selected items from the nutrient list on page 149.

What to Do

** At the onset of inflammation, the affected area should be completely rested for two or three days. This will usually end a problem that could otherwise last for weeks. Don't try to work through the pain.

** Use ice, ten minutes on, ten minutes off, if the joint is hot to the touch. If the joint is cool, try alternating cold and hot treatment.

• When the acute stage is over (after four or five days), replace cold treatment with heat and replace immobilization with exercise. Exercise of your overall body is very important to keep your circulation healthy.

• Take a mineral or salts bath once a week.

• Acupuncture or ultrasound therapy may help.

• *Topical treatment:* Try mullein hot packs. Boil three or four fresh mullein leaves in water for three minutes. Place the leaves over the joint. Wrap with a hot moist towel, then a dry towel. Leave on for twenty minutes, three times a day. Or try a castor oil pack.

- Rub the joint with MSM (methylsulfonylmethane) cream.

Nutrients

** Proteolytic enzymes, 1–3 g between meals two or three times a day for one to two weeks

** Vitamin C plus bioflavonoids, 1,000–3,000 mg per day in divided doses

** Injections of vitamin B_{12} (1,000 mcg per ml), especially for calcified shoulder bursitis, 1 ml intramuscularly daily for one to two weeks. As symptoms lessen, reduce to three times a week for two to three weeks, then once or twice a week for two to three weeks more. If your doctor doesn't offer B_{12} injections, try sublingual B_{12} dosages several times a day for a month. Injections do not have to be near the affected area.

- Apply DMSO (dimethylsulfoxide) to the skin two or three times a day for one to three weeks. First clean your hands and the skin over the bursitis thoroughly, and then apply vitamin E oil before applying the DMSO. It's best to obtain a 50–70 percent solution of DMSO from a compounding pharmacist. Ask if they can add minerals like magnesium, too.

C

CAFFEINE IN COFFEE AND TEA

Caffeinated foods include coffee, black and green tea, chocolate, cocoa, and many over-the-counter medications. Heavy caffeine consumption (six cups of coffee a day or eight cups of different caffeinated drinks) is linked to a number of problems. Postmenopausal women, especially those at risk for chronic heart disease and bone loss, should not overconsume caffeine. For pregnant women, heavy caffeine use has been linked to spontaneous abortions (especially during the second trimester and in women with nausea), adverse pregnancy outcomes, and developmental delays in newborns. Decaffeinated coffee has also been suspected to contribute to spontaneous abortion.

Caffeine can affect fertility. Two or more cups of caffeine a day have been linked to diseases of the fallopian tubes and endometriosis, both of which can cause infertility. One to three cups of coffee a day cut fertility by 50 percent, and the tannins in any kind of coffee (including decaf) and teas may also reduce fertility. Even half a cup of coffee a day may delay conception in women trying to get pregnant. If you are planning on getting pregnant, try not to drink more than one-half to one cup of caffeine a day; if you are having problems with conception or are pregnant, avoid caffeine entirely. One cup of decaffeinated a day is probably okay, unless you fail to conceive; then eliminate completely.

The good news is that coffee consumed twenty minutes after

brewing contains antioxidant properties and caffeine in general may help fight off cancer. Tea (black and green) may protect against heart disease, obesity, cataracts, and arthritis, as well as protect against inflammation (although not in smokers). Drinking one cup of tea elevates blood antioxidant levels, a healthy boost to start your day in the morning. Excessive tea drinking can contribute to iron deficiency. Coffee and tea do not cause dehydration as once believed. Coffee may protect against Parkinson's disease.

Caffeine abuse is a common undiagnosed cause of anxiety and insomnia. Caffeine can promote fibrocystic breasts and breast pain. Allergies to coffee and tea can be hard to diagnose and can manifest as a wide variety of health problems from phobias to heart disease, to chronic skin ulcers. This is well documented in scientific literature.

CALF CRAMPS

Cramps in the calves at night is a common complaint worldwide, especially in the elderly. Try calcium, 500 mg; magnesium, 200–500 mg; and potassium, 40 mg, at dinner and before bed. If these do not help, find a physical therapist or chiropractor who practices Dr. Janet Travell's myofascial trigger-point system to treat the calf muscle trigger points. This has been found to be more effective than quinine and works for a longer period of time without adverse side effects.

CANCER

Cancer is the unrestrained growth of abnormal cells in a body organ or tissues that results in malignant tumors. As the tumor grows, it spreads and infiltrates the tissues around it and may block passageways, destroy nerves, and erode bone. Metastasis occurs when cancerous cells have spread to other parts of the body via the blood vessels or lymphatic channels. Cancers that are specific to women include cancers of the cervix, ovaries, uterus, vulva, vagina, and fallopian tubes. Breast cancer can occur in both women and men, but much more rarely in men. Cancer now occurs in around one out of three Americans during their lifetime. Preventative measures are essential. See *Cancer Prevention*.

Once you develop cancer, take responsibility for decisions regarding your course of treatment and healing. Information is being accumulated too quickly for any one doctor to be on top of it. Go on the Internet, get many opinions, talk to

> See *Estrogen Dominance* for risk factors of lifetime exposure to higher than normal or unbalanced levels of estrogen. This is a must read for women with hormonal-driven cancers or those at high risk.

everyone. Many natural therapies can be used along with conventional therapies of surgery, radiation, and chemotherapy. Tell your doctor everything you are doing, since some alternative therapies inhibit conventional ones, and the timing of concurrent therapies is vital. Read *The Journey Through Cancer: An Oncologist's Seven-Level Program for Healing and Transforming the Whole Person* by Dr. Jeremy R. Geffen (Crown Publishers, 2000).

Breast Cancer

Fifteen million women see a doctor each year because they are worried about breast cancer, and 190,000 new cases are diagnosed annually. Approximately one out of every eight women (or 12.64 percent) will develop breast cancer by age ninety-five (most often in women over the age of seventy).

Types of Breast Cancer

There are many forms of breast cancer; some grow very slowly, while others are more aggressive. The size of the tumor is not always an indicator of virulence. The same type of cancer can act differently in different women.

In situ carcinoma is cancer that is contained entirely within a milk duct, with no invasion into the surrounding breast tissue. This type accounts for more than 15 percent of all breast cancers in the United States, especially in younger women.

Ductal carcinoma in situ (DCIS) is considered a precursor to invasive cancer. It is localized, but it becomes invasive if it is not treated. It is a common cause of small calcifications found on mammograms. DCIS accounts for 43 percent of breast cancers in women aged forty through forty-nine years old, and 92 percent of cases in women aged thirty through thirty-nine years old.

Lobular carcinoma in situ (LCIS) occurs mostly in premenopausal women and doesn't form a palpable mass, so it is hard to detect. Twenty to 25 percent of women with LCIS go on to develop invasive breast cancer, often up to forty years after finding the LCIS. Many doctors consider LCIS and atypical hyperplasia (abnormal but not cancerous cell changes sometimes found on breast biopsies) to signify that this woman has a *propensity* for breast cancer.

Invasive ductal and lobular breast cancers: Ninety percent of breast cancers start in the milk glands or milk ducts and 10 percent in the fatty or connective tissue. Women with less common types of breast cancer, such as pure mucinous adenocarcinoma, usually have a somewhat better prognosis. The prognosis becomes worse if the unusual form occurs not by itself, but rather alongside the more typical ductal and lobular forms.

Symptoms: Usually discovered when the woman feels a lump, which in most cases is not painful and does not become smaller after her period. Other symptoms can include an area of dimpled, creased skin on the breast; vague discomfort in the breast; indentation of the nipple; flaking, crusting, or "weeping" skin patches around the nipple; change in breast shape or color; a discharge (especially if bloody) from the nipple. If you notice any of these conditions, get a thorough breast exam and mammogram, even if your doctor thinks you just need antibiotics for a breast infection.

Risk Factors
- Age: Older women are more at risk, with the greatest risk after age seventy-five. However, younger and younger women are being diagnosed these days.
- Family history: If a first-degree relative in your family had breast cancer (parent, sibling, or child), this doubles or triples a woman's risk of getting the disease herself. A history of breast cancer in more distant relatives increases the risk slightly, but this slight risk may be bumped up if these distant relatives had breast cancer in both breasts or were diagnosed before menopause. When two or more first-degree relatives

---

BREAST SELF-EXAM

First, stand in front of a mirror, hands by your sides, and look for skin dimpling, nipple changes or discharge, redness, swelling, or other changes. Do the same with your hands lifted above your head, and then with your hands on your hips and elbows forward.

Next, examine your breasts:

- Lie down and place one arm behind your head, or perform the exam in the shower with soapy hands (which I think is the easiest way to feel for lumps).
- Use the pads of the three middle fingers of your hand to palpate the breast in the following three patterns:

    1. *Circular motion*—Move your fingers in circles spiraling toward the nipple.
    2. *Vertical stripes*—Trace up and down lines without lifting your fingers.
    3. *Wedge pattern*—From the outside edge of the breast, draw your fingers toward the nipple; repeat this pattern all the way around the breast.

For all tests, press firmly enough to feel different breast tissue textures.

- Completely examine the entire breast, up to the collarbone and down into the armpit. About half of breast cancers are found in the upper/outer part of the breast.

  - Squeeze the nipple to check for blood or a watery yellow or pink discharge.
  - Repeat the exam on the other breast using the opposite hand.

---

had breast cancer, the risk is five to six times higher. About 5 percent of women with breast cancer carry one of the two breast cancer genes (BRCA1 or BRCA2). What exact risk these genes carry is not known, but it increases the chances of disease by as much as 50 to 85 percent by age eighty. However, once women with these genes get breast cancer, they appear to have less risk of death from this disease, although they also have a higher risk of getting ovarian cancer.

- History of in situ or invasive breast cancer. The risk of getting breast cancer in the opposite breast increases by almost 0.5 to 1 percent a year.

- Early menarche, late menopause, or a late first pregnancy increases risk, as it increases lifetime exposure to estrogen.
- Women with a first-time pregnancy after age thirty are at a greater risk than women who have never had children.
- A history of fibrocystic breasts increases risk, but exactly by how much is not known. It is thought that women who have had multiple biopsies, or those found to have ductal proliferation or atypical hyperplasia (cells are changing, or overgrowing), have a modest increased risk. Women with numerous breast lumps, but without these definitive changes, should not be considered at higher risk. However, women with atypical hyperplasia and a first-degree family member who had breast cancer have nine times the risk of getting breast cancer.
- Overweight postmenopausal women are at increased risk due to the fact that fat produces estrogen. It is thought that 10 to 16 percent of postmenopausal breast cancers are due to obesity. Being overweight at twenty years of age increases the risk of postmenopausal breast cancer. If you have more than a twenty-five-pound variance from the lowest weight in your adult life to your present weight, this greatly increases your risk of breast cancer (some studies say up to 70 percent). Any *sustained* weight loss during premenopausal adult years decreases your risk by 20 percent.
- Radiation exposure before thirty years of age increases the risk.
- Diet and lifestyle factors. It is currently thought that a sedentary lifestyle with excess dietary fat may predispose a woman to breast cancer, but this has not been completely supported by research. It may not be so much the type of fat we eat as how we metabolize these fats into fatty acids, or perhaps the types of fats our moms ate while we swam in the womb, or what pollutants were in that fetal ocean. Premenopausal breast cancer is occurring at earlier ages, and so is DCIS, which points a suspicious finger at exposures in utero.
- Insulin resistance or elevated levels of insulin (see page 300). *Cancer Causes and Control* 7:605–25, 1999.
- Computer monitors have been found to make breast cancer cells grow (in the laboratory) and even to inactivate tamox-

ifen (a drug used to treat breast cancers that are driven by estrogen). So work in front of liquid crystal screens or use screen protectors.

- Smoking, active and passive, may increase the risk, especially that of premenopausal breast cancer.
- The role of alcohol is still being debated. It is known that heavy drinking can delay menopause by two years, so it must have some hormonal effect. Don't overdo it.
- Bouts of major depression and working night-shift jobs have been linked to subsequent breast cancer, which may be due to elevated levels of the hormone cortisol.

Tumor Markers. Cancer basically occurs when cells go crazy, so no cancer is entirely predictable. But identifying factors on the surface of cancer cells, called tumor markers, can give clues about how the tumor might act. For example, markers can tell if the tumor is growing fast or slow; if it is driven by estrogen (estrogen-receptor positive, which carries a better prognosis) or not driven by estrogen (estrogen-receptor negative, which carries a worse prognosis); or just how crazy and out of control your cancer is.

Oral contraceptives cause about 5 more cases of breast cancer per 100,000 women. An analysis of fifty-four studies showed that current users of birth control pills or those who have used them within the last five years are at higher risk. Women on progestin only or progestins plus estrogen are at modestly elevated risk.

If a woman started birth control pills before age twenty, the risk is slightly higher than if she had started when older, unless she has a fairly thin body type. Thin women between thirty-five and forty-five years of age on contraceptives seem to have a modest increased risk. Risk from contraceptives dwindles over the decade after cessation, but it is not known if this risk decreases for women who took the higher-dose forms of contraceptives widely used prior to 1975.

Women on birth control pills with a mother or sister who had breast cancer have three times the risk of getting breast cancer, and even higher if they took older forms. These women should be watched diligently.

However, a history of taking birth control pills *lowers* some women's risk of ovarian cancer.

Hormone replacement therapy (HRT) increases the risk moderately, especially after five to ten years or more of use. Synthetic progestins may increase this risk, though natural progesterone does not appear to have this adverse effect and may even have a protective effect (*Molecular and Cellular Biochemistry* 202:53–61, 1999).

The common progesterone added to Premarin is medroxyprogesterone, by the brand name of Provera. The combination of Premarin and Provera is the standard HRT practice today. Provera was added to minimize the risk of uterine cancer. But it has been shown to increase the risk of breast cancer by as much as 30 percent, meaning that for every 1,000 women taking this form of HRT, 30 will eventually develop breast cancer from taking it.

During surgery for cancer, the surgeon can put a sample of your tumor into a special vial and send this piece of tumor, with all the precious information it carries, to a special laboratory that can measure all kinds of tumor markers. This may help you and your doctor understand what type of cancer you are battling and help your doctor prescribe an optimal treatment regime. For example, these laboratories can test your tumor cells against eighteen various chemotherapeutic agents and find out which ones will kill your tumor and which ones won't work. It makes sense to find out which is the most effective poison for killing your cancer.

Two laboratories that perform these tests are: Weisenthall Cancer Group (704-894-0011) and Oncotech, Inc. (800-662-6832). Most oncologists are not aware of these laboratory tests, even though they have been around for almost twenty-five years. I highly recommend pushing to get your doctors to cooperate and pay for the fee if your insurance company won't cooperate, as this information can be extremely useful.

Get second and third opinions from pathologists who specialize in reading tumor slides to have the most up-to-date information. Excellent pathology specialists who offer second opinions include Dr. Michael Lagios in San Francisco and Dr. David Page at Vanderbilt University in Nashville, Tennessee.

What to Do

- Perform regular breast exams (see box on page 154). No one knows your breasts as well as you do. Examine your breasts each month at the same time, preferably during the week following your period, when hormonal influence is lowest. After menopause, pick a day of the month you will remember. If you find a lump or any changes in your breast, see your doctor at once. Twenty-five to 30 percent of breast cancers are not picked up by mammograms or ultrasounds.

- Always *add* alternative treatments on top of orthodox medical care. Women who relied solely on alternative methods had twice the risk of recurrence or death within the first five years after diagnosis. Ideally, work with several experts.

- *For bone metastases:* Ask your doctor about chlordronate or drugs related to bisphosphonates, which have been shown to be effective in reversing bone cancer, reducing pain, and reducing mortality.

- Ask, ask, ask. There are many therapies out there, and no one doctor knows about all of them. One study in Europe took fifty-nine late-stage breast cancer patients and brought more than 50 percent into remission (seventeen to eighty months) with heat therapy (hyperthermia—heat directed at the tumor and whole body), vaccines, thymus extracts, and nutrients (*Biomedicine and Pharmacotherapy*, 49:79–82, 1995).

- High fasting levels of insulin in the blood may be an independent risk factor. Get tested and see *Insulin Resistance*.

- *Prophylactic removal of ovaries:* If you have had an aggressive breast cancer, had a recurrence of an estrogen-receptor positive (ER+) breast cancer, or test positive for mutations and your ovaries are still making estrogen, you might ask your doctor about the protective measure of removing your ovaries. This has been suggested to increase survival for some women under fifty years of age. (Removal of the ovaries does not completely guarantee avoidance of ovarian cancer.)

- Ask your doctor about testing your *estrogen metabolite ratios*. Estrogen is metabolized into two competing compounds—

2-hydroxyestrone appears to be protective against cancer, and 16-alpha-hydroxyestrone appears to be associated with high cancer risk. Research suggests that altered estrogen metabolism (more 16-alpha than 2) exists before the onset of cancer, not as a result of cancer. This pathway can be modified by foods that improve this ratio of estrogen metabolites, including flaxseeds, raw cruciferous veggies (broccoli, cabbage, brussels sprouts, and kohlrabi, all of which may be more effective raw, though it remains to be seen), and supplements containing active ingredients in these vegetables (cruciferous vegetables contain high amounts of an anti-cancer compound called sulforaphane). Urinary tests of estrogen metabolite ratios can be used as monitors while on programs to reduce risks.

- Rule out hidden infections due to parasites, yeast, etc., to remove stressors from the immune system.
- Use tomato paste in cooking and drink tomato juice, as they contain high amounts of lycopene, a positive immune supporter.
- Use liquid crystal displays or radiation screens on computers.
- (Consider getting a blood test for pollutants. Elevated pollutants such as DDE (dichlordiphenylethylene) have been shown to be linked to poorer survival and a trend to more lymph node involvement (*Environmental Health Perspectives* 108(1):1–4, 2000). If you have very high levels, consider a detoxification program (*Cancer, Epidemiology, Biomarkers, and Prevention,* 9:161, 2000).
- Consider breast surgery during the second half of your menstrual cycle or with a pre-shot of progesterone, which is linked to better survival and outcomes.

Nutrients

** Melatonin, 3–20 mg before bed. Certain cancer patients take up to 20 mg a night. Melatonin is especially effective with various vaccines.

** Coenzyme Q-10, 90–390 mg per day; use the fat-soluble form and take with fatty meals.

TOO MANY SUPPLEMENTS?

Many supplements (like quercetin, turmeric, and indole-3-carbinol, etc.) have been suggested to be helpful. If you were to take them all separately, it's more than overwhelming on the wallet and the stomach. Dr. Davis Lamson has designed Supportive Care (4 capsules three times a day with meals). (The product is available through Thorne Research, 800-228-1966; a doctor must place the order.) Supportive Care is contraindicated if the patient is on methotrexate or has liver metastases.

- ** Vitamin E succinate and mixed tocopherols, 400 IU once a day
- ** Multivitamin/mineral supplement
- ** Indole-3-carbinol may reduce risk of metastasis (*Breast Cancer Research and Treatment* 63:147–52, 2000).
- ** Fish oil and evening primrose oil, 2–6 g per day of each in divided doses
- ** Zinc, 20 mg twice a day; balance with 2–3 mg copper
- • Phytosterols found in unrefined olive oil, peanuts, refined and unrefined peanut oil are excellent for boosting the immune system.
- • Avoid iron and cooking in iron unless you've been proven to be anemic.

Uterine Cancer

There are two distinct types of uterine cancer: cervical and endometrial. Most at risk are postmenopausal women who have never been pregnant or have had more than five births and those with a history of benign uterine fibroids. Serious vaginal infections are a warning sign.

Cervical Cancer

Malignant growth in the cervix. If not caught early enough, the cancer can spread into the tissues surrounding the uterus or into the vagina. It usually affects women between the ages of twenty and fifty-five, with the most common age being around fifty. One percent of cancers occur in pregnant or recently pregnant women.

Symptoms: Well-defined precancerous stages (see the section on dysplasia under *Cervical Problems*) are readily detected by an annual

EMERGING BREAST-CANCER TREATMENTS THAT CONSERVE YOUR ARM AND BREAST: ASK YOUR DOCTOR

Sentinel-Node Biopsy

Instead of having numerous lymph nodes removed, a dye injected into the breast shows which is the first lymph node that the breast drains into and is most likely to contain cancer cells. Only this lymph node is removed. This surgery is now offered throughout the United States. It protects women from a lifetime of concern about lymphedema. Find a surgeon who uses this technique. Doctors who don't know how to perform this won't necessarily recommend it.

RITA

This is a nonsurgical lumpectomy in which the breast is pierced with a stainless-steel probe that is heated. The cancer cells are killed by heating them to near boiling. This technique has been used for years in countries like Germany and should become mainstream in the United States by 2005.

Laser Lumpectomy

It is like the RITA, but a laser light kills the tumor. This technique will also become mainstream in the next several years.

Bone-Marrow Micrometastases

 This is another way to see how widely your cancer has spread by testing your bone marrow. It is now widely practiced but you may have to ask for it.

Pap smear and pelvic exam (though these tests are not infallible). Ask for the new ThinPrep Pap test, which is more sensitive. Precancerous and even cancerous stages cause no symptoms at all. Eventually a woman may notice vaginal bleeding or spotting between periods, after intercourse, or after menopause. Serious vaginal infections are a warning sign.

Risk Factors: Smokers and those exposed to secondhand smoke are at higher risk; their cervical mucus contains a large amount of nicotine. The greatest risk is intercourse with a man who has genital warts. One particular wart virus, HPV16, has been found in 90 percent of squamous-type cervical cancers and in 50–70 percent of precancerous conditions. Other risk factors include intercourse before age eighteen, a history of gonorrhea, multiple sex partners, and infertility. Low levels of vitamin A and folic acid might also put women more at risk. Estrogen metabolite imbalances may increase risk and may explain why cruciferous vegetables and their active substances seem to decrease risk and even help in treatment.

Endometrial Cancer

Malignant growth in the lining of the uterus. Unlike the great majority of cervical cancer cases, endometrial cancer may occur in women who have never had sexual intercourse.

Symptoms: Bleeding between periods, after intercourse, or after menopause; unusual discharge; painful or heavy menstrual periods.

Risk Factors: Never being pregnant, menopause after age fifty-two, a history of menstrual problems, exposure to high levels of estrogen, exposure to estrogen-only replacement therapy or tamoxifen therapy, obesity, diabetes, hypertension, and long-term use of hormone replacement therapy. At highest risk are women between the ages of fifty and sixty.

Ovarian Cancer

Malignant growth of the ovary. Most common after the age of fifty and in women who have had an excess of estrogen exposures in their lives. Using talc before a first pregnancy may be a risk factor.

Symptoms: Very hard to detect in its early stages. The first symptom is usually vague discomfort in the lower abdomen. Eventually the abdomen may swell and there may be pain in the pelvis, anemia, or loss of weight. If the tumor is large, it may push on other organs causing diarrhea, constipation, or frequent urination.

Risk Factors: Never being pregnant, first pregnancy after age thirty, obesity from high-fat diet, late menopause, long-term use of estrogen replacement therapy and possibly fertility drugs, BRCA1 and BRCA2 genes, family history, and a history of breast cancer. A history of taking birth control pills actually lowers the risk.

What to Do
- If you are a high-risk woman, read *Estrogen Dominance,* ask your doctor to measure the size of your ovaries with a baseline intravaginal ultrasound, and get a CA-125 blood test (although this only picks up common types of ovarian cancers and isn't foolproof). Repeat yearly. Doctors often don't think to recommend these tests. Request new prostasin test.

Prevention
- ** Add omega-3 flax oil, 2–6 g per day, ¼ tsp. of ground flaxseeds several times a week, and/or take evening primrose oil, 1,000–1,500 mg two or three times a day
- ** Alpha-linolenic acid, 100 mg twice a day (with a backup of biotin, 2.5 mg per day)
- ** Consider melatonin and indole-3-carbinol. See *Estrogen Dominance.*
- Avoid NutraSweet, especially in hot drinks.
- Use a talc-free condom during intercourse, don't dust baby bottoms with talcum powder, and don't use talcum powder yourself.
- Avoid exposure to asbestos and certain anti-inflammatory drugs (salicylates, nonsteroidals, and corticosteroids).
- Consume lots of veggies (especially raw cruciferous types), fruits, grains, nuts, and seeds. Drink green tea, use tomato paste, and drink tomato juice.
- Limit or avoid fatty meats, and eat organic eggs and butter. There is a high correlation between fatty meats and regular eggs and butter and cancer.
- Exercise reduces risk.

Cancer of the Vulva (Vaginal Lips)

This disease accounts for 3–4 percent of all cancers of the female reproductive system; usually occurs after menopause. It is predominantly a skin cancer near or at the opening of the vagina, although it may spread up into the body if left untreated.

Symptoms: Unusual lumps or sores near or at the opening of the vagina. May have scaly patches, discoloration, or puckering. Bleeding or a watery discharge ("weeping") may develop. It should be suspected in women over fifty when use of vaginal creams does not relieve chronic vaginal itching.

Cancer of the Vagina

This cancer accounts for only 1 percent of female cancers, with a peak incidence from age forty-five to sixty-five. *Frequent douching increases your risk of vaginal cancer.* Risk also increases with number of sexual partners, especially in young women, and may also be increased from cigarette smoking and a poor diet with low levels of nutrients (especially the B vitamins found in a whole-foods, fruit, and vegetable diet).

Symptoms: Sores that may bleed and become infected; watery discharge or bleeding and pain after intercourse; frequent urge to urinate and painful urination (occurs with large tumors).

A rare form of vaginal cancer (clear cell carcinoma) has been linked to in utero exposure to DES (diethylstilbestrol). It may be symptomless in its early stages, or a young woman may experience abnormal bleeding. Some doctors recommend that DES daughters minimize their exposure to estrogen from birth control pills, postmenopausal estrogen therapies, or post-intercourse contraceptives. Annual checkups should include both a regular Pap smear and a Pap smear of the upper vagina, as well as an iodine stain of the vagina and cervix to identify abnormal areas and possible abnormal glandular tissue.

Cancer of the Fallopian Tubes

This is the rarest of all female reproductive system cancers. Symptoms include vague abdominal discomfort and sometimes a watery or blood-tinged discharge. Usually diagnosed after a mass is removed from the pelvis.

CANCER PREVENTION

The good news is that the most common cause of cancer death in women is from lung cancer, which is mostly due to smoking and thus is usually preventable: Stop smoking and decrease your exposure to secondhand smoke.

The second-largest cause of cancer death in women between the ages of thirty-five and fifty-four is breast cancer. Many cases are thought to be due to factors that affect the balance of estrogen, our body's response to estrogen, or unknown factors that allow faulty cells to multiply rather than die. Environmental factors, especially exposure in the womb and during early life when the breast tissue is the most immature and thus the most vulnerable, are thought to be causing an increased incidence of estrogen-driven female cancers, especially premenopausal. We must work to identify and reduce these exposures. A study on 17,000 identical twins suggests that *most* cancers are made by environmental factors, not inborn genetics.

The Best Cancer-Fighting Foods
- Foods rich in protective carotenoids and lycopenes—carrots, yams, red/orange/yellow fruits, green vegetables, tomatoes (especially juice and paste)
- Foods rich in antioxidants—garlic, onions, broccoli, wheat germ, sea vegetables, leafy vegetables
- Cruciferous vegetables—broccoli, cabbage, cauliflower, brussels sprouts. Some researchers say the most protective substances occur in raw foods. (But who knows for sure now? No one.) But grate some into your salad (grating acts to break down the raw vegetables and make them more digestible), in addition to eating them cooked.
- Protease inhibitors—beans (especially soy), rice, potatoes, corn
- High fiber—whole grains (especially brown rice), fruits, and vegetables
- High lignin—flaxseeds; whole grains; soy, sunflower, and pumpkin seeds. Lignins are substances in whole foods that the body converts to biologically active forms that can fight carcinogens, bacteria, viruses, and act as weak hormones. They are thought to promote good health. Refined grains do not contain lignins.

THE TOP FIVE RULES OF CANCER PREVENTION

1. Don't smoke.

2. Avoid or limit consumption of alcohol.

3. Get regular exercise, at least three times a week.

4. Lose excess weight and eat less. Body fat increases the amount of estrogen in a woman's body. Excessive estrogenic stimulation causes cells to divide and is a causative factor in cervical, uterine, and breast cancer.

5. Eat a healthy diet, with a variety of foods:

   - Reduce intake of fat (especially animal and polyunsaturated fats like corn oil).
   - Increase quality fats (fish, olive, nuts, and seeds).
   - Reduce intake of red meats, fast foods, and fried foods.
   - Eat fruits and vegetables every day.
   - Take oral vitamin D and expose your skin to outdoor sunlight, for at least twenty minutes a day (not at the sun's hottest peak) while not wearing sunscreen. Then use sunscreen the rest of the day.
   - Eat organic foods, especially for foods high in fats, to avoid pesticide residues and added female and growth hormones.
   - Don't microwave in plastic.

- Flaxseeds improve the ratio of "good" estrogen (2-hydroxy-estrone) to the "harmful" estrogen (16-alpha-hydroxy-estrone), especially in post-menopausal women. Daily, grind ⅛ tsp. in a coffee grinder and put in smoothies, salads, casseroles, protein drinks, soups, and even baked pastries. Cooking does not reduce protective factors.

- For thousands of years, green tea (and its decaffeinated cousin) has been reputed to protect blood vessels, suppress cancer, and prolong life. Take green tea supplements if you don't like to drink the tea.

- Skim milk contains protective substances not available in milk with any amount of fat.

- Soy contains isoflavones, which may reduce excessive estrogenic signaling as well as block uncontrolled cancer cell growth and tumor blood supply. Isoflavones may, however, do the opposite in postmenopausal women who have had a history of estrogenic cancers and/or other estrogen-dominance problems, unless they are on some form of hormone replacement therapy. At this time we don't know the exact story. Do not consume soy if undergoing radiation (one week before, during, and one week after).

- See Anti-cancer Green Drink (page 465).
- Berries and berry juices (such as cranberry or blueberry) are excellent preventatives.

Avoid: Excessive consumption of processed oils, hydrogenated oils, polyunsaturated oils (like corn oil), simple and refined sugars and carbohydrates with high glycemic index (read Dr. Barry Sears's book *The Zone*, Regan Books, 1995, or Dr. Sears's *The Soy Zone*, Regan Books, 2000), natural foods and juices high in sugars, junk foods, fried foods, saturated fats, red meats, luncheon meats, cured or smoked meats, excessive alcohol, and peanuts (these legumes often harbor cancer-causing bacteria). Limit amounts of high-fat dairy products and try to consume low-fat or fat-free ones as much as possible.

Nutrients

To prevent estrogen-driven cancers, take these nutrients in dosages according to the severity of your risk and after consultation with your doctor:

- ** Indole-3-carbinol (the active ingredient in cruciferous vegetables that promotes optimal estrogen metabolism into less toxic and more protective metabolites). For a 120-pound woman, 200 mg twice a day; heavier woman, 300 mg three times a day. More isn't better. Or take diindolylmethane, 60 mg twice a day (available from Tyler at 800-869-9705).
- ** Melatonin, 1–3 mg before bed. Various clinicians report that more than 3 mg of melatonin nightly can reduce estrogen to the point of bringing on hot flashes or earlier menopause in some women. Long-term use of aspirin can reduce melatonin levels.
- ** Vitamin E succinate, up to 800 IU per day
- ** Vitamin D, 600–800 IU (discuss with your doctor, especially if you have had kidney stones or calcification problems)

** Selenium, 200 mcg per day
** Coenzyme Q-10, 100 mg per day in a fat-soluble form taken with a fatty meal
** Take evening primrose oil and fish oil capsules regularly (omega-3 fatty acids protect against breast and colon cancers).
** Use antioxidants such as alpha-lipoic acid as well as lycopenes and carotenoids (many of which come in high potency multivitamin/mineral preparations) on a regular basis.
- Vitamin A, 10,000 IU per day (more under a doctor's supervision)
- Breast-Guard is a multiple formula containing many of the nutrients mentioned above and is offered by Thorne Research to help women at high risk of getting breast cancer. Have your doctor call 800-228-1966. Take nine capsules a day with meals.
- Consume fish generously and use organic cold-pressed dark-green virgin olive oil freely.
- If high risk, add thymic polypeptides several times a week.
- Do not take iron tablets or cook in iron pots if you are at increased risk for getting cancer. Excess iron levels present an increased risk factor for developing cancer.
- Folic acid, 400–500 IU per day
- Ask your doctor about DHEA (dehydroepiandrosterone). Do not take without supervision if you have had cancer, and then take it only at very low dosages, if at all.

Herbs: Vitex is a slow-acting herb with effective results. It increases progesterone production and decreases prolactin. Take 40 drops of concentrated liquid extract in a glass of water in the morning for up to three months. Turmeric (curcumin) has powerful anti-inflammatory and anticarcinogenic properties. If you are at risk for breast cancer, try 300–500 mg two to three times a day. It is also in Breast-Guard.

Astragalus root, Siberian ginseng, and panax ginseng support the immune system and protect the liver during chemotherapy and radiation. Various mushroom extracts, colostrum, turmeric, garlic, green tea, quercetin, mistletoe extract, and transfer factor appear to either attack cancer cells or stimulate the immune system.

<u>Nutrients for Before and During Chemotherapy</u>

- Take Coenzyme Q-10, 100 mg fat-soluble twice a day. It protects the heart from developing problems (cardiomyopathy) when receiving chemotherapy like Adriamycin. So do antioxidants. Tell your women friends. Also, see *Lymphedema.*
- For enhanced benefit from chemotherapy eat a diet higher in omega-3 (fish) oils versus omega-6 (polyunsaturated) oils. A diet lower in saturated fats is linked to better prevention of cancer. With cancer, consume olive oil liberally, eat moderate amounts of fish and nuts, and lessen intake of animal fats. See *Fats and Essential Fatty Acids.*
- Astragalus root, Siberian ginseng, and panax ginseng *may* support the immune system and protect the liver during chemotherapy and radiation.
- Selenium, taken along with Taxol or doxorubicin (chemotherapy agents), enhanced action on estrogen-dependent breast cancer cells in one lab study.
- Antioxidants can reduce or prevent many side effects.
- Indole-3-carbinol, 200–300 mg twice a day, enhances the action of tamoxifen.
- Vitamin D (1, 25-dihydroxycholecalciferol) enhances paclitaxel.
- If you are on tamoxifen, ultrasound can monitor its effects on your uterus, and gamma-linolenic acid (GLA) *may* increase its benefits.
- If you are taking cisplatin, ask your doctor to add magnesium in pre- and post-treatment hydration fluids.
- For all on chemotherapy, intravenous (IV) or oral glutamine (1–2 g two to three times a day) helps protect intestinal lining and reduce numerous side effects and fatigue, especially paclitaxel-induced neuropathies. Chemo also causes bone loss; ask doctor.
- Find a doctor adept at mixing traditional and holistic care— for consultation and as an ally. Example: Dr. Keith Block (847-492-3040) integrates nutrition with chemo based on circadian timing of drugs shown to extend survival and reduce toxicity.

- Iscador (mistletoe) increases the survival time for some cancers, shown in a study on 10,226 cancer patients (*Alternative Therapies* 3:57–78, 2001).
- Look for nutrient combinations with turmeric and bioperine. To order, call Life Extension, at 800-544-4440.

CANKER SORES

Painful ulcer-like sores on the mucous membranes of the mouth, lips, and tongue. They may last several days to several weeks and are contagious. When canker sores keep recurring, the condition is called *recurrent apthous ulceration,* or RAU.

Symptoms: Sores have a white center with a red border and are painfully sensitive to pressure or spicy food. In RAU, a new sore may be forming before the last one is completely healed.

Causes: Emotional stress, severe illness, autoimmune problems, food allergies (especially to wheat and/or gluten, see pages 84, 493), local injury such as from dental work, wounds, or a burn from hot liquid. May be a hypersensitive reaction to certain bacteria. A detergent called *sodium lauryl sulfate* found in many toothpastes may destroy the natural protective coating that lines the oral cavity in sensitive folks and promote sores. Look for toothpastes without it in the health food store.

Uniquely Female: Canker sores occur more often in females, especially premenstrually. People with Crohn's disease are prone to them.

What to Do
- *For acute pain:* Rinse with tetracycline mouthwash. Or chew papaya enzymes and hold the macerated pulp on the canker sore with your tongue.
- Dab the powder from a capsule of colostrum onto the sores three or four times a day.
- Check for low stomach acid (page 469).

Diet: Consume lysine-rich foods, such as fresh fish, tuna fish, chicken, dairy, mung beans, soy, and eggs. Consume plenty of greens, vegetables, and nonacidic fruits (like bananas and apples), as well as lots of cultured products.

Avoid: Try avoiding gluten-containing foods (wheat, rye, and barley), dairy products (except for yogurt), citrus fruits, food additives and colorings, and high-arginine foods such as nuts, chocolate, coconut, buckwheat, chickpeas, brown rice, and wheat.

Nutrients

In addition to lysine and probiotics, try the following supplements:

- Antioxidant formula (one capsule twice a day) for several weeks
- Vitamins B_2, B_6, B_{12}, and folic acid have been shown to be helpful for some people with RAU.
- Vitamin B complex, twice a day, along with 100 mg thiamine, one to two times a day for several months, then reduce to one each for maintenance
- Zinc, 50 mg once a day, balanced with 2–4 mg copper at another time of day for three weeks. If there is no improvement, increase the zinc dosage to three times a day and take 6 mg copper. If you get nauseated, back down the amount. Only stay at this level for a few weeks.
- Iron, if deficient
- Ask your doctor about zinc oxide/glycine cream.

Use the same suggestions for canker sores for *Herpes simplex.*

WHEN YOU FEEL A CANKER SORE COMING ON

Start "loading" with 500–1,000 mg of the amino acid lysine four to six times a day and three to four capsules of probiotics four to six times a day. When you feel relief, reduce dosages of lysine to 1 g two to three times a day and the acidophilus mix to two capsules two to three times a day. If you are prone to recurrences, stay on 500 mg lysine and two capsules acidophilus mix once a day as prevention. Eat yogurt and live-culture products regularly.

CARPAL TUNNEL SYNDROME (CTS)

A disorder that occurs from pressure on the median nerve as it passes through the carpal tunnel, a narrow, hollow area in the wrist. Can involve the blood vessels, nerves, and tendons of one or both hands. Surgery for carpal tunnel is becoming the most common procedure in the United States; try natural remedies first before you undergo more serious treatment.

Symptoms: Numbness, tingling, and pain in the thumb, index, and middle fingers, wrist, or palm that often worsens at night. Other symptoms include stiffness of the wrist in the morning, cramping of the hands, inability to make a fist, weakness in the thumb, a feeling of burning in the fingers, and a tendency to drop things.

Causes: Repetitive actions that keep the wrists flexed up or down; sleeping in this position; wrist injury; diseases that cause swelling such as arthritis, diabetes, hypothyroidism, or alcoholism; tumors; and compression of the C6 nerve root due to malalignment of the neck or muscular spasm. Especially at risk are data processors, cashiers, assembly line workers, knitters and needleworkers, and those who drive for hours at a time. It affects one out of every ten Americans who work on computer terminals. Vitamin B_6 deficiencies (often caused by poor diet, various drugs, food colorings, and environmental pollutants) can cause CTS.

Uniquely Female: Women are twice as likely as men to suffer carpal tunnel syndrome, with an average age of onset between forty and sixty. Women's bones in this area are smaller, making the tunnel more prone to compression. Glandular imbalance in pregnancy or menopause can make women more prone to CTS; birth control pills can create vitamin B_6 deficiency, which has been linked to CTS. Also, fluid fluctuation during the middle and end of the menstrual cycle can cause pressure on this nerve. In this case, treating the premenstrual syndrome fluid problems may help the CTS. Fluid retention from food allergies or nutrient imbalances can also play a role and seems to affect women more than men. Certain thyroid medication contains a green dye that may compete with the activity of vitamin B_6, and women tak-

---

SELF-TEST FOR CTS

Hold out your right hand and tap the middle of your wrist (where it joins your hand) with your left index finger. If you get a tingling sensation or shooting pain down your fingers, you probably have carpal tunnel problems.

---

ing this medication may be more prone to CTS. They should ask their doctors about switching to medication that is free of colorings.

What to Do

- Do gentle exercises while working. Lift your hands off the keyboard and up into the air, rotating your arms and wrists. Move your hands around in circles for two minutes. Rotate your head for a few minutes, then turn your neck to look first over one shoulder then the other. Do these exercises at least four times a day.
- Yoga arm postures, such as putting the hands together in "namasté" prayer/greeting position, for several minutes twice a day, may help prevent and heal CTS.
- Get up from the computer at least once every hour and stretch.
- Gently squeezing the fingers can relieve the tingling feeling. Gently pull the fingers and the wrist and push apart your arm bones.
- Cold packs bring swelling down.
- Get physical therapy or evaluation of the joints above and below the wrist, including your shoulder and neck.
- Tingling and pain at night may be helped by a splint that keeps your wrist straight.
- Check thyroid function and medication. Low thyroid and certain medications can cause carpal tunnel symptoms.
- Ultrasound treatments have been reported to be as effective as surgery, so try this gentler program first. Find a chiropractor or physical therapist familiar with these protocols.

Avoid: Foods that deplete the body's level of vitamin B_6, such as excessive consumption of sugars, monosodium glutamate (MSG), and caffeine; processed grains and corn; yellow food dyes. Hard liquor and soft drinks bind magnesium; vitamin B_6 requires adequate levels of magnesium. Food allergies can cause swelling, which can affect pressure on this nerve. Identify and avoid.

Nutrients
** Vitamin B_6, 50–100 mg per day, helps many women after twelve weeks, though some women may need to go to 200 mg per day or use pyridoxal-5'-phosphate (predigested form), 50 mg twice a day.

** B complex, 100 mg per day, and 50 mg of riboflavin

• Proteolytic enzymes, 1,000 mg one to three times a day between meals on an empty stomach for two to three weeks

CELIAC DISEASE

A permanent intolerance to gluten (found in wheat, rye, and barley, and sometimes oats) that results in inflammation and damage to the intestinal tract. Overt celiac disease usually manifests itself with multiple digestive problems. However, hidden forms of celiac disease are being linked to an ever-widening array of medical conditions, from dental problems and bone disease to many autoimmune diseases like juvenile diabetes, thyroid disease, Sjögren's syndrome (dry eyes and mouth, and intestinal problems), as well as short stature, milk-sugar intolerance, infertility, recurrent pancreatitis, nonspecific abdominal pain, and cancer of the small intestine. It is one of the most common causes of overt or hidden malnutrition in young girls, affecting 1 out of 250 children, who have less lean muscle, poor growth, and abnormally low fat mass. Hidden celiac symptoms may occur outside the intestinal tract, in the form of various skin problems like chronic dermatitis. Anyone suffering from any chronic condition should be tested to determine if overt or hidden celiac disease is present. Avoidance of foods containing gluten often markedly improves these conditions and lowers the levels of substances that can attack various organs (autoantibodies). See page 493.

CERVICAL PROBLEMS (Benign)

The cervix is the lower part of the uterus, a hollow canal covered with layers of cells that projects into the vagina. The cells that line the canal secrete mucus, which prevents bacteria in the vagina from entering the uterus. The mucus becomes clear and elastic during ovulation so that sperm can swim through it, allowing fertilization.

Cervical Erosion

A condition in which the lining of the uterus spreads to cover the tip of the cervix, making it more likely to become inflamed or infected. Despite the name, there is no loss of tissue. May have increased mucus discharge from the vagina or unexplained vaginal bleeding. Risk increases with stress, repeated vaginal infections, and obesity. The cervix is especially vulnerable to erosion under the influence of estrogen at puberty and during pregnancy.

What to Do
- Don't douche.
- Treat any vaginal infection.
- Use pads instead of tampons.
- Take 5 mg per day of folic acid orally for two to three months, then reduce to 1–2 mg per day for several more months (this is especially helpful). Work with doctor.
- Squeeze a vitamin A capsule onto your finger and reach up inside as close as possible to dab on your cervix, once a day for a week.

Cervical Incompetence

In some women, the cervix is abnormally weak during pregnancy and stretches from the pressure of the fetus, usually leading to miscarriage. About one fifth of women who have had two or more miscarriages after the fourteenth week of pregnancy have cervical incompetence. When it is known that a woman has an incompetent cervix (from two or more miscarriages), the cervix can be stitched (in a procedure called *cervical cerclage*) to prevent labor from starting until the proper time.

Cervical Polyps

These small, bulbous growths on stalks protrude through the cervix from the lining inside the uterus. May be single or numerous. Usually benign, but rarely may represent early cancer of the cervix. More common in women who have not had children.

Symptoms: Spotting between periods or after intercourse or bowel movements; bleeding after menopause. Heavy, watery, bloody vaginal discharge.

Causes: Cervical inflammation from infection, erosion, or ulceration. Can accompany chronic infection in the vagina or cervix. Risk increases with diabetes or recurring vaginitis or cervicitis.

What to Do
- Wear cotton underwear.
- Use condoms to avoid sexually transmitted diseases (STDs).
- Don't douche, unless prescribed.
- Eat a high-fiber diet with no animal fats.
- Avoid fried and processed foods, caffeine, cigarettes, and alcohol.
- Reduce whole-milk products and consume skim milk.

Nutrients
- ** Vitamin D, 800 IU per day (ask your doctor if you have a history of kidney stones or calcification problems)
- ** Take 5 mg per day of folic acid for two months, then reduce to 1–2 mg per day for several months. Work with doctor.
- ** Indole-3-carbinol, 200–400 mg per day in divided doses, or DIM (diindolylmethane), 60 mg per day (two capsules twice a day), may *theoretically* help. See *Nutrition and Healing*, a newsletter written by Dr. Jonathan V. Wright, 410-223-2661.

- Calcium, 800–1,000 mg per day
- Vitamin A, 25,000 IU per day
- Vitamin C, 3,000 mg per day in divided doses

Cervicitis

Inflammation or infection of the cervix. Both acute and chronic cervicitis are contagious. It is the most frequent cause of bleeding after intercourse. Untreated, it may cause *endometritis* (infection of the lining of the uterus) or *salpingitis* (infection of the fallopian tubes). May infect a baby's eyes during delivery, resulting in blindness if not treated at the time of birth. Risk increases with multiple sexual partners or diabetes.

Symptoms: Chronic cervicitis may produce a slight vaginal discharge, bleeding from the vagina after sexual intercourse or between periods, and pain low in the abdomen felt during intercourse. Other symptoms include itching, a burning feeling upon urination, or belly or lower back pain. Acute cervicitis is often symptomless, or there may be a thick, yellow vaginal discharge (possibly with a bad smell).

Causes: Usually due to a vaginal infection or a sexually transmitted disease (chlamydia or gonorrhea). An IUD (intrauterine device), a forgotten tampon, or the chemicals in douches are sometimes at fault. May also follow injury to the cervix during childbirth or an operation on the uterus. Chronic cervicitis is caused by repeated episodes of acute cervicitis or a case that does not heal properly.

What to Do
- Wear cotton underwear.
- If you take antibiotics, eat yogurt or take acidophilus.
- Inform your sexual partner(s).
- Avoid sexual intercourse until healed.
- Use pads instead of tampons.
- Don't use commercial douches. A douche containing providone-iodine, used nightly for one week, will often clear up mild cervicitis.
- Use a barrier contraceptive.

Dysplasia (Cervical Intraepithelial Neoplasia, CIN)

A precancerous condition in the cervix, featuring cells that are abnormal in size, shape, and/or rate of multiplication. Can be mild, moderate, or severe. It is a sexually transmitted disease that is 100 percent treatable in early stages, but severe CIN can progress to cervical cancer.

<u>Symptoms:</u> Slow-growing and usually symptomless.

<u>Causes:</u> Exposure to human papilloma virus (HPV, the virus that produces condyloma) causes virtually all cases, although many women with HPV never get dysplasia. Risk factors include first intercourse before age eighteen, multiple sexual partners, giving birth before age twenty-two, smoking, possibly oral contraceptive use, and in utero exposure to DES (diethylstilbestrol). Elevated levels of homocysteine are associated with more severe dysplasia.

What to Do
- Use condoms to prevent contact with HPV.
- Don't smoke.
- If using oral contraceptives, take folic acid and B vitamins.
- Ask your doctor about capsaicin cream (0.075 percent) applied topically.

<u>Diet:</u> Add foods high in folic acid, such as lima beans, whole wheat, and brewer's yeast. Eat salmon and other cold-water fish and cruciferous veggies.

<u>Avoid:</u> Sugary junk foods. Reduce animal fats, caffeine, alcohol, and processed foods. Limit red meat consumption. Limit soy protein to 10 mg per day.

Nutrients
- ** Indole-3-carbinol, 200–400 mg per day in divided doses, or DIM (diindolylmethane), 60 mg per day (2 capsules twice a day) until you have a normal Pap smear (try for three to four months). Dr. Maria Bell demonstrated in a pilot study statistically significant evidence of regression of abnormal cervical

cells within twelve weeks after administering indole-3-carbinol (*Gynecologic Oncology* 78:123–9, 2000).

** Folic acid, 10 mg per day for three months. Ten milligrams of folic acid have improved the abnormal Pap smears only of women taking birth control pills. Work with doctor.

** Vitamin C, 1,000 mg two to three times a day.

• Vitamin A, 20,000–25,000 IU for two months; then reduce to 5,000 IU a day for maintenance. Or you can use vitamin A suppositories for six nights, alternating with herbal vaginal suppositories for six nights (work with a naturopathic or nutritionally oriented doctor).

• Vitamin E, 400 IU per day.

• Coenzyme Q 10, 20–60 mg once per day.

• Multivitamin/mineral supplement daily

Herbs: Myrrh, echinacea, and goldenseal.

Nabothian Cysts

Small cysts found under the surface of the cervix. They are harmless and can be left untreated. If bothersome, the cyst can be punctured by a doctor with a hot cautery needle.

CHOCOLATE

What is chocolate doing in this book? Most women love chocolate. Even though some people are allergic to it, or should avoid the caffeine-like substances in it (at least in excess), I thought you should know about the good personality traits of chocolate.

It appears as though high-quality chocolate and cocoa have powerful antioxidant action. And chocolate and cocoa powder contain three unsaturated N-acylethanolamines, which can act like *cannabinoid* (yes, that's correct—marijuana-like) substances in our brain. So chocolate does make us feel good and may be good for the free radicals that plague us. And rejoice! The fat in chocolate is especially high in stearic acid, which means it does not raise cholesterol levels. The moral of this story: Don't deny yourself the pleasure of chocolate, but be moderate. Deprivation increases desire, so buy a chocolate bar once in a while, take a few bites, and give the rest away, or try alternatives like nibbling on date or fruit-juice-sweetened chocolates. This is "satisfied moderation" in action.

Unfortunately, if you have osteoporosis, you need to avoid eating excessive chocolate as it binds up calcium. And much of non-organic chocolate may be laced with lindane, from pesticides on the bean. So buy organic chocolate and use it as a once-in-a-while treat.

CHOLESTEROL

Dietary cholesterol is what's contained in food, mostly in animal products. *Serum cholesterol* is a fat-related substance in your bloodstream; it's the cholesterol that's tested by your doctor and is divided (simplistically) into two parts—the "good" HDL (high-density lipoprotein) cholesterol, which seems to protect against arterial disease, and the "bad" LDL (low-density lipoprotein), which is the artery-clogging fat that increases your risk of developing arteriosclerosis (hardening of the arteries), which can lead to coronary heart disease or stroke. High cholesterol is also implicated in gallstones, mental impairment, and high blood pressure.

A "safe" level of cholesterol is considered to be a total count of less than 200 mg/dL (milligrams per deciliter), with those over 240 at high risk (although those with very low cholesterol [under 160] are more at risk of depression and/or suicide). A person with a total cholesterol level of 260 mg/dL increases the chance of heart attack by 500 percent. The normal adult HDL level for women is 50–60, with under 35 being considered risky. The average amount of HDL in women is approximately 10 percent higher than in men, since estrogen promotes HDL production. However, you can run a "high" total cholesterol that is actually above normal because your HDLs are high, which is good. Doctors must look at all the fractions of cholesterol and their ratios in your blood test to understand your total lipid picture.

Cholesterol is not evil. In fact, it is an essential part of all cell walls and important for nerve function and digestion. It becomes harmful when it is oxidized (as in nondairy creamers and powdered eggs). Cholesterol is the precursor in the body's production of sex and steroid hormones (cortisol, DHEA [dehydroepiandrosterone], estrogen, testosterone, and progesterone). And cholesterol is not the only indicator of heart disease risk. You can have low cholesterol and still get plaque in your arteries.

Symptoms: There are no real symptoms, but the following can be results of high cholesterol: plaque formation on artery walls, poor circulation, leg cramps and pain, high blood pressure, difficulty breathing, cold hands and feet, dry skin and hair, palpitations, allergies, and kidney problems.

Causes: About 70–80 percent of total body cholesterol is manufactured in the liver, while 20–30 percent is from food sources. So your cholesterol is not just from what you eat, but mostly from how quickly your body makes and eliminates the "bad" cholesterol. A healthy liver is a prime player in performing these actions.

Uniquely Female: Before menopause, women usually have higher HDLs and lower risk of heart disease as estrogen helps their body to make more HDLs and is thus cardioprotective. After menopause, women can get lower levels of HDLs and higher LDLs, putting them at more risk. After age fifty, women often have higher levels of cholesterol than men. Some studies suggest that women may not respond as much or as fast as men to decreasing saturated fat in the diet, but it's still worth the effort. See *Fats and Essential Fatty Acids. Eating more of the better fats is better than just reducing overall fat intake.*

The situation is more serious if your total count is above 250, with an LDL greater than 160 and/or an HDL below 40, and you suffer from angina, have had a heart attack, or there is a family history of premature heart disease. Women are more prone to hypothyroidism and subclinical hypothyroidism, both of which are linked to high cholesterol (*Clinical Endocrinology* 50:217–20, 1999).

What to Do

- Have your cholesterol monitored regularly so you know if your program is working.
- Lose excess weight. Every 2.2-pound increase in body weight elevates cholesterol levels by two points.

- Doctor should rule out or treat low thyroid.
- Have your DHEA tested, as low levels of this hormone may contribute to low levels of good cholesterol (HDL) and vice versa.
- Take a daily walk or engage in other aerobic exercise.
- Don't smoke. Nicotine raises cholesterol levels.
- Learn stress-reduction techniques, meditate, visualize. See pages 52–58.
- Check for food allergies.
- Lowering cholesterol is only one way to prevent hardening of the arteries. Other risk factors such as high blood pressure, elevated homocysteine levels, inadequate magnesium levels, inflammatory blood markers, smoking, obesity, and physical inactivity require as much attention.
- Aerobic activity and moderate alcohol consumption can slightly elevate HDLs but do not lower LDLs. Excessive drinking is a risk factor for numerous health problems, so doctors don't like to recommend alcoholic beverages, but one glass of red wine a day does reduce the risk of heart attack, if you can keep it to only one.
- Cholesterol may be less of a heart disease risk in women than in men. Specific tests of arteries suggest women suffer more from spasms of arteries than clots, perhaps due more to magnesium deficiency than to cholesterol. Try magnesium therapy first before going to cholesterol-lowering drugs, as these can cause problems themselves.

Diet: Essential fatty acids (fish, olive, flaxseed, nuts, and seeds) are very important in lowering cholesterol. Part of the problem with bad cholesterol (LDL) is caused when oxygen acts on it. Studies show that olive, fish, and hazelnut oils in particular prevent this. Liberal use of olive and fish oils is more effective than a low-fat high-carbohydrate diet in lowering triglycerides. See *Fats and Essential Fatty Acids.* Chicken, turkey, and fish contain about the same amount of cholesterol as lean red meats like beef, lamb, and pork. However, diets emphasizing fish and chicken appear to lower cholesterol better than diets allowing lean red meat. And diets that lean toward vegetarianism lower cholesterol more than any other. Emphasize soy products. A lower-fat vegetarian-based diet can reduce the need for cholesterol-lowering drugs and cardiac surgery in some patients (*Archives of Internal Medicine* 160:395, 2000).

Plant foods—nuts, seeds, vegetables, fruits, vegetable oils, olives, cereals, and grains—do not contain any cholesterol. Foods shown in studies to be especially helpful for lowering cholesterol are walnuts, pecans, hazelnuts, pistachios, brown or Chinese red rice (which is delicious, cooks like regular rice, and has been shown to significantly lower cholesterol), and olive and rice bran oils (though you must still lower *overall* fat in the diet).

Fiber lowers total and LDL cholesterol, especially oat bran and whole-oat groats and steel-cut rolled oats (precooked oatmeal may have some benefit), when combined with eating less total fat and improving the quality of fats. And consuming smaller meals, especially later in the day, along with high-fiber foods, reduces cholesterol. Drink Fiber Cocktails (page 464) or fiber drinks made from flaxseed or psyllium, guar gum, pectin (apples and grapefruits), soy fiber, legume fiber, and oat bran. Eat more beans than potatoes.

Other helpful foods are soy protein (try taking 2 heaping tsp. or 5–6 g every day), or snack on 1–2 Tbsp. roasted soy nuts, whole grains and whole-grain pasta, garlic, and green and black teas.

Studies on eggs and cholesterol are criticized for not taking into account confounding variables. One egg a day or two several times a week seems not to have an adverse effect on cholesterol if you are consuming a balanced diet generous with good fats.

Note for those with Syndrome X: Some people have higher levels of cholesterol because of insulin resistance. This means that by consuming carbohydrates with a high glycemic index (foods that are quickly converted to glucose), their bodies respond with elevating levels of cholesterol. If you are at risk of Syndrome X (page 300), reduce your natural and refined simple sugars, don't just concentrate on lowering fats.

Avoid: Major factors are hydrogenated and saturated fats and *overeating*. Foods highest in cholesterol are meat, poultry, seafood, dairy products, egg yolks, and organ meats. Egg yolks are more of a problem if they are broken when they are cooked, such as in scrambled eggs. This oxidizes the cholesterol they contain. Identify and avoid foods that trigger allergies. Reduce sugar, refined carbohydrates (eating fewer carbs can raise HDLs), processed lunch meats and sausage, and milk and dairy products (except for a limited amount of low- or nonfat ones). Nondairy creamers contain coconut oil, a highly saturated fat; use soy, rice, or almond milk. Avoid fast foods, many of which are fried in beef tallow, a fat that becomes poisonous in the deep-frying process. Margarine and partially hydrogenated vegetable oils also produce deadly fats when heated.

Drinking boiled or French-press coffee increases cholesterol levels. Using a paper filter traps the chemicals that elevate cholesterol, although it still can affect homocysteine. No one knows about decaffeinated coffee. High coffee intake (five to eight cups per day) may elevate cholesterol.

Nutrients

- ** Pantethine, 300 mg three to four times a day reduces total cholesterol, LDL, triglycerides and elevates HDL.
- ** Chromium, 200–500 mcg twice a day
- ** Niacin, 100 mg per day (women taking higher levels— 1,000–3,000 mg per day—should work with their doctor and get regular blood tests. Niacin at therapeutic dosages for lowering cholesterol can cause side effects like flushing and liver toxicity)
- ** Red Yeast Rice, 1,200 mg twice a day, starts to lower total and LDL cholesterol in eight weeks.
- ** Gugulipids, 140–500 mg daily
- ** Tocotrienols—often added to various formulas or vitamin E, several hundred IU per day
- ** Fish oil concentrate, 5–10 g per day
- ** Calcium, 800–1,200 mg per day

You can purchase, at most health food stores or through some holistic physicians, one inclusive formula that contains most of the items mentioned above. An excellent example is Guggul Plus by Naturopathic Formulas (1 capsule, three times per day). A multicholesterol-lowering formula like this, along with some fiber source emphasizing pectin (twice a day between meals), keeps your supplements down to a manageable level. The health food companies say that Red Yeast Rice does not aggravate candida complex problems, but there are formulas that do not contain this source if you want to avoid it. Some holistic practitioners recommend taking milk thistle several times a day while on Red Yeast Rice products, and others don't. The following list presents some other helpful items.

- Inositol hexanicotinate, 500–600 mg two to three times a day, is not as effective as niacin but does not cause flushing or liver toxicity.
- Friendly bacteria like *L. acidophilus* have been shown to lower LDL cholesterol. Consume live-culture products regularly.
- Magnesium, 300–500 mg per day
- Lecithin, 2 capsules (19 grains) three times a day
- Vitamin C, 1,000 mg three times a day
- Vitamin E, 400–800 IU, may raise HDL in younger folks with lower levels.
- Antioxidants daily to prevent oxidation of LDL
- If you have elevated platelets, add L-arginine. Foods high in it include roasted soybeans, light turkey and chicken meat, pumpkin seeds, salmon, chickpeas, tofu, hummus, and black beans. L-arginine supplements, 1,000 mg, should be taken once or twice a day on an empty stomach.

Herbs: Hawthorn/passionflower extract, 80–300 mg, two to three times a day; turmeric, 900–1,800 mg per day in divided doses. In one study Guggul lowered cholesterol more than the drug clofibrate and raised HDLs.

CHRONIC FATIGUE SYNDROME (CFS)

A serious and complex chronic illness characterized by unexplained persistent and debilitating fatigue that leads to a major reduction in activities for at least six months. CFS can last for many years. Most people respond to natural therapies and lifestyle changes in three to six months, and some are recovered after two years.

Symptoms: Symptoms may come and go. There are a host of possible symptoms, ranging from cognitive (impairment in short-term memory or concentration) and psychological problems to menstrual problems, including premenstrual syndrome and endometriosis, and weight changes without changes in diet. Others include blurred vision, nausea, anxiety, insomnia, mood swings, and noise intolerance. Various flu-like symptoms such as sore throat, tender lymph nodes, muscle and joint pain, low-grade fever, and headaches can occur.

Causes: CFS is a perplexing disorder that probably has many different causes. Chronic low-level chemical exposures have been directly linked to CFS as well as viral infections (including the polio virus). CFS has been associated with adrenal and thyroid deficiencies, food allergies, chemical sensitivities, parasites, intestinal yeast infections, and malabsorption. Hypoglycemia is often linked to CFS. Factors that contribute to the disease include the breakdown of the nervous and immune system from physical and emotional stress, heavy metals, smoking, heavy use of antibiotics or corticosteroid drugs, or a history of mononucleosis. Onset can be sudden or take the form of a steady decline. Some tests show certain sufferers have much smaller adrenal glands. One new surgical technique suggests that brain stem problems may cause some cases of CFS.

Uniquely Female: CFS affects more than three times as many women as men, usually women between the ages of twenty-five and fifty, who are active, independent overachievers. Among white women in this age group, it is more prevalent than lung cancer, breast cancer, and high blood pressure. Women with gynecological problems, such as irregular menstrual cycles, may be at higher risk. Some pregnant women report symptom remission from early in the pregnancy lasting until about six weeks after delivery. There is currently no evidence that babies born to parents with CFS are different from other babies.

What to Do

- Identify and avoid heavy-metal exposures, such as dental amalgams, dust from clay and pottery making, jewelry making, and nickel in jewelry and eyeglass frames.
- Decrease stress (pages 52–58).

- Avoid tobacco smoke, which contains dozens of toxic chemicals.
- Identify and avoid toxic chemical exposures, such as fumes from new carpeting, and mold exposure.
- Rule out *Candida albicans* yeast infections, mononucleosis, hepatitis, herpes virus, Epstein-Barr virus, and cytomegalovirus. Treat any chronic bacterial or fungal infections. Test for parasites.
- Identify and work with food allergies.
- Assess digestion and absorption to see if digestive aids are needed.
- Hormone therapy with cortisol (hydrocortisone, 1 mg three times a day), DHEA (dehydroepiandrosterone), and/or thyroid helps in some cases, as does amino acid therapy.
- Aerobic exercise. Begin with as little as three to five minutes of moderate exercise a day. T'ai chi ch'uan, light stretching, or short twenty-minute walks are noticeably effective when done every day.
- Acupuncture and massage may be helpful.
- Have your DHEA level tested and supplement if necessary with DHEA or licorice root.
- Have an MRI or CAT scan taken to judge adrenal size. If they are 50 percent or less of normal size, consider supplementation with multiple adrenal hormones and glandulars.
- Ask about allergy testing and desensitization toward your own hormones.
- See *Immune Enhancement*.
- If both adrenal and thyroid hormones are low and only the thyroid is treated, this can precipitate a health crisis. You must treat both.

Diet: Eat generously of fresh and some raw vegetables and fruits. Foods that build immunity include cruciferous vegetables, onions and garlic, wheat germ, sea vegetables, brown and red rice, prunes and bran, yogurt and miso, seafood, and whole grains. Some people respond well to high-protein diets that include meat, preferably organically grown.

Avoid: All processed foods, junk foods, refined flours, food additives, and fried foods. Limit sugary foods (including juices), white flour products, caffeine, soft drinks, alcohol, dairy, gluten, and chemical additives.

Nutrients

- ** Alpha-lipoic acid, 250 mg twice a day or more (take backup biotin, 2.5 mg per day)
- ** Intravenous (IV) Myer's Cocktail (page 471) relieves symptoms in 50 percent of cases according to Dr. Alan Gaby. Magnesium sulfate injections, 1 g once a week for six weeks and then as needed, may be substituted.
- ** Free-form amino acids, 7–15 g per day twice a day on an empty stomach (some labs run levels of amino acids and then customize a formula)
- ** Proteolytic enzymes, 1,000–1,500 mg between meals on an empty stomach for several weeks
- ** Pantothenic acid, 1,000 mg two to four times a day
- ** Vitamin B complex, 100 mg three times a day, with extra vitamin B_6
- ** Multivitamin/mineral supplement (high potency)
- ** Evaluate your need for digestive enzymes and/or bowel detoxification (page 468).
- ** Vitamin C or ester-C crystals with bioflavonoids, ¼ tsp. every half hour for ten days, then reduce to 3–5 g per day in divided doses. If you get gas or loose stools, lower the amount and dosage.
- • Acetyl-L-carnitine, 1,000 mg in the morning on an empty stomach (build up to two or three times a day) for several months
- • Adrenal glandulars, 2–5 tablets two to three times a day
- • Have your DHEA level tested.
- • Ask your doctor about injections of vitamin B_{12}, and ask about hydrocortisone. See *Adrenal Insufficiency and Adrenal Fatigue.*

Herbs: Licorice tincture, 6 drops twice a day for four to six weeks in place of hydrocortisone. Milk thistle, 420 mg per day for eight to twelve weeks; reduce with improvement to 280 mg per day for several more weeks. Olive leaf extract, 500 mg twice a day.

CIRCULATION

The heart and blood vessels (called the *cardiovascular system*) are responsible for the continuous flow of blood through the body, with *arteries* carrying blood away from the heart and the *veins* leading back to the heart. They provide all the tissues with a regular supply of oxygen and nutrients and carry away carbon dioxide and other waste products.

Symptoms: Many women frequently complain of having cold extremities, being cold, and not tolerating cold well. A healthy person should *not* have chronically cold feet and hands.

Causes: Low levels of nutrients secondary to poor diet or poor digestion (pages 208, 468), low thyroid function, food allergies, or dysbiosis (imbalance in intestinal bacteria) due to a variety of causes. Often, improving digestion and nutrient status improves circulation.

What to Do

For all circulatory conditions:
- Chiropractic manipulation and/or massage
- Increase exercise, although even those who regularly exercise, if they are not in nutritional balance, will experience chronically cold extremities, often called *cold intolerance.*

Diet: Eat foods with high mineral content such as leafy greens, veggies, nuts, and seeds, as well as foods high in bioflavonoids, such as various berries.

Avoid: Tobacco and secondhand smoke as well as fried and fatty foods, refined foods, and sugar.

Nutrients
- ** Magnesium, 250–400 mg, and B complex, 50 mg per day
- ** L-arginine, 1,000 mg two times a day, on an empty stomach

Herbs: Cayenne/ginger capsules, 2–8 per day, can be very helpful; or try butcher's broom, 1,000 mg three times a day for two to four weeks.

CLAUDICATION

Refers to blockage of blood flow in the legs because of arterial obstruction. As a result, the muscles don't get enough blood (a condition called *ischemia*). Lack of oxygen and buildup of waste products cause the muscles in the calf (and sometimes in the thigh, foot, hip, or buttocks) to become painful and tired.

Symptoms: Fatigue, pain, ache, or cramping during exercise, even after walking just a short distance and especially after walking fast or uphill. Eventually, the muscles may ache even when at rest. There also may be problems with cold and numb feet; dry and scaly skin over the lower extremities; and nails and hair may not grow well.

What to Do
- Stop smoking. This is essential.
- Walk, at least thirty to sixty minutes every day on a level surface. Leg pain from exertion is *not* dangerous.
- Take care of your legs and feet. Clean any break in the skin before it can get infected.
- Elevating the head of the bed four to six inches may help increase blood flow to the legs.
- Avoid extremes in temperature.
- Lose excess weight and lower cholesterol if it's high.
- Rule out heart disease and spinal stenosis.

Diet: Consume generous amounts of extra-virgin olive oil, nuts (especially walnuts and pistachios), seeds, and whole-grain and sprouted-grain products. See the recommended diet for heart disease, page 264.

Avoid: Sugars, refined carbohydrates, refined oils, alcohol, saturated fats, and high-cholesterol foods.

Nutrients
- ** L-carnitine, 1–4 g per day in divided doses
- ** Padma 28 (call PADMA AG at 877-877-2362), 760 mg twice a day for sixteen weeks. This is extremely effective.
- ** Folic acid, 5 mg per day. Work with doctor.
- ** Vitamin B complex, 50 mg per day
- ** Magnesium, 300–600 mg per day
- • Ginkgo biloba, 40 mg three times a day, is at least as effective as pentoxifylline, a conventional treatment.
- • Vitamin E, 400 IU two to four times a day
- • Zinc picolinate or citrate, 30 mg twice a day (balance with 2–4 mg copper); reduce zinc to 15–20 mg per day when symptoms improve.
- • Inositol hexanicotinate in high dosages—1–2 g twice a day. Does not cause flushing, but still needs to be monitored with periodic blood tests.

CONTRACEPTION
(Birth Control, Family Planning)

The control of fertility to prevent pregnancy. Women's rights to access birth control did not become legal until a Supreme Court decision in 1966 (Griswald *v.* Connecticut). Still, more than 50 percent of American pregnancies today are unintended (Brown and Eisenberg, eds., *The Best Intentions: Unintended Pregnancy and the Well-Being of Children and Families,* National Institute of Medicine, Washington, D.C., 1995). Selecting a method of birth control involves three questions: How effective is it? How safe is it for you? How acceptable is it to you?

Methods of Contraception
- • *Abstinence (natural family planning)*—Avoiding intercourse during the fertile part of the menstrual cycle either through the calendar rhythm method, temperature or mucus method, or symptothermal method (observing cervical mucus, basal

body temperature, and other symptoms, which is the most reliable abstinence approach). To be truly effective, this method requires no intercourse for more than half the cycle. Even though an unfertilized egg can live only twenty-four hours, fertilization can result from intercourse that takes place up to four days before the release of the egg. Not suitable for women who have *irregular* cycles.

- *Coitus interruptus*—Withdrawal before ejaculation; has a high failure rate.
- *Barrier methods*—Male or female condoms, diaphragm, cervical cap
- *Spermicides*—Vaginal foams, creams, gels, and suppositories
- *Hormonal methods*—Injectable progestogens, implants, the Pill. See the sections on hormone replacement therapy (page 272) and the Pill (page 361) for a full discussion.
- *Day-after pill*—A drug taken after the fact and used only in emergencies.
- *IUDs* (intrauterine devices)—Unlike older versions, today's IUDs are simple and cheap. Not good for women who tend to cramp during their periods.
- *Sterilization*—The fallopian tubes are sealed or cut to prevent the male sperm from reaching the egg. This is the most common method of fertility control, used by about 20 percent of couples and almost 50 percent of married couples.

Risks: Certain medications can interfere with the action of birth control pills and result in unwanted pregnancies. If you are taking barbiturates, carbamazepine, phenytoin, rifabutin, rifampin, or antibiotics, use additional contraceptive measures during this time.

Risk of stroke: Combined oral contraceptives, even with low-dose estrogen, along with progestins, especially desogestrel or gestrodene, have been associated with higher risk of stroke than oral contraceptives with levonorgestrel or noncombined ones. Although current users of combined oral contraceptives (estrogen and progestin) have a low risk of blood clots, the risk is still three to six times *higher* than for women who are not taking birth control pills. The risk is highest in the first year, less afterward, but persists until quitting, when the risk drops speedily to that of nonusers. There is little risk of blood clots for women on combined oral contraceptives containing less than 50 mcg of ethinylestradiol. The risk of blood clots from using oral contraceptives rises with increasing age, obesity, recent surgery, and some forms of thrombophilia. If you are at high risk for stroke, are over thirty-three, are a current smoker, have a history of pregnancy-related high blood pressure, or have had several children, you may be at risk for complications. Talk with your doctor. Consider running blood tests mentioned under coronary heart disease testing (p. 262), such as homocysteine, C-reactive protein, and lipid profiles, or go off the pill.

Oral contraceptives after miscarriage, abortion, and pregnancy: After a miscarriage or abortion occurring under twelve weeks, birth control pills can be taken immediately. Since pregnancy and oral contraceptives both increase the risk of stroke, women with pregnancies terminated between twelve and twenty-eight weeks should wait one week before starting birth control pills. Women who deliver after twenty-eight weeks and aren't breast-feeding should wait at least two weeks.

Combination contraceptives should *not* be used when breast-feeding, as the estrogen reduces milk production as well as levels of protein and fat in the milk.

- *Important!* Take B vitamins (25–50 mg per day) while on birth control pills, and even six months after. Oral contraceptives are notorious for making women deficient in B vitamins, especially folic acid. Folic acid is necessary during the first several weeks of conception (when most women have no clue that they have become pregnant) to avoid birth defects, such as neural tube defects. If you are on the pill, become deficient in folic acid, and get pregnant, your baby is at risk. Women on the pill who get depression might have low levels of tyrosine, and they may need to take extra tyrosine, plus vitamin B.

COUGH

Women who start taking any kind of hormones, including oral contraceptives, and suddenly develop a cough and chest pain may have clots in their lungs. This is a medical emergency! Older women with enlarged hearts or heart disease may have coughing and shortness of breath at night and after exertion from fluid buildup in the lungs. Coughs that worsen cyclically with the menstrual cycle could be related to hormonal imbalances such as unopposed estrogen, progesterone deficiency, and conditions like endometriosis. Premenopausal women with histories of allergies, asthma, or reactive airway disease may find that their symptoms worsen on a cyclical basis linked to the menses, especially if they suffer with severe premenstrual syndrome. Chronic coughing can be an early sign of lung disease; a reaction to medication; caused by food, mold, or inhalant allergies, heartburn, chemical fumes; or sometimes occur benignly after extreme exertion. Women with chronic coughs may develop urinary stress incontinence (urine leakage). Do Kegels (see page 433).

D

DEPRESSION

Intense feelings of sadness, hopelessness, pessimism, and a general loss of interest in life that may also be accompanied by wandering, indecisive train of thought. If depression occurs without any apparent cause, deepens, and persists, it may be a symptom of a wide range of psychiatric illnesses. Many of these illnesses have a biochemical basis, often linked to underlying health disorders. See your doctor for a complete physical checkup. An episode of depression can last for six to nine months. In 20 percent of depressed people, symptoms are milder but last for years (called *dysthymic disorder*). Depression is more common as we age and is often misdiagnosed.

Sadness is a natural response to loss, defeat, disappointment, trauma, or catastrophe. Grief or bereavement are reactions to the death of a loved one, divorce, or romantic disappointment. These normal emotional states don't usually cause persistent depression except in people who are predisposed to mood disorders.

Symptoms: In *vegetative depression,* the person tends to withdraw, speaks little, stops eating, and sleeps little; in *agitated depression,* the person is very restless, with compulsive talking and anxiety. In both disorders, symptoms may vary with time of day. There may also be various body pains, such as headache or chest pain, without measurable evidence of disease. Other symptoms may include slowed-down thinking, speech, and general activity; a preoccupation with intense feelings of guilt and worthlessness; the inability to concentrate; being indecisive and withdrawn; feeling progressively helpless and hopeless; difficulty falling asleep and awakening repeatedly, or excessive sleeping; loss of sexual desire or pleasure in general; poor appetite (except for overeating and weight gain seen in mild depression). Thoughts of death and/or suicide are the most serious symptom.

Risk Factors: Being a woman; a family history of depression or mood disorders; drug or alcohol abuse; highly dependent, compulsive, or rigid perfectionist personality type; very low cholesterol levels, maldigestion, and/or nutrient deficiencies, especially vitamin B_{12}; and possibly exposure to hormone disruptors, allergens, or toxic chemicals. Seasonal depression and/or mood changes may be related to low thyroid and/or lack of sunlight.

Causes: Biochemical brain imbalance; hormonal imbalance (excess progesterone can cause depression and is becoming a common side effect in women using too much progesterone cream); side effects of numerous prescription medications; traumatic events; anniversary reactions; nutritional deficiencies (especially B vitamins and magnesium); chemical sensitivities; allergies; and underlying conditions such as diabetes, low thyroid, heart disease, and chronic infections.

Uniquely Female: Twice as many women as men are likely to experience depression, which affects one in five women at some time in their lives. Changes in hormone levels can create mood swings, especially right before menstruation, after childbirth (see the section on postpartum depression under *Pregnancy*), and at menopause. Feelings of depression and disorientation are common when hormone levels start to change in the mid-forties. A miscarriage or abortion, rape, menopause, or a hysterectomy may trigger depression, as can

---

WARNING SIGNS THAT SOMEONE
MAY BE AT RISK FOR SUICIDE

Withdrawal from family and friends; neglect of personal appearance; mention of wanting to end it all or being a burden to others; manic or irresponsible behavior; having a suicide plan; sudden cheerfulness after prolonged despondency.

the use of oral contraceptives, endometriosis, or abnormal or subclinical thyroid function. Depression can also be a side effect when quitting smoking; nicotine acts on the serotonin system. Women are likely to cry, become withdrawn, and gain or lose weight, whereas men are more likely to abuse drugs and alcohol, work excessively, and/or become violent to themselves or others.

What to Do

- Refer to the *Physicians' Desk Reference* or ask your pharmacist if any of your medications may cause depression as a side effect.
- Have your doctor check for hypoglycemia, allergies, thyroid disorders, heavy metals, and maldigestion. Ask your doctor about T_3—one thyroid hormone that is helpful for depression and boosts the effect of antidepressants.
- Understand that feeling "blue" is temporary; don't get depressed because you feel sad.
- Turn off the TV and get out of the house.
- Get regular strenuous exercise. It is extremely helpful.
- Maintain a daily routine.
- Join a women's counseling or support group.
- Talk to friends and relatives who are supportive. If you are lonely and can't find someone to talk with, consider getting a pet, visiting Internet chat rooms, adopting a person in a nursing home, or starting a women's group in your house.
- Avoid heavy coffee drinking. Consumption of more than eight cups of coffee a day is linked to a greatly increased risk of suicide.
- Learn to control stress with deep breathing, muscle relaxation, massage, and meditation (pages 52–58). Hypnotherapy, biofeedback, and acupuncture have good success with chronic depression.
- Take two hours of morning sun, which can help lift depression.
- Avoid alcohol and recreational drugs if you are taking an antidepressant. Also watch for interactions with nutrients and certain foods (see appendices I, J, and K).

- Have your DHEA (dehydroepiandrosterone) level tested and treat if low.
- Avoid chemical fumes.
- If you have had a major depressive episode, have your tryptophan level tested (blood and/or urine). A low level suggests that you are at risk for recurrence.
- Realize that certain pharmaceutical antidepressants can stimulate the growth of cancer cells. If you presently have or have had cancer, ask your doctor to check which antidepressants have been linked to cancer, and avoid these if possible.
- Major depression can cause insulin resistance, so watch your diet. See *Insulin Resistance.*

Diet: Neurotransmitters in the brain (dopamine, serotonin, and norepinephrine), which regulate mood and behavior, are affected by what we eat. Eat more complex carbohydrates than protein if you are nervous and need to relax; eat more protein than carbohydrates if you are tired and need to be more alert. Proteins with essential fatty acids, such as salmon and white fish, are good choices. Fish are high in DHA (docosahexaenoic acid), which has been shown to improve depression. Eat foods rich in calcium, magnesium, and B vitamins.

Avoid: Excess processed fat. Fats inhibit the production of neurotransmitters. Reduce sugars, refined foods, caffeine, tobacco, and alcohol. Excess sugar from simple carbohydrates, such as fruit juice, results in fatigue and depression. Avoid food allergens. If taking MAO (monoamine oxidase) inhibitor drugs, avoid alcohol, cheese, red meat, yeast extract, and broad beans, foods rich in the amino acid tyrosine.

Nutrients

Your doctor must monitor your drug and nutrient intake to avoid adverse interactions, such as taking St. John's wort with some antidepressant medications.

- ** Vitamin B complex, 25–50 mg one to three times a day (the first sign of low tissue levels of B vitamins are mood changes and fatigue), with extra folic acid

** Inositol—start with 1 g twice a day and build up to 5 g per day for two weeks. When you start to see results, lower the dose until you find the lowest dose that maintains the benefit.

** SAMe (S-adenosyl-methionine, page 496)—Many psychiatrists are starting their patients on SAMe because it does not have the adverse side effects of many pharmaceutical antidepressants, is available at stores everywhere without prescription, and works for many people within two to fourteen days (page 485).

** Run blood level of DHEA and treat if low.

** Tryptophan (made by compounding pharmacists). Take either 2 or 3 g per day one hour before bed on an empty stomach or 1.5 mg twice a day, although some get sleepy taking it in the morning. Use trial and error to see what's best for you. Try tryptophan when nothing else works, and use only reputable (and expensive!) brands. Do not take with selective serotonin-reuptake inhibitors (SSRIs). Do not take higher levels of tryptophan, and make sure you eat whole-protein foods like eggs or protein powder during the day.

• If you've been taking antidepressants and not getting a response, ask your doctor to add 2 g tryptophan to your regime.

• Niacinamide, 500 mg three times a day (don't take at this dose if you have a history of liver disease; if you do take it, you must be monitored by periodic blood tests)

• Folic acid, 1–2 mg, and vitamin B_6, 25–50 mg once a day. Folic acid (500 mcg per day) has been shown to make Prozac and other such drugs more effective, but *only* in women.

• High-potency multivitamin/mineral supplement

• Ask your doctor about injections of vitamin B_{12} and magnesium, or take magnesium, 250–400 mg twice a day, and sublingual B_{12}. In *older women*, B_{12} deficiency is linked to a twofold increase in severe depression.

• Fish oil, 3–8 g per day in some cases. Fish and olive oil have mood-stabilizing actions.

• Melatonin, 1–5 mg at bedtime, improves the disturbed sleep of depression.

- Evaluate your need for digestive enzymes (page 468).
- If none of the above help, consider DLPA (D, L-phenylala-nine), 1,000 mg in the morning on an empty stomach and 500 mg midafternoon on an empty stomach, or L-tyrosine, 1,000 mg in the morning on an empty stomach.

Herbs: St. John's wort standardized to contain 0.3 percent hyper-icin, 300–350 mg three times a day for *mild* to *moderate* depression. (Caution: Do not take with MAOs or selective serotonin-reuptake in-hibitors like Prozac and Zoloft; the two together may cause excessive elevations of serotonin levels and side effects.) St. John's wort con-tains hyperforin, a natural SSRI. Don't take if you have a history of manic disorders or high blood pressure. Ginkgo biloba often works for depression in senior citizens; take 60–80 mg of extract two to three times a day.

DES DAUGHTERS

Women whose mothers were given DES (diethylstilbestrol, the first synthetic estrogen and the most powerful hormone disruptor ever manufactured) while pregnant between 1938 and 1971 are especially prone to developing hormonally related conditions, such as those re-lated to estrogen dominance (see page 227). Up to 80 percent of DES daughters have benign changes of the cervix or vagina, and some may experience malformed uteri and infertility. There is a definite link between DES exposure in utero and one form of vaginal cancer as well as infertility. DES mothers have a higher-than-average rate of breast cancer. The possibility of DES daughters developing female cancers, precancers such as cervical dysplasia, and other problems linked to excessive estrogenic stimulation is high, and they should be monitored. Some DES daughters have increased risk of various im-mune disorders as well as recurrent upper respiratory infections.

If you are a DES daughter who has experienced a lifetime of prob-lems related to estrogen dominance, then you need to do a lot of re-search before taking any kind of synthetic hormones. However, DES daughters should be evaluated for progesterone deficiency and consider natural hormone therapy, as some can suffer effects from unopposed estrogen for decades of their lives.

It is recommended that DES daughters minimize their exposure to estrogen in birth control pills or estrogen rings (especially if they have a history of cervical dysplasia), postmenopausal estrogen therapies, or contraceptives used after intercourse. Annual checkups should include both a regular Pap smear and a Pap smear of the upper vagina, as well as an iodine stain of the vagina and cervix to identify abnormal areas and possible adenosis. If you are a DES daughter with breast cancer, there *may* be some questions about whether it's safe for you to take tamoxifen.

If you suspect you might be a DES daughter, send away for hospital records to see if you were exposed in utero. DES was manufactured under hundreds of different names (see the appendix in my book *Hormone Deception*, Contemporary/McGraw Hill, 2000). Some DES daughters with histories of several cancers, precancers, or unopposed estrogen disorders (such as fibroids, tubular and ovarian cysts, premenstrual syndrome, and endometriosis), should discuss with their doctors the use of yearly prophylactic intravaginal ultrasounds and CA-125 blood tests. See *Estrogen Dominance*. Join and contribute to DES ACTION, 800-DES-9288. DES-L is an online support group for DES daughters at *http://www.surrogacy.com/online_support/des/*.

DHEA (Dehydroepiandrosterone), see *Hormones*

DIABETES MELLITUS

To get energy from the starches and sugar we eat, we need insulin, a hormone produced by the pancreas. In diabetes, a person either does not make enough insulin or is unable to use the insulin he or she does produce. See *Insulin Resistance*. Without insulin, sugar builds up in the blood and can lead to a host of serious problems, such as damage to the heart, kidneys, eyes, blood vessels, and nerves. Diabetes is a stronger predictor of coronary disease in women than in men. Diabetes is the third leading cause of death in the United States.

Insulin-Dependent (Type 1) Diabetes

The more severe form, it first appears in people under the age of thirty-five and develops rapidly. People with type 1 diabetes usually require regular injections of insulin.

Symptoms: Irritability, frequent urination, abnormal thirst, nausea or vomiting, weakness, fatigue, and unusual hunger. May have weight loss even with increased eating.

Non-Insulin-Dependent (Type 2) Diabetes

A gradually developing chronic degenerative disease that occurs mainly in people over the age of forty (though it may have been developing insidiously for decades). More than 11 million Americans have adult-onset diabetes and many are undiagnosed. The pancreas continues to manufacture insulin, but the body develops resistance and fails to make use of it. A combination of diet and nutrition, weight control, exercise, and sometimes oral medication manages the condition. African Americans, Native Americans, and Hispanics have a two to three times higher risk of developing diabetes than the rest of the population. The disorder tends to run in families and is more common in those with Syndrome X (elevated total cholesterol, triglycerides, blood pressure; low HDL cholesterol; and overweight, especially around the abdomen). See *Insulin Resistance.*

Symptoms: Extreme hunger and unusual thirst, frequent urination, severe fatigue and weakness, weight loss, frequent infections, blurred vision, dry itching skin, obesity, slow healing, easy to bruise, ketotic breath, and tingling or numbness in the feet. Other signs include lingering flu-like symptoms, multiple skin tags (small bits of pedunculated skin at the armpits, neck, and torso), loss of hair on the legs, increased facial hair, small yellow bumps anywhere on the body. High levels of sugar in the blood and urine can also lead to urinary tract infections such as cystitis, vaginal and intestinal yeast infections (candidiasis), and recurrent skin infections. Chronic yeast infections may be the first sign of diabetes in women.

A SELF-TEST TO DETECT
YOUR ABILITY TO TASTE SWEETS

Often, type 2 diabetics are not able to perceive sweet tastes and thus consume more sugary foods. Most people will perceive a sweet taste with 1 tsp. or less of sugar mixed in a cup of water. Many with type 2 diabetes will not perceive sweetness until they have tasted 1½ to 2 tsp. sugar in the water.

- Don't take any caffeine or sweets for one hour before the test.
- Label seven identical glasses: one with no sugar and one each with ¼ tsp., ½ tsp., 1 tsp, 1½ tsp., 2 tsp., and 3 tsp. of sugar. Fill each glass with 8 oz. of water and add the labeled amount of sugar. Have someone hide the labels and mix up the glasses.

- Sip through a straw from each glass (rinsing your mouth out with water in between each taste test), and mark which amount of sugar you think is in each.

Causes: Type 1 is thought to be an autoimmune disease. Early formula feeding (before three months), early cow's milk introduction, and heavier weight between one and seven months in girl infants are associated with higher risk of type 1. There is controversy over the role of mumps vaccinations and milk consumption in early childhood linked to type 1. Type 2 may be due to diet, obesity, lifestyle, and genetic predisposition. If diabetes runs in your family, discuss with your doctor vaccinations against diabetes and a six-hour glucose-tolerance test and an insulin level test, and look up information on the web. Currently, the role of hormonal pollutants interacting with insulin receptors and contributing to the severe rise in diabetes is being investigated. Nitrates in smoked and cured meats have been weakly linked to diabetes.

Uniquely Female: A small number of women get *gestational diabetes* during pregnancy, usually identified in the last three months when increased glucose is found in the urine or the baby is bigger than expected. Increased risk is from overweight, being over thirty years old, having had a previous stillborn delivery, having a family history of diabetes, or taking excessive iron during pregnancy. Gestational diabetes usually disappears with the delivery of the baby, but it can be a sign of future diabetes or heart disease in up to three fourths of these mothers. It's essential to control your blood sugar level if you develop this disease during pregnancy.

Preexisting diabetes is associated with higher-than-average rates of birth defects, stillbirth, preterm labor, and problems in the new-born. These mothers may have increased rates of high blood pressure and difficulty in controlling blood sugar levels and must be carefully monitored. Type 1 diabetics may require early delivery planned at around thirty-eight weeks. If you don't wish to become pregnant but insulin control is difficult, don't take combination birth control pills.

What to Do

- Losing excess weight can improve your blood sugar levels. *Losing ten pounds reduces your risk of getting type 2 diabetes by 70 percent.*
- Exercise at least thirty minutes three times a week, especially brisk walking, jogging, swimming, rowing, or bicycling. Up to 8 percent of cases of diabetes in inactive older women might be prevented if they began regular physical activity.
- Don't skip or delay meals. Always carry some form of sugar to take if you develop symptoms of mild low blood sugar (numbness in the mouth, cool wet skin, a fluttery feeling in the chest, sweating, trembling), or grab some orange juice.
- Reduce stress.
- Don't smoke. Smoking worsens diabetes and promotes earlier death; nicotine increases desire for sugar.
- Have your homocysteine levels tested. Elevated levels increase risk of death especially in type 2 diabetics, and levels can be lowered by taking folic acid, vitamin B_{12}, and vitamin B_6 along with vitamin B complex. Have your homocysteine levels monitored two times a year.
- Check for food allergies, particularly to cow's milk for type 1 diabetics.
- Use stevia herb instead of sugar or artificial sweeteners.
- It's important for all diabetics to have high blood pressure monitored and treated.
- Drink tea, not coffee. Tea has substances that reduce diabetic complications (aldose reductase inhibitors).

- Avoid hot tubs (they can worsen heart conditions and increase your risk of pseudomonas infections).

Diet: In the past, most diabetic women have been advised to lower fat intake and increase carbohydrates. But unless there is an adequate balance between protein and carbohydrates with the right types of fats, and unless whole complex carbohydrates are substituted for simple refined ones, this diet can actually cause more problems than it solves. It's best to increase complex carbohydrates (nonprocessed food sources like whole grains and beans); lower animal fat but increase fish and flaxseed oil intake. Work with your doctor and a nutritionist. High fiber lowers insulin levels and protects against obesity and heart disease, which is rampant in diabetics. Those with insulin resistance may do better with a lower-carb diet (25 percent of calories) or one in which carbohydrates are balanced with protein, like the Zone diet.

Consume small, frequent, largely vegetarian meals (although some diabetics do better with some meat) with an emphasis on *beans*. Eat lots of salads and grate in all kinds of veggies, not just the same old ones. Fried onions and onion soup are good sources of quercetin and help prevent problems in eyes and nerves. Emphasize foods rich in chromium—whole grains, brewer's yeast, string beans, cucumbers, soy foods, organic liver and organ meats, onions and garlic, fruit, shiitake mushrooms, and wheat germ. Diet may be so effective in lowering insulin requirements that you need to be carefully monitored. Limit eggs to two per week, more if you're just eating the whites. As much as possible, bake and poach chicken and fish (be creative, poach in various broths, water and a touch of wine, or soy sauce). Grilled and broiled protein has more AGEs (advanced glycation end products), which hasten kidney and heart problems in diabetics. Emphasize beneficial fats like olive oils, nuts, seeds, and fish, but use in moderation.

Type 1 diabetics should consume monounsaturated fats generously, such as olive oil, olives, macadamia nuts, and high-oleic oils. Consume sauces made from tomato paste and drink tomato juice.

Avoid: All refined sugars (including fructose), refined carbohydrates, excessive saturated fatty foods and fried foods. Limit caffeine and alcohol. Some studies suggest that a few drinks a week are linked to less disease in women with diabetes. Strictly avoiding dairy products in *early* type 1 diabetics may stop the further destruction of pancreatic islet cells. Also avoid large amounts of PABA (para-aminobenzoic acid), salt, and large doses of cysteine and aspartame (NutraSweet, etc.).

Nutrients: Dietary changes cannot cure type 1 diabetes. In type 2, changes in the diet can have a profoundly positive influence. All dietary changes should be medically supervised. This is a very large list; don't take all of these supplements. Check the nutrient charts (pages 35–39) to see which nutrients you're lacking.

- ** High-potency multivitamin/mineral formula with trace minerals, *without* iron
- ** Chromium, 500 mcg twice a day as aspartate or polynicotinate. If taking chromium while eating a high-fiber diet, your blood sugar can get too low if your doctor doesn't lower your insulin. Higher doses of chromium are more effective.
- ** Niacin, 30–100 mg per day may increase the benefit of chromium in type 2 patients. But excessive doses of niacin can worsen blood sugar problems.
- ** Niacinamide, 500 mg three times a day in early type 1 diabetics protects pancreas cells.
- ** Magnesium, 200–500 mg per day. Magnesium blood levels are inversely related to insulin resistance. Optimal levels are associated with better glucose handling, while low levels are associated with problems.
- ** Potassium, 99 mg per day, and 600–1,000 mg per day of calcium in divided doses. These help prevent glucose from being driven into the wrong tissues and causing various diabetic problems.
- • Lipoic acid, 100–250 mg once or twice a day
- • Evaluate digestive enzymes, especially pancreatic (page 468)
- • Vitamin B_6, 50 mg twice a day
- • Vitamin C, 1,000 mg two to three times a day
- • To prevent bone loss from poor sugar control, add vitamin D, 400–1,000 IU per day.
- • Taurine, 500 mg two to three times a day

EARLY DIAGNOSIS CAN PREVENT FUTURE DIABETES!

Early diagnosis of blood sugar intolerance can *prevent* the occurrence of type 2 diabetes years down the road. All women, even young ones, should have a glucose-tolerance test if there is a family history of diabetes; multiple skin tags; a history of gaining weight easily (especially around the abdomen); low-blood-sugar problems; high blood pressure (above 140/90); high total cholesterol and high triglycerides (above 250 mg/dL), or low HDL cholesterol (below 35 mg/dL), even if the fasting blood sugar is normal. Also, African American, Native American, and Hispanic women are at greater risk and should be tested—especially if they have any of the other risk factors—as should any woman who has delivered a baby weighing more than nine pounds. It's a good idea for any woman over the age of forty-five to get tested. If you have an abnormal glucose-tolerance test, then do the following to prevent getting diabetes: lose weight, take vitamin supplements, exercise, and improve your blood fats and blood pressure.

- Biotin, 1,000 mcg three to six times a day (certain cases may need 8–16 mg per day)
- Zinc, 20 mg twice a day, balanced with copper, 2–4 mg per day
- Manganese, 10 mg twice a day
- Ask an informed doctor about: lotension, a drug that slows down kidney damage and enhances mortality; also vanadium; and, for severe cases, chelation therapy, if at risk of losing a limb. Some patients have recovered from grim gangrene with chelation.

For Diabetic Neuropathies

These nerve complications, which can occur in various extremities, can be helped by supplementation:

** Vitamin B_6, 50 mg three times a day

** Alpha-lipoic acid, 100–1,800 mg per day (average dose is 600–800 mg per day) to reduce oxidative stress (take backup biotin, 3–5 mg per day)

** Evening primrose or borage oil, 4–6 g per day in divided doses for six to twelve months

** Acetyl-L-carnitine, 500 mg twice a day. High amounts of car-nitine have been shown to reduce pain from diabetic nerve damage.

- Injectable vitamin B_{12}, 1,000 mcg of hydroxocobalamin twice a week for a six- to eight-week trial. If it helps, over time re-duce to a dosage that maintains a therapeutic effect; if not, stop.

- Ask your doctor about capsaicin cream (0.075 percent) ap-plied topically.

For Diabetic Retinopathy or Nephropathy
- Quercetin, 500 mg twice a day
- Bilberry, 80 mg twice a day
- Have your homocysteine levels tested (page 269).
- Ask your doctor about *continuous* insulin delivery, which one study showed stopped and reversed these complications.
- Avoid artificial tanning agents containing canthaxanthin.

Herbs: Burdock tea, 2 cups per day for three months, helps your body manufacture insulin. American ginseng, 300 mg per day, re-duces type 2 blood sugar elevation after eating.

DIGESTIVE DISORDERS

Hormone receptors (cells that "read" hormonal e-mail messages) line the intestinal tract, so we know that hormonal signals can affect intes-tinal functioning. Note on your menstrual calendar (page 328) if your symptoms of maldigestion, constipation, or loose stools occur or get worse on a regular basis anywhere from midcycle through the first several days of your period. If this is the case for more than three months in a row, testing and treating your hormonal imbalance may be an integral part of improving your digestion or healing a digestive disorder. Read my book *Healthy Digestion the Natural Way* (John Wiley, 2000) for an in-depth discussion of nutrition and mind-body tools to heal more than fifty digestive illnesses, as well as detailed sections on digestive enzymes. See appendix F.

Maldigestion

Inadequate absorption of nutrients into the body's cells, so even though you eat well, your cells starve.

Symptoms: May have no symptoms, or you could have bloating, gas, burping, fatigue, mood swings, or upset stomach within two hours of eating. Other symptoms may include feeling better if you don't eat, chronic loose stools or constipation, intestinal pains, heaviness or fullness not associated with disease, frequently seeing undigested food in your stools, chronically coated tongue and/or bad breath, not sleeping well and waking up tired, chronically cold extremities, bruising for no reason, severe food cravings, being overly stressed, problems with dentures and/or mouth pain, or having an elevated pulse (increasing by 20 to 25 beats) within fifteen minutes after eating. Eighty percent of the body's immune system lives in the intestines. Chronic maldigestion can create imbalances in flora and increase toxic substances within the intestinal tract than can impede optimal immune functioning.

Maldigestion and the need for digestive enzymes should be evaluated in *any* chronic health condition. As a matter of fact, just as our skin thins with aging, so does the lining of the intestinal tract, often leading to inadequate secretion of stomach acid. Routine testing of stomach acid should be done in all women past the age of forty (see appendix F).

Causes: Gas, belching, bloating, or maldigestion symptoms after fatty meals, especially with pain in the right shoulder and back area, suggest gallbladder problems and possibly food allergies (page 84). An often undiagnosed cause is inadequate digestive enzymes (low stomach acidity and/or pancreatic enzymes). See appendix F. Maldigestion after starting a nutritional program and/or herbs suggest starting too many things at one time or inadequate levels of digestive enzymes. Bloating and fluid retention in various parts of the body such as eyes or fingers suggests food allergies, low thyroid functioning, or inadequate digestive enzymes.

Uniquely Female: Maldigestion can worsen anytime from midcycle to several days into the period. The intestinal tract is richly lined with receptors, receiving stations for the messages that hormones, like estrogen, deliver. Thus the intestinal tract is ultrasensitive to hormonal fluxes. In some women, this can affect fluid shifts, which can, in turn, cause cyclic diarrhea or constipation in relation to the menstrual cycle. See *Menstrual Calendar*. Women, especially those over age seventy, suffer from low stomach acid more than men.

What to Do
- Eat slowly, chew, chew, chew, and don't overeat.
- Don't smoke, especially close to mealtimes.
- Drink fewer bubbly liquids, such as soda or beer.
- Cut back on carbohydrates and see if there is improvement.
- Check for food allergies.

Nutrients

If maldigestion occurs cyclically with your menstrual cycle, consider taking the following for several months:
- ** Multivitamin/mineral supplement
- ** Digestive enzymes along with added vitamin B_6, 50–100 mg per day
- ** Vitamin B complex, 25–100 mg per day
- ** Magnesium, 250 mg once or twice a day
- Flaxseed oil, 1 tsp. once a day
- Vitamin E, 400 IU per day
- Pantothenic acid, 600 mg in the evening, to relieve constipation

Heartburn (Gastroesophageal Reflux Disease, GERD)

Heartburn occurs when stomach acid flows back into the esophagus, the tube connecting the mouth to the stomach. With time, the stomach acid can irritate your esophagus and cause problems, such as ulcers.

Symptoms: Burning in your chest, especially at night. Other signs of esophagitis may be burping, trouble swallowing, a sour or acid taste in the mouth, a sore throat, hoarse voice, or indigestion.

Causes: Spicy foods, excessive alcohol, food allergies and sensitivities, caffeine, and tobacco. Certain drugs (aspirin or antiarthritics) are well-known causes of heartburn. Chronic use of nonsteroidal anti-inflammatory drugs (NSAIDs) can result in stomach ulceration.

Overdose of progesterone can cause relaxation of the valve between the stomach and esophagus, allowing stomach contents and acid to back up and cause symptoms.

Uniquely Female: The most common conditions associated with heartburn are peptic ulcers and gallbladder problems, which affect more women than men, particularly those over the age of forty with a fair complexion and who are overweight. Women on birth control pills have a greater frequency of gallbladder disease and heartburn symptoms. Heartburn affects 60 percent of pregnant women, usually starting midway through the pregnancy as the growing uterus impinges on the stomach and as levels of progesterone increase. Peptic ulcers are rare in pregnancy because acid secretion in the stomach actually decreases. Synthetic hormone replacement therapy (HRT) causes gallbladder problems in 40 percent of women taking these medications.

Note: Asthma and its associated medications can easily exacerbate heartburn symptoms. Adult women are prone to asthma, more so if they are on hormone replacement therapy. Asthma sufferers should elevate the heads of their beds and talk to their doctors about altering their asthma medication to reduce the risk of reflux and break the cycle. Up to 90 percent of asthmatics experience complete relief of symptoms if they adhere to antireflux lifestyle and dietary changes.

What to Do
- ** Identify and eliminate food allergies (page 84), especially to gluten.
- ** Don't eat or drink anything one to two hours before bed.
- ** Take ½ tsp. arrowroot powder in ½ glass water.
- ** Rule out stomach acid deficiency (you can get symptoms of heartburn even when actually deficient in stomach acid) or inadequate pancreatic enzymes. Sometimes getting the food to digest properly reduces problems. See appendix F.
- • Rule out infection with a bacteria (*H. pylori*) and check for parasites. *H. pylori* infection can cause nausea, maldigestion, acid and ulcer symptoms, and/or loss of appetite.
- • To help prevent heartburn at night, place four- to six-inch blocks under the head of your bed to keep your head and

esophagus higher than your stomach. If you can't use blocks, sleep with several pillows under your head and shoulders.

- Avoid bending over, especially after eating. Also avoid straining during bowel movements, or when you're urinating or lifting things.
- Don't wear clothing that constricts your chest or stomach.
- Don't smoke. Smoking often causes the stomach to make more acid.
- If you are overweight, lose weight.
- Rule out lactose intolerance.
- Especially during pregnancy, decrease the size and increase the frequency of meals, and avoid spicy foods.

Diet: Whenever you have heartburn, eat six small meals a day instead of three big ones. This keeps your stomach from getting too full. Eat slowly. Try the enzyme-rich fresh fruits papaya and pineapple before meals or between courses to aid digestion. If *H. pylori* is the problem, drink cranberry juice, use mastic gum herb, and read about this bug (D. Lindsey Berkson, *Healthy Digestion the Natural Way*, John Wiley, 2000).

Avoid Sugar, refined carbohydrates, alcohol, and caffeinated foods and beverages—colas, coffee (even decaffeinated coffee can cause problems), chocolate, and tea. Colas are a triple threat with their caffeine, carbonation, and acidity, all of which directly irritate the esophagus. Also avoid excessive intake of fatty foods, which may cause the stomach to release cholecystokinin, a hormone that loosens the muscular valve which is supposed to prevent the backup of stomach juices. Other culprits include citrus fruits, peppermint, spearmint, onions, peppers, tomato-based products, spicy foods, and any other foods and drinks that seem to increase heartburn. Avoid these foods for one month to see if you get better, and reintroduce them one a day to see which ones aggravate your symptoms. Stop smoking and try to limit your use of aspirin and similar pain relievers.

Nutrients

- ** DGL (deglycyrrhizinated licorice), 1–2 380-mg tablets chewed three to four times a day, twenty minutes before meals

**   Probiotics several times a day
**   Aloe vera juice, 2 Tbsp.–½ cup in a glass of water on waking
     and several times a day
**   Digestive enzymes if necessary
•   Ask your doctor about enterically coated peppermint and
     caraway oil products if you have heartburn associated with a
     lot of gas or colicky pains.

Herbs: Angelica (several drops of oil in hot water) or chamomile
tea sipped throughout meals to soothe esophageal irritation.

DIZZINESS/VERTIGO

Dizziness or light-headedness is a vague spaced-out feeling, especially after suddenly standing up or after sitting or lying down. *Vertigo* is the sensation of objects spinning around you, or the false
sensation that you are moving or spinning, usually accompanied by
nausea and loss of balance. Persistent dizziness with vertigo needs to
be evaluated by a doctor.

Symptoms: Light-headedness; a sense of falling, losing your balance, or floating; a feeling that you are moving from one direction to
another; or a conviction that you are going to faint. Your stomach may
become upset. You may lose your balance and fall. Headaches,
slurred speech, double vision, weakness in the limbs, and uncoordi-
nated movements usually mean the vertigo is caused by a neurologic
brain disorder.

Causes

Dizziness or Light-headedness (or Near Fainting): Insufficient blood
reaches the brain for various reasons, such as a brief fall in blood pressure from changes in posture; vision problems; a head injury; a quick
movement of the head; or motion sickness. More serious causes include internal bleeding, high blood pressure, and low blood sugar.

Vertigo: May be caused by an inner ear infection or disease, or by
neurologic damage in the brain usually caused by hardening of the
arteries at the base of the brain (usually in elderly women).

Other Causes: Hidden food allergies (especially in Ménière's disease) and drugs (tranquilizers, antihistamines, aspirin, and diuretics). Stress, anxiety, and vitamin B and magnesium deficiency may play a role. Chemical sensitivities can cause both dizziness and vertigo.

Uniquely Female: Chronic blood loss from heavy menstrual periods or rapid loss of blood in ectopic pregnancy can produce dizziness. Dizziness is more common in pregnancy because the growing uterus compresses the blood vessels to and from the heart. Fibroids can cause heavy periods, which can lead to anemia and dizziness. It can also occur in women taking blood pressure medication.

What to Do

** Rule out any diseases, and have your serum ferritin and iron levels checked to rule out iron deficiency. If you are iron deficient, your doctor must determine the sources of blood loss.

** Check blood pressure.

** If you have vertigo, have a neurologic exam.

- If you are feeling dizzy, lie down until the feeling passes.

- Rise slowly from a prone to a sitting position or from a sitting to a standing position if you are prone to dizziness. Especially when pregnant, roll to the side and slowly push up with your arms to get out of bed.

- Avoid sweets, especially if you are prone to hypoglycemia. Do not skip meals, especially breakfast.

- Avoid dehydration.

- Stay away from drugs such as alcohol, marijuana, methamphetamines, cocaine, and hallucinogens, which can alter your sense of balance.

- Chiropractic adjustments and shiatsu massage may help.

- If your dizziness is the result of motion sickness, taking ginger capsules, 500 mg every one to two hours or several times a day until symptoms are eased, can help.

Nutrients

** Magnesium, 250 mg per day, and a multivitamin/mineral supplement

** B complex, 25 mg twice a day

** Iron supplementation if a blood test shows you have low iron or low ferritin levels
- Vitamin B_{12}, 1,000–2,000 mcg, sublingually
- Vitamin E, 800 IU per day

If Your Dizziness Is Linked to Low Blood Pressure

** Pantothenic acid, 500 mg per day or more
- Vitamin C with bioflavonoids, 1,000–3,000 mg per day in divided doses
- Adrenal glandulars, 2–3 tablets several times a day
- Licorice root extract, 250–500 mg twice a day for two weeks

Herbs: Ginger powder, 2–4 g per day.

E

EATING DISORDERS

Include anorexia nervosa and bulimia. In both disorders, there is a disturbed sense of body image and relationship to food. There can be associated mood disturbances or obsessive-compulsive features. Eating disorders are rare in men.

Binge Eating Disorder

In this newly identified disorder, a person binges without purging afterward. More common in obese older people, more than half of whom are women. About 50 percent of obese binge eaters are depressed. Psychotherapy seems to have better results than appetite suppressants or antidepressants.

Anorexia Nervosa

A disorder characterized by a distorted body image, an extreme fear of getting fat, and a rejection of food, with a relentless pursuit of thinness. To reach an "ideal" weight, a female may follow increasingly restrictive diets, often accompanied by hours of aerobics, weight training, calisthenics, or running. Food becomes a major preoccupation. The woman fails to realize there's a problem even as her body wastes away. Around 30 percent of anorectics have this problem for their whole lives, and almost that many have at least one life-threatening bout. Many die prematurely, and at least 5–18 percent of those hospitalized with anorexia later die of starvation or suicide.

Symptoms: Loss of 15 percent or more of original body weight; abuse of laxatives, diuretics, enemas, and self-induced vomiting; menstrual periods may cease. Sufferers see themselves as fat even when emaciated. Many are meticulous and compulsive high achievers.

The symptoms of malnutrition that accompany anorexia include constipation, digestive discomfort, and bloating; dehydration, muscle cramps, and tremors; downy body hair on the face, back, or arms; flattened breasts; dull, brittle, thinning hair; cracked or dry skin; icy hands and feet; irregular heartbeat; and depression and anxiety.

Causes: Unknown, but cultural attitudes toward beauty and thinness and emotional problems are important. Two thirds of all adolescent girls diet to control their weight, although only a small percentage become anorectic. There is a high correlation between sexual abuse and eating disorders. Frequently there is a very difficult mother-daughter relationship. Zinc deficiency and sometimes food allergies and maldigestion can contribute to anorexia, and repleting with zinc and nutrients and avoidance of food allergens along with psychotherapy has been found to be very successful.

Uniquely Female: Ninety-five percent of those with this disorder are middle- to upper-class females. Usually starts in adolescence or the early twenties, and one out of every hundred young, middle-class women has anorectic symptoms, with five times that number at risk. Anorexia causes reduced levels of estrogen and thyroid hormones, increased levels of cortisol, and often loss of normal menstruation (amenorrhea).

SUSPECT A PROBLEM IF YOU:

- Have lost at least 15 percent of your original weight, without a physical illness, and still think of yourself as fat.
- Have not had your period for three months in a row.

  - Fear being overweight and losing control of your diet.
  - Feel that staying hungry is the only way to keep your weight under control.

What to Do

** Work with a specialist.

** Consume more calories.

** Identify and avoid food allergies.

- Learn about celiac disease (problems with gluten sensitivity), which can worsen anorexia; have your AGA antibodies tested. If elevated, eliminate gluten foods (pages 174, 493).
- Enjoy some mild exercise every day.
- Have regular massage therapy.
- Do anything that builds self-esteem.
- Eat breakfast.
- Eat slowly and chew well. Have small meals.
- Have your doctor run amino acid screens. Persistent dieting can deplete tryptophan, which may encourage relapses.

Diet: Regular eating patterns are necessary: either small frequent meals throughout the day or three meals daily, whichever is realistic and the individual will follow.

Avoid: Refined sugar, white flour, heavy starches, and fruit juice or caffeinated beverages, as they disrupt normal body chemistry. Avoid allergic foods.

Nutrients

** Zinc, 20 mg two to three times a day as lozenges or capsules for several months. Low tissue levels of zinc contribute to eating disorders and supplementation can help stabilize the condition. Balance with 2–3 mg per day of copper.

** Tryptophan (from compounding pharmacies), 2 g before bed on an empty stomach, raises serotonin levels, which helps some anorexics, as does SAMe (S-adenosyl-methione).

** Multivitamin/mineral supplement, once or twice a day. The minerals that are lost through vomiting are the ones that help control weight—potassium and iodine stimulate the thyroid to keep metabolism (calorie-burning) strong. Excessive use of laxatives also depletes potassium and magnesium.

- Vitamin B_{12} internasal gel; sublingual B_{12}, 200–250 mcg per day; or folic acid with B_{12}, 400–600 mcg per day

- Vitamin B complex, 25–50 mg per day
- Vitamin C, 500–2,000 mg a day in divided doses
- Lactobacillus multiformula, twice a day
- Evaluate for digestive enzymes (page 468), but don't supplement if you are an active bulimic, as vomiting up stomach acid can harm your teeth.
- Glutamine, 1–2 g per day to rebuild the gut lining. If vomiting was regularly induced, the gut wall becomes traumatized, and gut flora may be imbalanced.

Herbs: Appetite stimulants—ginger root, ginseng, gotu kola, peppermint.

Bulimia

An irresistible craving for food, leading to repeated bouts of binge eating (at least twice a week for three months), followed by purging (self-induced vomiting, misuse of laxatives, diuretics, and/or enemas), fasting, or excessive exercise. Often accompanies anorexia nervosa, where after months or years of barely eating, an anorectic develops a constant craving for food and begins to binge. Binges (during which someone can consume up to ten times the normal amount of food) may be carefully planned and are almost always undertaken in secrecy. Binges may occur frequently and last a few hours, or may last for a day or longer. Bingeing and purging may occur once or several times a day. Bulimics either maintain normal weight by following binges with strict diet and exercise, or have wide variations in weight. Although bulimia is rarely life-threatening, it can eventually cause serious health problems, such as kidney damage or ruptured esophagus or stomach.

Symptoms: The gastric acid in vomit may damage teeth, which may look brown and eroded. Excessive use of laxatives can result in constipation, indigestion, cramps, bloating, and gas. Patients may display belligerent, aggressive behavior. Other possibilities include broken blood vessels in the face and bags under the eyes from vomiting, scarred knuckles from inducing vomiting, and rapid or irregular heartbeat. Severe cases of bulimia lead to dehydration and loss of potassium, causing weakness and muscle cramps. Psychological distress about compulsive behavior can lead to guilt, shame, depression, and suicide.

Causes: Dancers, actors, models, and athletes sometimes adopt this abnormal eating pattern for professional reasons. For others, anxiety and depression may trigger the binges.

Uniquely Female: Most sufferers are girls or women between the ages of fifteen and thirty, often with a history of obesity in the family. The odds of young women developing bulimia are estimated between 1 in 10 and 1 in 20.

What to Do

- Learn stress-reduction techniques such as deep breathing, muscle relaxation, meditation, or biofeedback (pages 52–58).
- Keep a calendar to record when and how you eat, how often you induce vomiting or use purgatives or laxatives. Awareness of what is actually happening is the first step toward changing behavior.
- Professional counseling is usually necessary.
- Group therapy or an informal support group can help you cope.

Diet and Nutrients, see diet and nutrient sections for anorexia nervosa (page 218).

EDEMA, see Bloating

ENDOMETRIOSIS

A condition in which small patches of the lining of the uterus (endometrium) grow in the wrong places, such as in the ovaries, fallopian tubes, vagina, abdomen, deep inside the uterine muscle (adenomyosis), or even in other parts of the body. Misplaced tissue can grow and cause trouble anywhere. It can grow between organs and cause them to stick together. The extra tissue gets red, swollen, and may cause pain, especially during menses. Adhesions may form that can block or interfere with the functioning of organs. The only way to diagnose endometriosis is through a surgical procedure that goes inside and takes a look, called *laparoscopy*. Diagnosis can take years to figure out.

Endometriosis is most prevalent in women between the ages of twenty-five and forty-four and affects as many as 10–15 percent of reproductive-age women. Around 30 percent of women with endometriosis are infertile. More than 500,000 surgeries are performed each year for endometriosis, and 40 percent of these women experience recurrence as well as continued pain and disability (see *Adhesions*). The disease subsides after menopause, when the ovaries stop making estrogen, or goes away after surgical removal of both ovaries. Endometriosis does not seem to swell in response to hormone replacement therapy as it does in response to the body's own hormones.

Symptoms: Because the misplaced endometrial tissue responds to the same hormones as the uterus, it may bleed during menstruation; can cause cramps, pain, and irritation; and can form scar tissue wherever these occur. Symptoms vary widely, with the most common being irregular or heavy menstrual bleeding. Women may have severe abdominal and/or lower back pain and diarrhea during menstruation, especially toward the end of a period; they may have pain deep in the pelvis during sexual intercourse or midcycle bleeding. Sometimes there are no symptoms, but the severity of the symptoms has no relation to the extent of the disease. Large areas of disease may be painless, while small areas of endometriosis can be very painful. Endometriosis increases the risk for uterine fibroids or breast cysts and may be accompanied or followed by severe fatigue, chronic fatigue syndrome, or fibromyalgia.

Causes: Backward bleeding, called "retrograde menstruation" (bleeding that goes up into the uterus), is thought to be the leading cause. There are many theories about what causes endometriosis, some saying it is an autoimmune disease, but none have been proven. Environmental pollutants, such as dioxin, may play a role, and a suspicous finger has been pointed to bleached tampons with pollutant residues.

Risk Factors: Having a mother or sister with the disease; giving birth for the first time after age thirty; having long menstrual cycles with a shorter than normal time between cycles; excess estrogen or unopposed estrogen (page 226); being Caucasian; having an abnormal uterus; stress; and high-fat diets. Risk increases for adult women who never become pregnant. Women who have been smokers from an early age have less risk, as smoking decreases estrogen levels and perhaps alters estrogen metabolism (I am not advocating smoking).

What to Do
- Endometriosis can cause infertility. Consider having children before the disease does excessive damage.
- Don't use an intrauterine device (IUD).
- Avoid pesticides, heating food in plastic containers, bleached tampons, and other sources of environmental estrogens. Read my book *Hormone Deception* (Contemporary/McGraw-Hill, 2000).
- Keep a menstrual calendar (page 328) and note if symptoms are better or worse in relation to what you eat and how much you exercise.
- Moist heat or a heating pad may relieve cramps in your abdomen. Try a cold pack if heat doesn't work.
- Moderate exercise such as brisk walking increases the body's production of endorphins, the natural pain relievers.
- Find a support group.
- Ask your doctor about the pill RU486.
- If you want to avoid surgery, certain specialized doctors do immune therapy by finding out which hormones you're allergic to and desensitizing you to them.

Diet: Eat a high-fiber diet. Drink filtered water. Eat organic as much as possible.

Avoid: Eliminating specific foods doesn't seem to help much. However, the foods that are best to limit are fried foods, shellfish, and fatty red meats.

Nutrients
- ** Gamma-linolenic or alpha-linolenic oil, 300 mg one to three times a day
- ** Magnesium, 250–400 mg per day
- ** Vitamin B complex, 50–100 mg per day
- ** Proteolytic enzymes, 2–3 g twice a day between meals for one month
- Lipotropic formulas, two to four times a day
- Identify and treat candida-related complex (page 457).
- Melatonin, 1–2 mg each night before bed may *theoretically* help. Chew and let the tablet dissolve under your tongue as slowly as possible.
- DIM (diindolylmethane, an active metabolite of indole-3-carbinol), 60 mg twice a day. Improves estrogen ratios, which *theoretically* may help reduce cell overgrowth of endometriosis.

Herbs: Tincture for acute pelvic pain: 1 oz. each of black cohosh, wild yam, cramp bark, and valerian, ½–1 tsp. every two to four hours. Tincture for long-term problem: 1 oz. each of chaste tree, dandelion, prickly ash, motherwort, ½ tsp. three times a day.

ENERGY

The capacity to do work or effect a physical change—oomph! There are many different forms of energy—light, sound, heat, chemical, electrical, and kinetic—most of which play a role in the body. For example, muscles use chemical energy obtained from food to produce movement and heat, the two most important forms of energy in the body. Most of us aren't concerned with energy unless we don't have enough!

Causes of Low Energy: Fatigue and/or mood changes are often the first signs that we are low in nutrients like B vitamins and magnesium, either from poor diets (low in fruits, vegetables, and whole foods and too high in sugars, which rinse out these nutrients) or from maldigestion. Stress can use up many of these nutrients, and inadequate tissue levels put our bodies in jeopardy of low energy. Other causes: low thyroid, anemia, depression, food allergies, chemical sensitivities, undiagnosed illness, chronic infection including possible parasites, hormone imbalance, and lack of sufficient rest and/or insomnia.

Uniquely Female: Women's bodies go through vast hormonal fluxes each month. If you are the slightest bit out of nutritional balance, working both at home and at an outside job, or emotionally stressed, these changes can be as exhausting as producing a rock concert every thirty days. Even more energy is needed during pregnancy and lactation in order to meet the baby's needs as well as the mother's. Heavy menstrual bleeding can cause iron deficiencies, which in turn can cause fatigue, and women are more prone to thyroid disorders than men, which can also deplete energy. It sure isn't easy being a woman! Hot flashes, insomnia, and low hormones are a classic cause of fatigue in peri- and postmenopausal women.

What to Do

- Exercise. Most women don't exercise because they are too tired, but ironically, exercise helps the energy-producing machines (mitochondria) inside our body. To reap the benefits, you may have to struggle through the first six or more weeks of an exercise program, but it's worth it.
- Brisk walking or aerobic exercise every day helps oxygenate the tissues. Stretch to release energy blocks.
- Get evaluated for iron, thyroid, and ferritin blood levels and digestive enzymes (page 468).
- Massage can help.
- Alternating hot and cold water (showers, whirlpool, steam, or sauna/cold plunge) can increase circulation.
- Get a good night's sleep. If you have trouble sleeping, try chewing melatonin, 1–2 mg per night before bed, and letting it dissolve under your tongue for thirty seconds.
- Have your adrenal and thyroid glands and DHEA (dehydroepiandrosterone) level, estrogen, progesterone, and testosterone levels evaluated.

Diet: Foods that are rich in potassium and magnesium fight fatigue, as do complex carbohydrates, foods high in vitamins B and C, and iron-rich foods. Try Green Drinks four to seven times a week (page 465).

Avoid: Caffeine, sodas, or sugar; they give a temporary lift but result in nervousness and restlessness. Overuse of chemical stimulants leads to dependency, irritability, and lethargy.

Nutrients
- ** Digestive enzymes if indicated, as optimal digestion is essential
- ** B complex, 50 mg twice a day
- ** Potassium/magnesium aspartate, 1–2 capsules two to three times a day (2 g per day of both minerals combined) for two to six months, or try 2–3 capsules before bed; reduce amount if you get loose stools.
- ** Multivitamin/mineral supplement
- ** Pantothenic acid, 500–1,000 mg two to three times a day
- • Alpha-lipoic acid, 100–250 mg once a day
- • Vitamin B_1, 50 mg once a day
- • Chromium, 200 mcg per day
- • Free amino acids, 1,000 mg per day on an empty stomach

Herbs: Butiao, 500 mg twice a day for two weeks before your period for six months.

ENVIRONMENTAL ILLNESS,
see *Multiple Chemical Sensitivities*

EPSTEIN-BARR VIRUS

A herpes-like virus, twice as common in women as in men, that causes infectious mononucleosis. It is associated with lethargy that lasts for six months or more, with swollen lymph glands, muscle weakness, joint pain, and insomnia. Initially suspected as a possible cause of chronic fatigue syndrome, there is little evidence to support this theory. Ninety percent of American adults have been exposed to the Epstein-Barr virus (EBV) at some time in their lives, and it is not clear if antibody tests show an active infection or past exposure. EBV may be associated with fibromyalgia. Antiviral agents include elderberry extract (1 dropperful every hour while awake for two weeks), high doses of vitamin A (work with your doctor), olive leaf extract (500 mg twice a day for one month), and transfer factor (2 capsules twice a day for several weeks—call 4Life Research at 310-914-5191 to order). When EBV plus the pollutants polychlorinated biphenyls (PCBs) are elevated together in the blood, this increases the risk of non-Hodgkin's lymphoma by twenty times.

ESTROGEN DOMINANCE
(Unopposed Estrogen)

Contemporary Western women can have higher levels of estrogen during their premenopausal (reproductively active) years when compared to women from other cultures or from other times in history. American women menstruate 350 to 400 times during their lifetime, as compared to the 100 menstrual periods usual for indigenous women of African tribes (who have more pregnancies and spend more time breast-feeding). The first week of every menstrual cycle occurs with unopposed estrogen, followed by a surge of estrogen that releases LH (luteinizing hormone) from the pituitary, which in turn causes ovulation to occur. Thus, the more cycles of menstruation, the more estrogen surges. Increased exposure throughout a woman's life to estrogen or estrogenic chemical compounds results in an increased estrogen body burden that then elevates the risk of estrogen-dominant conditions.

Under ideal conditions, immediately after a premenopausal woman releases an egg (ovulation) during the middle of her cycle, levels of both estrogen and progesterone (and some DHEA—dehydroepiandrosterone) start to rise and continue to do so until the menstrual flow begins. During this time (approximately two weeks), progesterone acts as an antagonist to estrogen. A variety of estrogen-dominant conditions arise if there is no adequate supply of progesterone (and some DHEA) to counteract the adverse effects of estrogen.

Estrogen-dominant conditions include:

- Benign breast disorders, especially with a history of two or more biopsies (even if they were normal)
- Heavy menstrual bleeding, especially necessitating treatment and/or surgery
- Severe pain with menstruation and/or midcycle
- Fibroids
- Thyroid problems (high estrogen is antagonistic to thyroid; conversely, taking too much thyroid hormone can lower progesterone levels)
- Moderate to severe premenstrual syndrome (PMS)
- Endometrial polyps
- Moderate to severe endometriosis or adenomyosis (endometriosis confined to *inside* the uterus)
- Recurrent ovarian and/or tubular cysts
- Severe symptoms with menopause
- Infertility problems, especially due to fibroids, adenomyosis, or endometriosis
- Tumor formation resulting in breast, uterine, or ovarian cancer
- Autoimmune disorders such as lupus, diabetes, rheumatoid arthritis, and thyroiditis (Hashimoto's) *may* suggest estrogen dominance.
- Other problems include: low blood sugar problems; blood clotting problems; increased blood and fat levels; allergic reactions; loss of zinc and reduced oxygen levels in cells; recurrent periods of feeling extremely weak, with swelling for no specific reason; and copper retention

Risk Factors: The following risk factors are clues that you may have been exposed to excess estrogen or estrogenic growth factors at some time in your life. Some unopposed estrogen conditions are in themselves risk factors. The factors below play a real role in your risk, even though doctors and nurses may not be aware of them. The more risk factors, the greater the preventive action you should take to ward off unopposed estrogenic disorders (also see *Cancer Prevention*).

Menstrual and Reproductive History

- Puberty at ten years or younger. When young girls start to menstruate, they bleed but do not ovulate (see section on precocious puberty under *Puberty*). The body produces progesterone during ovulation, so no ovulation means no progesterone. Thus, vulnerable preteen uterine and breast tissues are stimulated by estrogen without the protection of progesterone.
- History of short cycles (closer to every three weeks than to every four)
- No children, first child born after thirty, or last child born when mother is in her forties
- Late menopause (fifty-five years or older)
- During the transitional premenopausal years, from the late thirties through the early fifties, most eggs get used up and a woman stops ovulating, and once again no progesterone is being made. However, estrogen is still produced during anovulatory cycles, resulting in persistent unopposed estrogen stimulation. Environmental pollutants may be increasing the number of years women have anovulatory cycles.

Family and Clinical History

- Mother, sister, or aunts with hormonally driven diseases like breast, uterine, or ovarian cancer
- History of two or more breast biopsies (even if results are benign)
- History of breast biopsy with atypical hyperplasia
- History of any epithelial cancer, precancer (such as cervical dysplasia), or cervical, thyroid, or colon cancer
- Recurrent breast pain, especially noncyclic and in one breast

- History of fibroids, especially those causing heavy bleeding, requiring treatment and/or surgery
- History of chronic midcycle pain and/or spotting
- History of recurrent ovarian cysts
- History of moderate to severe PMS
- History of moderate to severe abnormal menstrual bleeding
- History of ten-year or current use of synthetic hormones, such as hormone replacement therapies or fertility drugs
- History of high blood estrogen or metabolizing estrogen into "bad" (16-alpha-hydroxyestrone) rather than into "good" (2-hydroxyestrone) metabolites. This may depend on genetics and/or factors such as diet and alcohol consumption. Certain laboratories now will test for ratios of "good" to "bad" metabolites of estrogen.
- Race: African American women may be more at risk than Caucasians.
- High levels of cholesterol
- History of asthma
- History of low levels of progesterone and DHEA
- History of thinning, fine hair during reproductive years
- Exposure in the womb to estrogenic substances, such as certain pesticides, plasticizers, or pharmaceutical DES (diethylstilbestrol)

Dietary and Lifestyle History
- Chronic obesity. Almost 50 percent of women in America are overweight. Fat cells make estrogen. The more fat cells a woman has, the more estrogen she makes. Aromatase is an enzyme that helps produce estrone locally within the fat cells. The estrone fools the pituitary gland into believing that there is too much estrogen in the body, and it shuts down the production of estrogen in the ovaries, even though it was really the fat making the estrogen. Shutting down the ovaries closes the progesterone factory, and thus we again have a situation of unopposed estrogen. Obesity is also associated with elevated levels of testosterone and lower levels of protective

hormone-binding proteins, both of which can lead to more available free estrogen.

- Yo-yoing weight throughout your life
- Carrying five or more extra pounds around your waist throughout the majority of your life
- Consuming a diet high in red meat (may be due to hormones and pesticides and not the meat itself)
- Excess intake of *animal* fats, which stimulate the growth of specific bacteria, transforming the deactivated estrogen back into its active form and allowing it to become readily reab-sorbed back into the body. Animal fats encourage prosta-glandin F2-alpha, which decreases the production of proges-terone.
- A diet low in high-fiber foods that further helps deactivate estrogen and move it on through the gut
- Excessive consumption of sugars, refined carbohydrates, and carbohydrates with a high glycemic index. Elevated release of insulin and growth factors may contribute to abnormal cell growth.
- The regular consumption of alcoholic beverages has been linked to increased estrogen levels in women due to its effect on the liver. In postmenopausal women, one drink a day in-creases estrogen 16–20 percent, and two to three drinks per day increases it by 30 percent. In premenopausal women, moderate drinking (two to three drinks per day) reduces lev-els of progesterone while increasing levels of both natural and synthetic hormones.
- Soy foods and flaxseeds are known to promote healthy metabolites of estrogen. However, these plant estrogens ap-pear to stimulate estrogen-sensitive tissues in the breast and uterus. This can be beneficial if you are menopausal and de-sire more estrogen, or may be harmful if you have had an estrogen-dependent illness. To soy or not to soy presently is a real conundrum (see *Soy*).
- Stress (physical and emotional) elevates cortisol and lowers progesterone, which is used to make cortisol.

- Body's inability to break down and remove excess estrogen because the liver is overloaded from clearing out alcohol, pharmaceuticals, recreational drugs, and/or environmental pollutants
- Deficiency of vitamin B_6 and magnesium, nutrients that are needed to help the liver deactivate estrogen and produce progesterone
- Inadequate production of progesterone due to nutrient deficiencies
- Estrogen supplementation without additional progesterone supplementation
- Long-term use of aspirin can reduce melatonin levels. Healthy levels of melatonin appear to counterbalance levels of estrogen.

Environmental Factors

- Environmental substances, such as pesticides, some components of plastics, dioxins, etc., may be acting in our body as estrogens or blocking the metabolism of our own estrogens. Many pesticides can make estrogen-sensitive fibroid and breast cancer cells grow in the laboratory.
- Estrogenic additives are given to the animals we eat (cows, pigs, and chickens) to hasten their growth and make production more profitable. DES is one pharmaceutical estrogen that was used in the 1950s and 1960s as a cattle-fattening agent. Although its use was banned in 1971 because it was proven to cause a rare vaginal cancer in women, DES was found in exported U.S. meat as recently as 1999. Given these concerns, it seems best to eat organic meat.

Nutrients

** Fiber (pages 44, 464)

** Indole-3-carbinol (or its metabolite DIM—diindolylmethane), 200 mg twice per day, *theoretically* should help. Breast-Guard (200 mg twice a day) is a product with many of these protective nutrients (call Thorne Research at 800-228-1966).

** Iodine (prescription)—ask your doctor about the dose.
** Vitamin B$_6$, 25–50 mg per day; magnesium, 250–400 mg per day; essential fatty acids (several grams per day)
** Vitamin B complex, 25 mg per day
** Have your hormone levels tested, especially progesterone.
** Your liver is the main organ responsible for estrogen metabolism. See *Liver Health*.
• Melatonin, low dose before bed (2–3 mg per night can cause hot flashes in some women), should *theoretically* help.

Herbs: Vitex helps, but use while under the care of a doctor. It increases progesterone and balances prolactin (often elevated along with excess estrogen); 40 drops in a glass of water in the morning for anywhere from six weeks to several months.

F

FAINTING (Syncope)

A temporary drop in pulse rate and blood pressure accompanied by a brief loss of consciousness.

Symptoms: Warning signs typically include light-headedness and a sudden feeling that you are going to pass out, often accompanied by sweating, weakness, dizziness, nausea, and possibly rapid breathing and a fast heartbeat.

Causes: Occurs when there is insufficient blood to the head. The vagus nerve controls blood pressure. When this nerve is stimulated through pain or overwhelming stress or fright, blood pressure can suddenly drop, causing fainting. Blackouts can also be caused by low blood sugar, standing up too quickly from lying down, dehydration, or diabetes.

Uniquely Female: Fainting is common in early pregnancy and is associated with low blood sugar or vomiting.

WHAT TO DO IF YOU FEEL FAINT

Lie down or sit with your head between your knees. Inhale smelling salts or spirits of ammonia. If you faint easily, always rise slowly. Avoid sudden turning of your head or wearing clothes that are tight around your neck. If you hyperventilate, breathe into a paper bag to prevent fainting. When pregnant, eat frequent small meals to prevent rapid changes in blood sugar.

FATS and ESSENTIAL FATTY ACIDS

Fats are not bad. They serve the body in many healthful ways. Fat molecules are made of *fatty acids*, which make up all our cell membranes. Fats also influence the production of important chemicals—called *prostaglandins*—which appear to affect many aspects of female health.

Fatty acids are basically chains of carbon atoms. If they contain the maximum number of hydrogen atoms, the fat is *saturated* (butter, animal fats, coconut oil, palm kernel oil, and cocoa butter). A fatty acid with fewer pairs of hydrogen atoms is called *polyunsaturated* (such as in fish, veggies, seeds, and nuts). If it's only missing one pair of hydrogen atoms, it's *monounsaturated* (omega-9, or oleic acid, found mainly in olives, olive oil, and avocados). Monounsaturated fats are inversely related to the risk of breast and uterine cancers. Macadamia nuts are 75 percent fat, of which 80 percent is monunsaturated. Almonds, pecans, and walnuts also have a fair amount of monounsaturated fats.

Bad Fats

Processed fats (on the label it will say *hydrogenated* or *partially hydrogenated*) are unhealthy. The more refined (heated and processed) any oil is, the less healthy it is. Buy cooking and salad oils that are cold-pressed (not heated) and darker in color (less processed). *Trans fatty acids* come from hydrogenated vegetable oils, margarines, and frying fats. They are not healthy; they lower protective cholesterol (high-density lipoprotein, or HDL). In the near future, the Food and Drug Administration (FDA) will be requiring labels on products to state the amount of trans fats and suggest consumption limits.

Good Fats

Our bodies can't make *essential fatty acids*, but they are essential for our health, so we must get them from our foods. There are two kinds of essential fatty acids, and theoretically it is the balance between the two that is important for health. The typical American diet contains far too much *omega-6* in relation to *omega-3* oils. This imbalance contributes to many health conditions, from heart disease to endometriosis, learning disabilities, hyperactivity, premenstrual syndrome, and cancer.

Omega-3 Oils

Found in fish, flaxseed, walnuts, and, to a lesser extent, in soy oil. These oils suppress inflammation (which is usually a good thing). GLA (gamma-linolenic acid), found in borage (highest source), evening primrose, and black current oils, also protects against inflammation. Omega-3 oils also block arachidonic acid, a chemical substance that promotes inflammatory processes and uncontrolled cell growth (not a good thing). If taking GLA, take some fish oil with it.

Omega-6 Oils

These oils, such as corn, sunflower, safflower, and soy oil, are polyunsaturated. When we consume more omega-6 oils than omega-3 oils, this encourages inflammatory and other unhealthy processes.

Eating fish is healthy because fish contain two protective omega-3 oils: *EPA (eicosapentaenoic acid)* and *DHA (docosahexaenoic acid)*. These oils lower triglycerides, protect the heart, keep blood from clotting too quickly, reduce inflammation (which is thought to be more linked to heart disease than even cholesterol), and may help heal and prevent numerous health disorders from painful periods and inflammatory bowel problems to heart arrhythmias, schizophrenia, depression, and high blood pressure.

High in protective oils are salmon, sardines, albacore tuna, black cod, herring, mackerel, anchovies, whitefish, scrod, and sturgeon. (Wild game meats also have these oils.) Some of the oil found in flaxseed can be converted by the body into omega-3 oils.

Some studies say farmed fish may have just as much essential fatty acid as wild fish, except for some commercially grown catfish (more economical to grow when fed with soy and veggie oils, which changes the oils their flesh contains). Cod liver oil is a good source of both DHA and EPA, but it also contains high amounts of vitamins A and D. Make sure you are not taking too much of these nutrients. *Women who want to become or are pregnant should not take cod liver oil without the guidance of a nutritionally oriented doctor.*

CLA (conjugated linoleic acid) is a mixture of beneficial *trans* fats that enhance immunity, help with heart disease, and help lose weight. It's naturally found, ironically, in animal fats like beef and dairy (*Science News* 159:136–37, 2001).

> The oils we eat from our food (outside) affect our prostaglandin ratios (inside). Just adding good fats won't help. You must avoid bad fats for your body to preferentially use good ones.

FIBROIDS (Uterine Myomas, Leiomyomas)

Benign tumors of any layer of the wall of the uterus, varying in size from a pea to that of a grapefruit. In most cases, several fibroids of varying sizes grow together. They occur in about 20–25 percent of women, most often between the ages of thirty-five and forty-five, and have been found microscopically in 70–90 percent of elderly women. There is a three to nine times higher incidence in African Americans. Fibroids are the number-one cause of heavy and irregular uterine bleeding and are responsible for numerous hysterectomies.

Symptoms: Most fibroids cause no symptoms. If a fibroid protrudes into the uterine cavity, it may cause heavy or prolonged menstrual periods, usually with blood clots, cramplike pains, and shorter cycles. Other symptoms include a feeling of pressure or heaviness, bloating, pain during vaginal sex, urinary frequency, and backache. Severe bleeding can lead to iron-deficiency anemia. Large fibroids can exert pressure on the bladder, causing urinary discomfort or frequency, or on the bowel, causing backache or constipation. Fibroids can be a cause of recurrent miscarriage or infertility. Pregnancy and estrogen replacement therapy can cause fibroids to enlarge. Fibroids often reduce in size after menopause.

Causes: Fibroids are thought to be a response to elevated estrogens or secondary to estrogen dominance (page 226). Estrogenic chemicals like certain pesticides, and perhaps even plant estrogens like those found in soy, may stimulate their growth. They appear more frequently in heavier women.

What to Do

- If fibroids cause severe problems, the only effective remedy is surgery. Hysterectomy (removal of uterus) is the conventional treatment. But there are safe alternatives (often not mentioned to women) that allow a doctor to remove the fibroids while keeping your uterus and maintaining your ability to have children (see box on page 74). Laser myomectomy techniques can remove multiple fibroids as well as the seedlings that later can grow larger. Embolization techniques tie off blood supply to the affected parts of the uterus and can often be done through the navel. However, tying off the blood supply often affects healthy uterine tissue as well, making it more prone to infection, and smaller seedlings, which can cause recurrent problems within several years, aren't removed by this technique. Embolization also requires large doses of painkillers and a longer recovery time than women realize.
- Use ice or heat on your abdomen for fifteen to twenty minutes out of every hour for pain reduction. Do not sleep on the heating pad or ice pack.
- Lose excess weight. Obesity leads to higher levels of estrogen in the body.
- It's very important to have all of your hormone levels evaluated with saliva and/or twenty-four-hour urine testing. Consider estrogen metabolite tests.
- Exercise lowers excess estrogen in some women.

Diet: Nutrients and dietary changes have not been as successful with fibroids as with other female problems, so these suggestions are only for early stage fibroids (when most women don't even know they have them). It is unclear whether dietary phytoestrogens (soy, flax) stimulate the growth of fibroids in some women. It may be that the higher the levels of estrogen a woman has, the more these isoflavones and lignins have an antiestrogenic effect. More research is needed. Eat whole grains, high-fiber foods, and legumes to lower your estrogen. Eat ground flaxseeds (⅛ tsp. a day). Fibroids are linked to the consumption of beef and ham (possibly due more to estrogenic chemicals consumed by the animals than to the meats themselves), whereas greens seem to be protective.

Avoid: Saturated animal fats, sugar, caffeine, alcohol, and junk foods, which interfere with the liver's ability to metabolize hormones. Avoid hormone-laden red meats, greatly restrict all meats, and avoid full-fat dairy products.

Nutrients
- ** Lipotropic factors, 1–2 capsules twice a day with meals
- ** Proteolytic enzymes, 1–3 g two to three times a day between meals on an empty stomach for four weeks
- ** Essential fatty acid oil, several grams each day in divided doses
- ** Have thyroid, estrogen, and progesterone levels evaluated.
- • Iodine (available by prescription)

Herbs: Echinacea/red root compound, 30 drops three times a day; gelsemium/phytolacca compound, 5 drops three times a day. Milk thistle or phyllanthus for liver function. Avoid straight dong quai extract, which may increase bleeding. Chinese botanical Gui (2 tablets three times a day before meals) has a strong study in 100 women suggesting its effectiveness. Call the Tahoma Clinic dispensary at 888-893-6878 for more information.

FIBROMYALGIA (Myofascial Pain Syndrome, Fibromyositis)

A group of disorders characterized by aching, pain, and stiffness in muscles, tendons, and joints, either in a specific area or all over the body. See *Autoimmune Disorders*. People who have fibromyalgia are not at greater risk for any other musculoskeletal disease.

Symptoms: Diagnosis is based on the exclusion of other diseases along with the presence of muscle pains and stiffness at three or more places in the body for three or more months. There are at least several (often six to ten) small, distinct sites of very tender points, such as the top of the shoulder blade, the outside of the upper buttock and hip joint, and the inside of the knee. The pain is usually worse when a person is trying to relax, and is less noticeable during activities or exercise. Recurrent sore throat, headache, low fever, sleep disturbance, and depression are also common. Other symptoms include daytime tiredness, headaches, alternating diarrhea and constipation, numbness and tingling in the hands and feet, memory difficulties, and dizziness. Like chronic fatigue syndrome, fibromyalgia is chronic and difficult to cure.

Causes: Unknown, but thought to be related to immune dysfunction. Some symptoms are triggered by physical or mental stress, injury, exposure to dampness or cold, certain infections, food and/or mold allergies, chemical exposures, and sometimes by rheumatoid arthritis. Lack of sleep means your body doesn't produce the chemicals needed to control or regulate pain, resulting in tenderness in the upper back and forearms, leading to symptoms of fibromyalgia. Some believe it is a variant of chronic fatigue syndrome that endures for five years and changes its main symptom from fatigue to muscle pain. Many symptoms overlap with the profile of multiple chemical sensitivities.

Uniquely Female: Affects women far more than men, especially in midlife.

What to Do
- Rule out Lyme disease, lupus, and rheumatoid arthritis.
- Check for underlying thyroid disorders (low thyroid or resistance to thyroid hormone), including subclinical hypothyroidism.
- Have your DHEA (dehydroepiandrosterone) level tested.
- Try stress-reduction and relaxation techniques to relieve muscle tension.
- Mind-body therapies, like meditation and visualization, have been shown to be effective. See pages 52–58.
- Exercising for thirty minutes three times a week improves cardiovascular (heart and lung) health, especially brisk walking, biking, swimming, and water aerobics. Remember to

stretch. A six-month program of exercises in a temperate pool has been shown to help.

- Gentle massage or acupuncture on a regular basis has good success.
- Gentle heat applications can relieve discomfort.
- Check for food allergies and avoid chemical exposures.
- Don't smoke.
- Lose excess weight.

Diet: Eat foods that build the immune system, such as wheat germ, sea vegetables, lots of various veggies, brown rice, prunes and bran, yogurt and miso, and eat organic as much as possible. Some women are helped with a strict vegetarian diet, while others need meat.

Avoid: Foods high in salicylates (page 112), alcohol, and tobacco, and reduce caffeine.

Nutrients

- ** SAMe (S-adenosyl-methione), 200–800 mg per day (page 496). Try for up to one month to improve depression as well as reduce chronic pain.
- ** Multivitamin/mineral supplement and antioxidants
- ** Magnesium, 250–400 mg once or twice a day along with malic acid
- ** Evaluate for digestive enzymes (page 468).
- ** Bromelain, 500 mg between meals two to three times a day for six weeks (stop earlier if there's no pain reduction)
- ** Vitamin B complex, 25–50 mg one to two times a day
- Reduced L-glutathione, 400 mg per day
- Relaxin. The first female hormone identified, even before estrogen, it relaxes muscles and is available by prescription. Try 20 mcg once a day for one week, then twice a day for several months. Your doctor can order it from the Tahoma Clinic dispensary, at 888-893-6878. Try Biz injections.
- Melatonin, 1–3 mg before bed, chewed and then held under your tongue until dissolved. It has been shown to improve

sleep, fatigue, and pain but measure your blood levels first—it may be elevated in some women with fibromyalgia.

- Some subtle forms of vitamin D deficiency can cause muscle problems. Try 800–1,000 IU per day for six weeks. You may need higher amounts; if so, work with your doctor.
- Ask your health practitioner about Metagenics UltraInflamX, a medical food that can reduce inflammation.

Herbs: Two cups of burdock tea daily; wood betony for headaches; turmeric, 300–500 mg two to three times a day.

G

GALLSTONES

The gallbladder is a small, pear-shaped sac that stores bile made by the liver until it is needed during digestion to break down the fats in food. One principal disorder of the gallbladder is the formation of *gallstones*, crystals that are made mostly of cholesterol, though some are from calcium salts or bile pigments. Up to 20 percent of Americans over the age of forty have gallstones. Gallstones may be found in the gallbladder *(cholelithiasis)* or in the bile ducts *(choledocholithiasis)*. There may be one or many stones, varying in size from 1 to 25 mm. Complications can include inflammation of the gallbladder *(cholecystitis)* or bile duct obstruction that leads to jaundice. Gallbladder inflammation and spasming often occurs without stone formation and is another common disorder of the gallbladder. The digestive system can function normally (but not always optimally) without a gallbladder if it is surgically removed.

Symptoms
Gallstones: "Silent" gallstones stay in the gallbladder or pass through without causing problems. However, if one gets stuck on its way out, or if there is swelling and inflammation in the duct even without stone formation, intense colicky pain can result in the upper middle and/or upper right side of the abdomen, often radiating to the lower right shoulder blade. Pain usually occurs two hours after eating (especially fatty foods) and is typically constant, with pain pro-

gressively rising and then falling gradually over several hours. Other symptoms include nausea and vomiting, and, if there is infection, fever, chills, and jaundice (yellow skin or eyes). You may also feel bloated, be unable to eat fatty foods, and burp more than usual. However, the symptoms of gallstones can vary.

Gallbladder Inflammation: Recurrent colicky pain in 75 percent of sufferers, often radiating to the right shoulder.

Causes: Stones are linked to diets high in cholesterol and saturated and processed fats, inadequate vegetables and fiber, constipation, or a low-grade infection of the gallbladder. Diets high in refined sugars increase the amount of bile acids in the colon, which reduces the solubility of cholesterol in the bile. This keeps cholesterol from breaking down inside the gallbladder, which can lead to the formation of gallstones. Gallbladder attacks and inflammation (not stones themselves) have been linked to food allergies (especially eggs) and/or inadequate stomach acid.

Risk Factors: Obesity, drinking too much alcohol, estrogen dominance, a high-fat/high-sugar diet, active Crohn's disease, and genetic predisposition. Native Americans have high risk.

Uniquely Female: Women are affected four times as often as men, especially fair-skinned, overweight women over forty years old. Higher risk with use of hormones, such as in birth control pills and hormone replacement therapy (some studies suggest that up to 40 percent of healthy women on hormone replacement therapy develop gallbladder problems). Risk increases if a woman has had many children or experienced sudden extreme weight loss. Chronic gallbladder problems can contribute to poor fat digestion, which in turn can cause inadequate absorption of protein and minerals, which in turn can contribute to osteoporosis, maldigestion, and various symptoms like fatigue and depression. Women with low levels of vitamin C have higher risk of gallbladder disease.

What to Do
** Identify and eliminate food allergies, especially eggs and dairy.
** Check levels of stomach acid (page 468). Half of those with gallstones don't make enough stomach acid.

** Lose excess weight *slowly* by reasonable methods.

- Apply a castor oil pack to the abdominal area for pain. Cut a piece of flannel to the size of your abdomen. Soak with castor oil (not enough to cause dripping). Place over abdomen and cover with a plastic bag. Put a heating pad over the plastic on low setting for fifteen minutes. Be careful not to burn yourself.
- Regular mild exercise can help.
- Acupuncture and acupressure are helpful.
- Get your thyroid function checked. There is a link between low thyroid and bile duct stones.
- Coffee may decrease the pain from gallstones in some women.
- See my book *Healthy Digestion the Natural Way* (John Wiley, 2000) for a gallbladder flush.

Diet: Asymptomatic gallstones can often be managed by dietary adjustment, primarily by reducing the intake of dietary fats; consuming more vegetables, fruits, and whole grains; and avoiding foods that trigger allergies. Eat beets—shredded in salads, steamed, and in soups—and steamed or sautéed beet greens. Also good are garlic, soy products, tomato juice, artichokes, pears, and apples. Coffee may help prevent gallbladder symptoms (wow!).

Avoid: Refined sugar and carbohydrates, processed and hydrogenated fats, dairy products except cultured ones like yogurt. Eat small, frequent meals.

Nutrients

** Evaluate digestive enzymes, especially stomach acid (page 468).

** Vitamin C, 1,000–3,000 mg per day in divided doses. Reduce if diarrhea or abdominal pain occur.

** Lecithin, 8–9 g twice a day or 1 tsp. liquid twice a day before meals, or a purified extract called phosphatidylcholine, 300–2,000 mg per day in two divided doses

** Magnesium, 250 mg once or twice a day

** Iodine (available by prescription) helps keep cholesterol in solution.
- Vitamin A, 10,000 IU per day for several weeks, then 5,000 IU per day. Only take a dose higher than 5,000 IU per day with a doctor's supervision.
- Ask your doctor about peppermint oil, 5 drops three times a day.

Herbs: Five to seven cups of gravel root tea daily for a month, or 600 mg milk thistle divided in two doses to help dissolve stones. Artichoke leaf, 250–500 mg two to three times a day, and dandelion root, 250 mg two to three times a day for six weeks (you may use artichoke or dandelion by itself, or together), stop for one month, then repeat. Attacks and stone dissolution: Drink 3–4 cups of strong peppermint tea between meals or take peppermint tablets, 2–6 g per day.

GINGIVITIS (Sore Gums)

Normal gums (*gingivae*) are firm, pink, fit well around teeth, and don't bleed easily. Gingivitis is inflammation of the gums.

Symptoms: Swelling, redness, puffiness, and easy bleeding.

Causes: The most common cause is lack of sufficient brushing and flossing, which causes plaque to accumulate and irritate gums. Other factors are poor dental bite, calcium deposits, sensitivity or allergy to metal in a crown (even if the dentist says this is not possible), food getting caught between teeth, and faulty dental restorations. However, chronic gingivitis also can occur because of systemic problems such as hormonal changes, oral herpes, nutrient deficiencies (especially vitamins C and B complex), allergies, heavy-metal toxicity such as to lead, diabetes, or severe illnesses like leukemia and AIDS. After the mid-thirties, gingivitis is more responsible for tooth loss than cavities. Certain drugs (like Dilantin) can cause gingivitis and overgrowth of the gums.

Uniquely Female: Hormones greatly affect gums. Gingivitis commonly occurs at puberty, during the menstrual period, or during the first trimester of pregnancy, when it may worsen, and it may or may not stop after delivery. Oral contraceptives may cause or aggravate gingivitis. During menopause, a woman may be dismayed to discover that her mouth ages just like her skin and vagina (not fun). Many women develop problems with gums and teeth during menopause. Sequential administration of estrogens and progesterone, natural or synthetic, may be helpful. Ten percent of women have undiagnosed nickel allergies, and gums can be chronically irritated by nickel alloys in some crowns.

What to Do

** Get professional cleanings frequently (every three to four months), have pockets around teeth regularly monitored, and have scaling done if necessary. Have X rays and an exam by a specialist to check the status of your tooth roots. Severe gum disease can increase the risk of heart attack by raising blood levels of an inflammatory substance (C-reactive protein).

** Brush with an ultrasonic toothbrush, and floss twice a day until problems go away, then continue to floss at least once a day. Rinse for thirty seconds to several minutes with 5 ml liquid folic acid (0.1 percent solution) or use herbal tea tree oil mouth rinses twice a day for one to two months.

• When eating out, rinse your mouth with water after eating.

• Get expert advice on how to floss correctly.

• If menopausal, consider hormonal therapy. See *Menopause*.

• Crowns can irritate the gums if they fit poorly, have metal portions in contact with the gums, or are broken.

• Check side effects of medications you may be taking.

Nutrients

** Folic acid, 400–800 mcg per day, plus vitamin B complex, 25–50 mg per day

** Coenzyme Q-10, 50 mg per day

** Vitamin C plus bioflavonoids, 100–500 mg of each per day

• Calcium, 500 mg twice a day

• Vitamin K, 2–5 mg per day

<u>Avoid:</u> Toothpastes with sodium lauryl sulfate.

H

HAIR

Hair is composed of dead cells filled with keratin, the protein that makes up nails and the outer layer of skin.

Brittle hair, which breaks easily and splits at the ends, may be the result of too much shampooing, combing, or blow-drying, but sometimes indicates nutritional deficiencies such as low levels of essential fatty acids, mineral deficiencies, inadequate stomach acid, inadequate progesterone (which is a natural anti-androgen agent), and hypothyroidism. Try biotin, 2–5 mg per day for several months. *Very dry hair* may come from excessive use of hot rollers or curling irons, frequent perming, dying, or bleaching, or can be a sign of malnutrition, maldigestion, and/or lack or imbalance of essential fatty acids. *Dandruff* is an irritating condition in which dead skin is shed from the scalp in unsightly white flakes. The usual cause is seborrheic dermatitis, an itchy, scaly rash on the scalp. See the section on dandruff under *Skin*. Focus on vitamin B_6, 25 mg per day; magnesium, 250 mg per day; and essential fatty acids, several grams per day.

See *Baldness* for hair loss. Remember, it's normal to lose up to one hundred hairs a day.

Hirsutism

A condition of excessive hairiness that commonly affects women and can cause significant emotional distress. It is relatively common in women of Mediterranean or East Indian ancestry and runs in families of dark-haired women. Usually it is not a sign of any underlying disorder.

Symptoms: The hair is coarse, like a man's, and grows in a male pattern on the face, trunk, and limbs. If a hirsute woman also has an enlarged clitoris, a deepening voice, a lack of menstruation, and receding hair, then the condition is called *virilism* and requires medical treatment.

Causes: Usually hereditary, but also occurs when levels of the male hormone testosterone in the blood are abnormally high (such as can occur in polycystic ovary syndrome) or if the woman is particularly sensitive to testosterone. Higher androgen and lower estrogen and progesterone levels is a hormone imbalance that can be triggered by stress, irregular periods, acne, obesity, infertility, and excessive intake of DHEA (dehydroepiandrosterone). Estrogens act in the opposite manner to androgens, slowing growth and producing finer, less highly pigmented hair.

Uniquely Female: Certain enzymes activate the testosterone in the skin, and these enzymes are present at higher levels in women who have excess body and facial hair. Changing hair growth patterns normally accompany puberty, pregnancy, and menopause. After menopause, when estrogen levels drop and androgen levels rise, excess hair can grow on the face, around the nipples, and on the chest and belly button area, while hair on the head can thin.

What to Do
- Excess hair growth that comes with puberty, pregnancy, or menopause may be mild and temporary and requires no treatment.
- Test hormones, including testosterone and DHEA.
- Birth control pills or nutrients can be used to balance hormones, although this may not always help in losing unwanted hair.
- Cosmetic treatments include bleaching solutions that lighten the hair, depilatory creams, and wax treatments. The only potentially permanent solution are forms of electrolysis.

HAY FEVER (Allergic Rhinitis)

Hay fever refers to a condition that can be triggered by any inhaled substance, not just hay. So a better name is *allergic rhinitis.* Seasonal allergic rhinitis occurs only at certain times of the year (for example, the spring or fall), while nonseasonal allergic rhinitis can affect susceptible people at any time. Treatment of symptoms can bring relief but no cure. For that, the cause of the allergies needs to be addressed.

Symptoms: Sneezing; an itchy, runny, or stuffy nose; itchy, red, swollen, burning, or watery eyes. Other symptoms include an itchy throat, coughing, and headache.

Causes: Seasonal hay fever is caused by plants that produce pollen at certain times of the year. House dust, feathers, mold, dust mites, and animal dander cause nonseasonal rhinitis. Tobacco smoke, air pollution, and sudden changes in temperature also cause allergic rhinitis.

Uniquely Female: Women can experience heightened allergy symptoms two weeks before their periods or at menopause, when their bodies are changing. Keep a menstrual calendar (page 328). If symptoms worsen with each period, consider vitamin B complex, 25 mg per day; vitamin B_6, 25–50 mg per day; magnesium, 250–400 mg per day; and essential fatty acids, several grams per day, along with evaluating digestive enzymes and identifying and avoiding food and inhalant allergens and chemical irritants. See *Allergies* for treatment.

HEADACHES, CHRONIC

The pain of a headache comes from a spasm of the head and/or neck muscles *(tension headaches)* or from swelling in the brain due to dilated blood vessels *(migraines).* Forty-five million Americans suffer from chronic and recurrent headaches.

Tension Headaches

These headaches are caused by muscle tension in the neck, shoulders, and head. They usually begin in the morning or early afternoon and worsen during the day, with a steady, moderately severe pain above the eyes or in the back of the head. It may spread over the whole head and down into the neck and shoulders.

Causes: Many headaches are the body's response to hunger, fatigue, a change in the weather, emotional distress, or biomechanical stress such as talking with the phone cocked on one shoulder, sitting in front of the computer, or having a problem originating from the lack of normal motion in your spine (called a *fixated spinal unit* or *subluxation*). Chronic headaches can be triggered by premenstrual syndrome (PMS), estrogen dominance, nutrient deficiencies, eye or muscle strain, depression, colds and flu, alcohol, caffeine, certain medicines, low blood sugar, poor posture, a noisy or stuffy environment, excessive sleep, or allergic reactions to certain foods or food additives like monosodium glutamate (MSG) or to chemical fumes. Other causes include toothache, ear or sinus infection, or head injury. Rare causes of headache are brain tumor, hypertension, or aneurysms.

Uniquely Female: Women seek care for headaches four times as often as do men. Changes in hormone levels during a woman's monthly cycle can be to blame. Fluid shifts in the last two weeks of the cycle can cause or heighten headaches. It is common for women with inadequate levels of magnesium or unopposed estrogen to develop muscle strain and tightness anywhere from midcycle to the beginning of the menses. Birth control pills can cause tension headaches or migraines.

What to Do

** Keep a menstrual calendar (page 328). If you see a pattern of cyclic headaches, take vitamin B$_6$, 50–100 mg per day; magnesium, 250 mg per day; and omega-3 fatty acids, 2–5 g per day.

** See a chiropractor or osteopath.

** Stretch and massage the muscles in your shoulders, neck, jaw, and scalp. An ice pack on the neck may stop a headache from getting worse.

• Take a hot bath, except for cluster headaches (headaches that last from fifteen minutes to three hours, are severe, one-sided, located around the eyes, and occur up to eight times a day), which get worse with increased body heat (including from exercise or sex).

• Put a drop of tea tree oil on each temple; use Olbas Analgesic Oil in a vaporizer.

• Rest in a quiet, darkened room with a warm or cold wet cloth over the aching area.

• Don't skip or delay meals. Drink plenty of liquids, including between meals.

• Don't drink too much alcohol; hangovers make for nasty headaches.

• Don't smoke; cigarettes often make a headache worse.

• Test for food and inhalant allergies.

• Get a good night's sleep.

• Check for temporomandibular joint (TMJ) syndrome, a problem in the jaw joint.

• Make sure your pillows are not too high, and consider purchasing proper orthopedic ones.

• Try a clear-water or coffee enema.

• Acupuncture helps some cases of recurrent headaches.

• For headache from neck tension (slept wrong, stress, computer work, etc.), do neck exercises twice a day.

• For nonresponsive headaches, ask your chiropractor or doctor about PENS (percutaneous electrical nerve stimulation).

<u>Diet:</u> Low-protein diets help some cases of migraines.

<u>Avoid:</u> Tyramine and aspartame (amino acids found in some sweeteners and nitrites). Tryptophan (found in high-protein foods like turkey) can worsen headaches. Also avoid chewing gum, ice cream, iced beverages, salt, and possibly too much sunlight. Some chronic sufferers link headaches to chocolate.

Nutrients

At the Onset of Headache

** Magnesium, 250 mg twice a day

** Niacin, 50 mg per day (may cause some skin flushing)

** Bromelain, 100–500 mg two to three times a day on an empty stomach

For Headaches During the Second Half of Your Cycle

- Take vitamin B$_6$, B complex, 25–50 mg per day; magnesium, 25 mg per day; and omega-3 fatty acids, 2–3 g per day.

For Cluster Headaches

- Melatonin, 10 mg in the evenings for two weeks, then stop. If this doesn't work, try oxygen therapy. Have your doctor order an oxygen tank. When you feel a headache coming on, turn the tank on, put the clip on your nose, and slowly breathe oxygen for three to five minutes. Some doctors prescribe the drug lidocaine in nosedrop form for cluster headaches.

For Chronic Tension Headaches

- Try L-5-hydroxytryptophan, 300 mg per day for two months, or vitamin B complex, 50–100 mg per day, as a prophylactic.

Herbs: Try a paste of ginger root applied to the forehead.

Migraines

Headaches with recurring, throbbing, intense pain, associated with nausea, vomiting, and light sensitivity, usually beginning in and around the eye or temple on one side of the head, often spreading throughout the face and head. They can last anywhere from a few hours to a few days and can occur weekly or less than once a year. The average is two or three times a month. Migraines usually begin between the teen years and the age of forty and often run in families.

Symptoms: Classic migraines begin with flashing lights or colors, tunnel vision, loss of appetite, nausea, vomiting, or sensitivity to noise, light, or smells. These warning signs last about fifteen to thirty minutes and are followed by headache pain. With common migraines, you may feel tired, depressed, or restless for two or three days before the headache starts.

Causes: Allergies to certain foods (alcohol, citrus, chocolate, aged cheeses, excessive caffeine) and food additives (such as MSG and the nitrates in cold cuts and hot dogs) frequently cause migraines. Liver malfunction, constipation, stress, environmental allergies, and chemical sensitivities can be underlying causes. Migraines can be triggered by tension, bright lights, loud noises, strong smells, weather changes, fatigue, missed meals, and emotional upset. Artificial sweeteners can trigger a migraine. Lack of exercise can worsen the problem.

Uniquely Female: Seventy percent of those who have migraines are women. After puberty, changing levels of estrogen can trigger migraines. Many women get the headaches before or during their monthly period. In some women, migraines disappear during pregnancy but can return later. Migraines in late pregnancy may come from elevated blood pressure, rapid weight gain, and fluid retention. During menopause, migraines may disappear or may occur for the first time. Migraines before the onset of your period may be helped with vitamin B_6, 25–50 mg per day, and magnesium, 250–400 mg per day.

What to Do

- Test for blood sugar problems, TMJ syndrome, spinal problems, bowel problems, and candidiasis.
- At the first sign of a migraine, sit in a hot bath and apply cold compresses or ice packs to your head, or splash cold water on your face; lie down in a quiet, dark room for several hours, but don't read or watch TV. Another option is to drink one or two cups of strong coffee (only if you are not a regular coffee drinker).
- If the headaches first appeared after you began taking birth control pills, talk to your doctor about using another method of birth control.
- At the start of a migraine, immediately soak your hands and forearms or feet in water as hot as you can stand it. The extremities can get very cold at the onset of a migraine, and this will help release the constricted energy.

- Another option at the start of a migraine: Take tryptophan, 500 mg; niacin, 100 mg; calcium, 500 mg; and two tablets of Anacin with water or ½ cup milk. Avoid high-potassium foods (bananas, nuts, oranges, tomato juice, dried fruit, and magnesium supplements). If needed, repeat the supplements four hours later.
- An intravenous (IV) Myer's cocktail (see appendix G) in a doctor's office may stop a migraine within a few minutes.
- Ask your doctor about oxygen (see section on cluster headaches, page 252).

To Help Prevent Migraines
- Get regular aerobic exercise.
- Check for food and/or chemical allergies, especially to sulfites (used to keep veggies nice looking in salad bars).
- Keep a record of what you ate before each headache. Avoid foods that seem to cause an attack. Don't skip or delay meals.
- Try to keep your life as free of stress as possible. Learn to pace yourself. Yoga, biofeedback, or relaxation therapy may be helpful (see page 52).
- Don't smoke.

Diet: Foods high in magnesium reduce throbbing and contractions. Eat dark leafy greens, fresh fish and sea vegetables, nuts, whole grains, molasses, almonds and almond milk, watercress, parsley, fennel, garlic, and gentle green drinks. Follow a hypoglycemic diet. Eat small, frequent meals to stabilize your blood sugar and avoid excessive protein.

Avoid: Refined sugars, caffeine, and alcohol. Work with food allergies, especially to all dairy products, primarily milk and cheese, chocolate, citrus fruits, red wine, and nitrate-containing foods such as shellfish and pickled fish, and aged and smoked meats. Migraine sufferers are often deficient in the intestinal enzyme that breaks down phenols and phenyls in foods like chocolate and in chemical additives, so strictly avoid these foods.

Foods rich in the amino acid tyramine may cause problems for people who suffer migraines. Tyramine, a blood vessel dilator, may prompt headaches in people who are taking certain types of antidepressants. Avoid foods rich in this amino acid, such as fermented products, pickled products, bananas, figs, prunes, pineapples, raisins, and cheese.

Blood Sugar and Headaches: Low blood sugar can trigger migraines. Refined and simple sugars promote excess insulin release, which can drop blood sugar below normal. This causes stress hormones to be released, which can cause headaches. Excessive consumption of caffeine in coffee, tea, and cola may trigger low blood sugar and headaches.

Nutrients
   ** Magnesium, 300–600 mg per day (at onset)
   ** Vitamin B_2, 400 mg in the morning, and vitamin B complex, 25 mg once per day
   ** Cod liver oil, 15 ml once or twice a day, balanced with vitamin E, 400 IU
   • IV magnesium sulfate has been shown to stop and/or reduce migraines in a number of studies. Drs. Jonathan V. Wright and Alan Gaby recommend magnesium plus B vitamins, vitamin C, and calcium (page 471).
   • If all else fails, try 200 mg of SAMe (S-adenosyl-methionine) on an empty stomach once a day for at least several weeks (page 485).

Herbs: For prevention, not treatment, try feverfew, 50–125 mg per day for up to six weeks to see if it works. Don't take if pregnant or breast-feeding. Take 500–600 mg of powdered ginger in water at the onset of the attack and repeat at four-hour intervals, a maximum of two more times that day. Continue for three to four days.

HEART ATTACK (Myocardial Infarction, MI)

A medical emergency that occurs when a blockage in a coronary artery restricts or cuts off the blood supply to a region of the heart. It is the leading cause of death in America.

Symptoms: The classic symptom is intense chest pain not relieved by rest. The pain may feel crushing, tight, or heavy and may spread to the neck, jaw, shoulders, back, or left arm. It may also feel like indigestion or burning under the breastbone. The person may also become cold, sweat profusely, feel weak and nauseated, or even lose consciousness. Both angina and heart attack may lead to arrhythmias. Some people have no symptoms at all. This is called a "silent" MI. Women may have nonclassic symptoms (see below).

Causes: Most heart attacks are caused by a clot blocking an artery or a spasm in an artery, resulting in reduced blood flow. Cocaine, certain chemical fumes, and certain nutritional deficiencies, such as inadequate levels of magnesium or the amino acid arginine, can cause coronary arterial spasms. Taking iron when you don't need it also increases risk. Location seems to count as well. Women over thirty-five who live in Mississippi, New York, and West Virginia are more likely to die of heart disease than women anywhere else in the United States.

Uniquely Female: Women die more often in the hospital after a heart attack and during the first year after a heart attack than do men, and women are more likely to experience a second heart attack. Women's heart disease progresses differently from men's—often more subtly, over a longer period of time, and with different or no symptoms—so women may be more ill by the time they arrive in the emergency room with a heart attack. Most important, because women's symptoms of heart attack are different, they are often misdiagnosed even by emergency room doctors. Women may have just one or two symptoms, perhaps only for a short time, and those symptoms may occur without any chest pain, making them difficult to link to the heart. A woman under the age of fifty is twice as likely to die as a man of the same age because the woman will tend to wait longer before going to the hospital.

Women's Symptoms of Heart Disease and Heart Attack

A woman may have only one or two of the symptoms on the list, or she may have them all.

- Upper abdominal pain mimicking indigestion
- Back pain

(docosahexaenoic acid—the active oil component in fish) reduces death risk by 50 percent. Fish oil reduces the risk of heart attack, lowers triglycerides, and reduces the risk of blood clots and cardiac arrhythmias. DHA is high in fatty fish such as salmon, tuna, and mackerel and very low in meat and eggs.

Consider eating less carbohydrates (especially refined) and more quality protein like soy, eggs, and organic chicken. Replacing carbs with protein (but not overdoing it) has been shown to lower the risk of heart disease. The flavonoids in tea (both green and black) protect the heart.

Light to moderate alcohol consumption in women thirty-five years or older reduces overall risk of heart attack with as little as one drink a week. Wine, beer, and spirits have equal effects. Increasing this to one drink a day does *not* improve the benefit. Alcohol abuse increases risk of stroke.

Nutrients

** Magnesium, 200–500 mg per day. Magnesium levels have been found to be inversely associated with death from heart attacks. If you have had a heart attack, discuss magnesium and intravenous (IV) vitamin B with your doctor as well as taking these nutrients orally. Magnesium administered through an IV immediately after a heart attack decreases the incidence of arrhythmia, pump dysfunction, and death. It is safe, cheap, and effective. See *American Heart Journal* 139 (4):e2:703, 2000. According to Alan R. Gaby, M.D., intravenous magnesium has proven more effective in dissolving clots in coronary arteries during the early stages of heart disease than commonly used drugs. IV magnesium reduced the mortality rate by 70 percent, but it has to be administered in exactly the right dose at the right time (page 471), or it can worsen the situation.

** Low levels of selenium are associated with MIs.

** Cod liver oil, 1 Tbsp. once or twice a day (balance with vitamin E, 800 IU per day)

** Multivitamin/mineral supplement

** See nutrients under *Heart Disease*.

HOW TO SURVIVE A HEART ATTACK
WHEN YOU'RE ALONE

Many people are alone when they suffer a heart attack. Without help
son whose heart stops beating properly and who begins to feel faint
time left before losing consciousness. However, these people can he
selves by *coughing repeatedly and very vigorously.* A deep breath s
taken before each cough, and the cough must be deep and prolonged,
producing sputum from deep inside the chest. A breath and a cough
repeated about every two seconds without letup until help arrives, or
heart is felt to be beating normally again. Deep breaths get oxygen
lungs, and coughing movements squeeze the heart and keep the blood
ing. The squeezing pressure on the heart also helps it regain normal rh
this way, heart attack victims can get to a phone and, between breaths
help.

Tell as many other people as possible about this; it could save their
you are not alone, teach everyone in your house to give an aspirin as fas
sible to the person having the heart attack.

From *Health Cares,* Rochester General Hospital, via Chapte
And the Beat Goes On . . .

- Nausea
- Fatigue (can be overwhelming and perhaps only short
- Difficulty breathing (hard to catch your breath, may wa
  you up at night gasping)
- Dizziness (unexplained light-headedness, even blackou
- Rapid or fluttering heartbeats
- Swelling, especially in ankles and/or lower legs
- Angina (chest pain)—a tightness in the chest often radia
  into your jaw or down your left arm

What to Do

See the recommendations for prevention under *Heart Diseas*
Diet: Just lowering total fat and increasing carbohydrates
ens heart health, especially in women. You need to increase the
types of fats, like those in fish. Fish consumption is inversely re
to sudden death from heart attack. Two hundred mg per day of l

Aspirin: Aspirin lowers risk for MI, but read pages 106 and 473. Other beneficial antiplatelet aggregate substances are bromelain (taken on an empty stomach) and/or turmeric and arginine.

Avoid: Cocaine—one forth of nonfatal heart attacks among those eighteen to forty-five years of age comes from using this drug. Stop smoking. Smoking cessation after heart attack significantly reduces risk of death. One large study suggests an increased risk of MIs within an hour of smoking marijuana.

Congestive Heart Failure

Congestive heart failure often follows a heart attack. It's a problem with the heart that causes fluid accumulation in the lungs, abdominal organs, and other tissues that produces a whole series of body reactions, such as stress on the kidneys.

Follow general heart rules in this section. Check DHEA (dehydroepiandrosterone), as lower levels are linked to oxidative stress and greater severity of this condition. Check testosterone too, as the heart is a giant muscle and testosterone helps it get stronger. Evaluate digestive enzymes (page 468) and supplement minerals lost through the use of diuretics. Avoid salt.

Nutrients

** If using diuretics, get more vitamins B_1 and B_{12}, magnesium, and potassium. Ideally, ask your doctor for slow IV magnesium pushes. Ironically, diuretics can lower B_{12} levels, and B_{12} deficiency symptoms can aggravate or mimic congestive heart failure. Omeprazole and lansoprazole may inhibit B_{12} absorption. Discuss supplementation with your doctor.

** Fat-soluble coenzyme Q-10, 100 mg two to three times a day with fatty meals

** L-arginine, 2–5 g per day

** Taurine, 1,500 mg twice a day on an empty stomach

** Vitamin B complex, 25–50 mg once or twice a day with extra B_1 and a multivitamin/mineral supplement

** Hawthorn berry extract, 80–300 mg two to three times a day, and garlic, 500 mg twice a day

** L-carnitine, 1,000 mg twice a day

HEART DISEASE
(Coronary Heart Disease, CHD)

Coronary heart disease is damage to or malfunction of the heart caused by narrowing or blockage of the coronary arteries (called *arteriosclerosis*, or hardening of the arteries), which supply blood to the heart muscle. It's found often in people with high cholesterol. When the arteries that bring the blood supply to the brain harden, this can cause a stroke, just as common a cause of death as cancer. When the arteries that supply the heart harden, a heart attack may occur. Most deaths from CHD are in people over sixty-five, but the foundation for the disease is laid in the teens and early adult life. *Plaque* refers to the fatty deposits along the walls of arteries that can cause blood clots to form; plaque deposition usually increases with age.

The best treatment for arteriosclerosis is prevention, before complications such as angina, heart attack, arrhythmias, heart failure, kidney failure, stroke, or obstructed peripheral arteries develop. Read books by Dr. Dean Ornish for guidelines on diet and lifestyle changes.

Symptoms: Arteriosclerosis produces no symptoms until the damage to the arteries is severe enough to restrict blood flow. Symptoms depend on where the arteriosclerosis develops, such as angina (chest pain) due to lack of oxygen to the heart or leg cramps while walking (intermittent claudication) due to lack of oxygen to the legs.

The following are symptoms of some of the major heart conditions:

Chest Pain: When muscles don't get enough blood (called *ischemia*), cramping results. *Angina* is a sensation of tightness or squeezing in the chest that comes when the heart, which is a muscle, doesn't get enough blood. (See *Angina Pectoris.*) *Pericarditis* is an inflammation of the sac that surrounds the heart, which causes pain that worsens when lying down and improves when sitting up and leaning forward. An *aneurysm* occurs when part of the aorta (the main heart artery) bulges out or tears, causing sudden severe pain, often felt in the back of the neck, between the shoulder blades, down the back, or in the abdomen. If the valve between parts of the heart bulges, there can be stabbing or needlelike pain centered below the left breast.

Shortness of Breath: In the early stages of heart failure, someone may be short of breath during physical exertion; as it worsens, shortness of breath occurs with less and less activity until it finally occurs at rest.

Fatigue: When the heart is pumping less efficiently, there is not enough blood flow to the muscles and a person feels weak and tired.

Palpitations and Heart Arrhythmias: The muscle fibers in the heart contract on a regular basis, controlled by a rhythmic electrical discharge that happens at a steady speed. A normal heart rate is usually between 52 and 70 beats per minute, although it can be lower in physically fit young adults. Heart rate is also influenced by circulating hormones—adrenaline, noradrenaline, and thyroid. *Tachycardia* means the heart rate is greater than 70 beats per minute; *bradycardia* means that the heart rate is less than 52 beats per minute. *Arrhythmias* happen when the electrical impulses travel in abnormal pathways, leading to abnormal heart rhythm (see *Arrhythmias*). *Atrial fibrillation* is an episodic or continuous racing of the heart. It may represent a predisposition to stroke. *Atrial tachycardia* means that the heart suddenly contracts too rapidly. It is associated with coronary artery disease.

Light-headedness and Fainting: A result of not enough blood flowing to the brain, often caused by an abnormal heart rate or rhythm, or if the pumping ability of the heart is impaired.

Causes: Arteriosclerosis causes plaque to form on artery walls, which become thicker and less elastic as a result. This is what narrows the channel and impairs blood flow. Risk factors include cigarette smoking, obesity (mid torso), high blood pressure, consistently low HDL (high-density lipoprotein) levels and/or high LDL (low-density lipoprotein), elevated triglycerides in association with low HDL, higher than normal blood sugar levels, physical inactivity, diabetes, Syndrome X (see page 300), insulin resistance, family history of coronary artery disease, and an anxious or aggressive personality.

Uniquely Female: Coronary heart disease (*atherosclerosis,* which is a form of arteriosclerosis) is the leading cause of death in women. Women in their reproductive years have a much lower risk of heart disease than men; in fact, their risk of death is equal to that of men ten years younger. This changes in menopausal woman, with heart disease becoming the number one cause of death. Overweight women, especially those who are "apple" shaped rather than "pear" shaped, are at greater risk. A woman's risk for heart disease increases if her father had a heart attack or stroke before the age of fifty or if her mother had one before age sixty-five. After menopause, a woman's HDL levels decrease and LDL levels go up, increasing the risk of high blood pressure and heart disease.

During pregnancy, the heart has to work harder to move an increased volume of blood at a faster rate through the blood vessels. The heart beats faster to do this. The additional strain begins at the eighth week of pregnancy and reaches a maximum at the thirtieth week. Symptoms that need to be checked by a doctor: becoming breathless, especially at night; excessive tiredness; coughing. Palpitations are common in pregnancy, especially when lying down. Palpitations of any kind can increase any time from midcycle to the first few days of the period due to hormonal fluctuations.

What to Do

- Determine your risk for heart disease through medical history, physical exams, and tests. Insist your doctor run the following tests before you start taking birth control pills or hormone replacement therapy (HRT) as predictors of CHD, heart attack (myocardial infarction), and stroke:

1. Lipid profile (good and bad cholesterol and their ratio)—very important
2. Homocysteine blood levels (page 269), very important. A 5 μmol/l increase in homocysteine is associated with a 70 percent increased risk of CHD and with a five-year mortality risk for CHD. High levels can be due to genetics or to low levels or deficiencies of vitamin B_{12}, folic acid, or vitamin B_6. Chronic diuretic use also increases homocysteine. HRT does lower levels, but it also raises C-reactive protein. Homocysteine levels can be normalized within a short period of time just by taking high-potency multivitamins!

ORAL CONTRACEPTIVE PILLS AND HORMONE REPLACEMENT THERAPY

There is a slight trend for increased levels of cholesterol, triglycerides, and bad (LDL) cholesterol in oral contraceptive users, which may not be as marked with the newer third-generation Pill. Women between the ages of thirty-five and fifty-four tend to have higher levels of most lipids when they're taking the Pill. Women between the ages of fifty-five and seventy-four on hormone replacement therapy (HRT) tend to have lower total cholesterol and LDL and higher HDL, but still have more clots and strokes and adverse cardiac events (especially in the first year of supplementation) than women not on HRT.

3. C-reactive protein (a marker of inflammation, which is now thought to be the initial promoter of artery damage). C-reactive protein was the strongest marker in a study of 28,263 women on the Pill and hormone replacement therapy.
4. Plasma fibrinogen

In addition:
- Have your blood pressure, cholesterol, and blood sugar monitored annually, or two to three times a year if abnormal.
- Have your thyroid function evaluated, and rule out subclinical hypothyroidism or hyperthyroidism. Low thyroid greatly increases the risk of clogged arteries and heart attacks in elderly women. But giving thyroid to heart disease patients can cause angina or heart attacks, so start low and build up slowly with strict supervision.
- After menopause, evaluate your need for hormonal therapy.
- Quit smoking. It decreases good cholesterol (HDL) and increases the bad (LDL); raises the level of carbon monoxide in the blood, which increases injury to the lining of the artery walls; constricts arteries; and increases the blood's tendency to clot.
- Exercise to make your heart stronger and lower your blood pressure, at least one hour of moderate exercise three times a week. Don't do heavy exercise after large meals, which in-

creases the risk of heart attack. Long-term moderate exercise like walking and resistance training improves heart function and quality of life for those with chronic heart failure.

- Lose excess weight. Obesity makes the heart work harder.
- If you are at high risk for heart disease, don't take HRT.
- Have your DHEA (dehydroepiandrosterone) level tested, as low levels make your lipids more prone to oxidation, but elevated levels may predispose you to heart disease.
- Alternate hot and cold showers to increase circulation.
- Laugh, and you may live longer. Those less likely to see the humor in life have higher risk of contracting heart disease.
- Women's hearts seem to be more vulnerable to stress than men's. Learn stress-management techniques, and do at least fifteen minutes a day of meditation or relaxation exercises (pages 52–58).

Diet: *Changing your diet and lifestyle can improve your blood levels of fats within three weeks.* Eat a lower fat diet with less animal and hydrogenated fats and more monounsaturated fats such as from olives and avocados. Consume lots of vegetables, fruits, and more fish. Take fish oil supplements, with an emphasis on DHA (docosahexaenoic acid)—the principle active component in fish oil for heart protection. One doctor in Scotland hands his heart patients tubs of marinated herring to eat. A Mediterranean-type diet (high in fish, legumes, vegetables, and monounsaturated fats like olive oil and low in saturated fats and animal foods) offers the greatest protection. See the section on diet under *Heart Attack.* Monounsaturated oils (like olive oil) together with fish and flaxseed oils help prevent oxidation of "bad" LDL cholesterol. Increase fiber intake, especially from whole-grain cereals for breakfast, as side dishes with main meals, and as whole-grain or sprouted-grain breads. Low fiber intake is associated with higher insulin levels, weight gain, and other CHD risk factors. Flavonoids (found in colorful foods like berries, vegetables, teas, and wine) reduce a woman's risk of death from CHD.

Eat foods rich in magnesium and potassium, such as fresh greens, sea vegetables, fruits, green tea, seafoods, brown rice, whole grains, garlic, and onions. Drink eight glasses of bottled or filtered water each day; chlorination destroys vitamin E in the body. Purple grape juice protects arteries and prevents oxidation of bad cholesterol. The Food and Drug Administration (FDA) has approved the health claim that soy is good for the heart. Eat sauces from tomato paste and drink tomato juice. Read about the *Pritikin* and *Ornish* diets if your case is severe.

Avoid: Salt, junk foods, refined or processed foods, hydrogenated oils (including margarine), coffee, tea, alcohol, red meat, homogenized milk, spicy foods. Cut down sugar and juices with added sugars to help lower blood triglyceride levels. Do not overconsume carbohydrates, even healthy ones. High egg consumption (two to three eggs daily) is under suspicion, especially in women with elevated blood sugar. If you eat eggs, cook them so the yolks don't break (this oxidizes the cholesterol), like in soft-boiled, hard-cooked, or poached eggs. Do not take iron unless you are anemic. Excess iron may be an important factor in starting the process of arterial plaquing. Do *not* reduce fats too low, which can actually increase the risk of heart disease (*Science News* 155:181, 1999). Remember, *the type of fats you eat is more important than reducing overall fat intake.*

Nutrients

- ** Taking a multivitamin/mineral supplement daily can reduce CHD by 25 percent, mostly because the B vitamins keep homocysteine levels normal. Make sure your supplement contains trace minerals like zinc, copper, selenium, chromium, and manganese.
- ** Vitamin E, 400–1,000 IU per day. Blood plasma levels of vitamin E are inversely related to plaquing of arteries, and adding vitamin E to a multivitamin supplement reduces CHD by 40 percent.
- ** Magnesium, 250 mg twice a day
- ** Vitamin B complex, should contain at least 50 mg vitamin B_6, and vitamin B_{12}, 400–1,000 mcg twice a day
- ** Fish oil (EPA [eicosapentaenoic acid] and DHA), 1–3 g per day in divided doses with meals
- ** Folic acid, 800 mcg–5 mg per day protects blood vessels.
- • Mixed carotenoids (some multivitamin/mineral supplements now come with carotenoids, so read labels)

- Vitamin A, 10,000 IU per day; vitamin A makes a hormone that regulates heart circadian rhythms (*Science News*, July 14:22, 2001).
- Coenzyme Q-10, 50–150 mg per day
- Vitamin C, 500–1,000 mg two or three times a day. Build up from low to higher doses. Keeps vessels flexible.
- Consider 1–3 mg melatonin at night.
- Ask your doctor about intravenous (IV) magnesium (page 471). Heart patients should *not* get IV calcium.
- For angina: take 1 g of astragalus twice a day, but not during acute phases of any kind of infection you may have.
- Arginine, 1–3 grams per day, acts as a natural blood thinner by reducing platelet stickiness.

Good Cholesterol: These are the high-density lipoproteins that protect your heart and arteries. A low glycemic diet (see *Insulin Resistance*) is directly related to optimal levels of HDLs. To help elevate HDLs, take pantethine, 300 mg two to four times a day; vitamin C, 2–3 g per day; magnesium, 300–500 mg per day; niacin, 100 mg per day; and lecithin, 2 capsules (19 grains each) three times a day.

Herbs: Hawthorn berry, 80–300 mg two to three times a day, or as liquid extract, ¼ tsp. twice a day, can be very helpful. Hawthorn and/or passionflower extract, along with exercise, reduces breathing difficulties. Hawthorn lowers cholesterol and may help reduce arrhythmia, increase circulation, decrease tension in blood vessels, and decrease platelet stickiness. Also ginkgo biloba, 60–80 mg twice a day, wheat germ oil caps, one raw clove of garlic a day in food, or 4,000 mcg allicin per day (garlic both prevents and regresses plaque).

Mitral Valve Prolapse (MVP)

A common diagnosis among healthy people in their thirties and forties, more frequent in women then men. Can cause palpitations and occasional dull chest pain, especially with fatigue or stress, although many women have no symptoms. Many of those with MVP have a heart murmur. MVP has been linked with a higher incidence of candidiasis-related complex and magnesium deficiency, and the three occurring together form a sort of syndrome. Turmeric (curcumin), 300–600 mg three times a day, helps lower levels of fibrinogen (thought to damage blood vessels) and prevent platelets from forming clots, as does 1–3 g of arginine a day.

What to Do
- ** Magnesium, 250 mg three to four times a day or more (less if stools get loose)
- ** Coenzyme Q-10, 10–60 mg two to three times a day
- ** Vitamin B complex, 50–100 mg per day
- ** L-carnitine, 500 mg two to three times a day
- ** Have an echocardiogram to rule out *valve regurgitation.* If you have this condition, take antibiotics before any dental procedures.
- ** Rule out overactive thyroid.
- ** Rule out candida-related complex.
- ** Have a chiropractor or osteopath check for problems with your musculoskeletal and nervous systems.
- • Get enough sleep.
- • Develop good stress-management skills; see mind-body techniques (pages 52–58).

HEMORRHOIDS (Piles)

Varicose veins in the lining of the anus, either near the beginning of the anal canal *(internal hemorrhoids)* or at the anal opening *(external hemorrhoids).* Sometimes the internal hemorrhoids protrude outside the anus *(prolapsing hemorrhoids).*

Symptoms: Swelling or a soft lump at the anus, sometimes accompanied by pain and itching; passing mucus after a bowel movement; streaks of bright-red blood on the toilet paper or on the stool. The water in the toilet may also be reddish from blood.

Causes: Constipation; excessive straining during bowel movements; sitting too long on hard surfaces; sedentary lifestyle; eating too many sweets and not enough fiber; abdominal muscle strain; excess weight; liver problems; genetics.

Uniquely Female: Very common during pregnancy and immediately after childbirth due to increased pressure in the veins of the anus. To prevent or relieve hemorrhoids during pregnancy, lie on your left side for twenty minutes every four to six hours to decrease the pressure on the main vein draining the lower half of the body. Constipation is reported twice as often by women as by men.

What to Do

- Rest with your legs and pelvis higher than your heart.
- To relieve pain, take a hot sitz bath (soaking in a tub of hot water that covers the hips and abdomen) for twenty minutes three times a day. Add yarrow to the bathwater.
- To relieve itching, bathe anal area in infusion of chervil (one handful per quart of water).
- Apply an ice pack to the anal area if the hemorrhoid is swollen and painful.
- Clean the anal area gently with soft, moist toilet paper after each bowel movement.
- Soak a cotton ball in chilled witch hazel and apply to the anus—one of the best remedies for external hemorrhoids, especially if they bleed.
- Avoid sitting or standing for long periods of time. If the hemorrhoid is painful, lie down as much as possible.
- Try to establish a regular pattern of bowel movements at the same time every day.
- Don't try to hurry bowel movements and don't strain. Use a stool softener if necessary.
- Lose excess weight.
- Exercise regularly.
- Hemorrhoids that bleed profusely or are extremely painful may require surgery.

Diet: High-fiber diet with fresh fruits and vegetables, oat and bran cereal, whole-grain bread, and brown rice. Drink plenty of water, at least six to eight glasses a day. Drink Fiber Cocktail (page 464) twice a day for two weeks, then reduce to once a day.

Avoid: Excess caffeine, refined foods, and spicy foods. *Laxatives to avoid during pregnancy:* Castor oil, Ex-Lax, Phillip's M-O, mineral oil, Peri-Colace, and Purge. See my book *Healthy Digestion the Natural Way* (John Wiley, 2000) for more details.

Nutrients
- ** Flaxseed oil, 1 Tbsp. per day. Balance with vitamin E, 400 IU per day.
- ** Rutin, 500 mg twice a day
- Aloe (in the form of liquid aloe extract), ½ cup two or three times a day
- Magnesium, 250 mg three times a day
- Vitamin B complex, 50 mg twice a day

Herbs: For recurrent hemorrhoids, take liver decongestants (milk thistle, 280–420 mg per day, and/or yellow dock, 2 capsules two to three times a day for one month). Horse chestnut, 50–75 mg twice a day. Ointments and suppositories that include butcher's broom are helpful.

HERPES

Herpes simplex is a common viral disease in two forms: *Type I,* associated with infections of the lips, mouth, and face (see *Canker Sores*) and *Type II,* associated with infections of the genitals (see *Sexually Transmitted Diseases*). Both are contagious and spread by direct contact with the lesions or the fluid from the lesions. *Herpes zoster* is an infection of the nerves that supply certain areas of the skin (see *Shingles*) and comes from the chicken pox virus.

HOMOCYSTEINE

A sulfur amino acid normally produced within our bodies from the essential amino acid methionine. In a healthy body, homocysteine is recycled back into methionine or broken down further into cystathionine. In some, these mechanisms are genetically impaired, or certain nutrients (B vitamins) that enhance these processes are lacking. Elevated levels of homocysteine (above 14 μmol/l) are being connected to coronary heart disease, stroke, diabetes (especially with increased risk of death in type 2), hypertension, underactive thyroid, cognitive problems, venous clots, bone loss, severity of cervical dysplasia, epilepsy, problems during pregnancy (especially neural tube defects), bowel diseases such as Crohn's disease and ulcerative colitis, as well as Alzheimer's disease. Homocysteine can be measured by a blood test.

Causes: Abnormally high levels of homocysteine occur from missing certain genes or from B vitamin deficiencies (vitamin B_{12}, folic acid, and vitamin B_6), as well as various stressors: alcohol abuse, smoking, taking niacin or SAMe (S-adenosyl-methione) without other B vitamins, underactive thyroid, chronic diuretic use, and possibly excessive consumption of coffee. These stressors block the body's normal methods of detoxifying homocysteine. Anger and hostility have been linked to increased homocysteine levels and may be one way personality traits are linked to heart disease risk. Higher levels of homocysteine may occur more often in some patients with untreated low thyroid.

Uniquely Female: Blood levels of homocysteine should be tested on women as part of their yearly checkup (along with lipid profiles) to monitor heart disease

> Insist your doctor test homocysteine levels as part of your annual checkup and during pregnancy.

risk, and before oral contraceptives or hormone replacement therapy is prescribed. Elevated levels of homocysteine may be a side effect of taking synthetic hormones as well as a predictor of complications of pregnancy such as preeclampsia, spontaneous abortion, and placental abruption. These events are linked to nearly 30,000 infant deaths before age one in the United States as well as birth defects. Moderately high levels of homocysteine in the general population are linked to plaquing in arteries and thickened arterial walls, which are not good.

Diet: Eat foods that help metabolize homocysteine, such as green veggies, unrefined and unprocessed grains, and brewer's yeast. A balanced diet with generous amounts of fruits and vegetables lowers homocysteine levels.

Nutrients: Homocysteine levels can be rapidly reduced to normal through supplementation with B vitamins (found in B complexes, 25–50 mg per day), vitamin B_{12}, folic acid, and vitamin B_6, and by avoiding the above-mentioned stressors. When these measures don't work, betaine (3–6 g per day) and choline (1 g twice a day) can help.

HORMONE DISRUPTORS

Chemicals from outside the body that can mimic or alter the action of our own hormones and cause various irreversible adverse health effects in some children and adults. Mixtures of chemicals or the breakdown products of chemical metabolism in our bodies may also disrupt our natural hormones. Presently recognized as hormone disruptors are some components of plastics (phthalates, bisphenol A); some ingredients in detergents (APEs and NPEs) and personal care products; persistent organic pollutants, such as dioxins; polychlorinated biphenyls (PCBs); polyvinyl chloride; many pesticides and fungicides; PAHs (polycyclic aromatic hydrocarbons) from incomplete combustion of petrochemical products, wood, arsenic, and tobacco; and metals, such as lead, cadmium, mercury, and arsenic (semi-metal).

The science investigating hormone disruption is new. *We presently think that the most significant exposure to hormone disrupting chemicals occurs to the unborn child in the womb (especially at the end of the first trimester).* This exposure comes from the chemicals in the body of the mother, and what she has been exposed to through daily living. Certain populations may be more sensitive to chemicals that mimic hormones, such as those with underlying thyroid disease and the elderly.

Hormone disruptors are being examined in relation to various diseases and conditions, such as Parkinson's disease, diabetes, hormonal cancers, the age of onset of puberty and menarche; behavior in children, such as hyperactivity, stress-coping skills, academic performance; IQ; sperm count; infertility; female disorders, such as endometriosis and fibroids; and autoimmune diseases.

Uniquely Female: Environmental estrogens in particular may have adverse effects on women who already have ample if not excessive levels of estrogen in their systems. See *Estrogen Dominance*. Many natural and man-made chemicals can act to increase estrogen-like activity or can block the other hormones that help maintain normal estrogen levels. In order to have a thorough understanding of your own hormonal situation before embarking on any hormonal treatments, you need to take into account your exposure to hormone disruptors. This information is particularly important if you are planning to become pregnant or are thinking about taking birth control pills, fertility treatments, or hormone replacement therapy. Hormone disruptors are now being identified in the amniotic fluid of healthy pregnant women.

Our constant exposure to chemicals overloads our systems, leaving us more susceptible to hormonal fluctuations and the effect of stress. Avoid exposure as much as possible. Read my book *Hormone Deception* (Contemporary/McGraw-Hill, 2000) for more information.

HORMONE REPLACEMENT THERAPY

When hormones start lowering and/or going out of balance in menopause or perimenopause and women start experiencing uncomfortable symptoms, they have choices about treatments. The first level revolves around lifestyle changes, including exercise, diet, nutrition, and herbs (see *Menopause*). The next level is using natural hormone replacement therapy, or, for women who don't respond to that, standard hormone replacement therapy.

When considering hormonal therapy, either natural or synthetic, doctors should first take a detailed history of how the woman feels, then run a baseline test of her hormones before starting supplementation (see appendix A). After six to eight weeks of taking supplemental hormones, a woman should see her doctor again, report how she feels, and, ideally, rerun the same test. This is proper monitoring.

Why do this? Women vary widely in how much of a hormone they require to feel their best and vary considerably in their response to treatment. For example, most women on progesterone supplemen-

Note that if you insist on having your replacement therapy covered by insurance, you will probably need to choose traditional hormonal pharmaceuticals. If you have a history of any kind of liver disease or risk of cancers, you may opt not to take creams, since they must come in higher dosages and mildly stress the liver.

The doctor's job is to protect you from unopposed estrogen. Don't take estrogen by itself, even if you no longer have a uterus. Progesterone and DHEA are estrogen's natural balancers, so have levels of progesterone run in saliva tests and DHEA tests.

Never go off hormones cold-turkey; taper off over several months.

tation will experience improvement of their progesterone-to-estrogen ratios and will feel better. However, a few actually will have increased estrogenic stimulation after taking progesterone, meaning progesterone isn't good for this particular woman. This would be found only with competent monitoring. Remember that no laboratory test is perfect, certainly not in the field of hormone testing. *Women should always be treated by how they feel, along with test monitoring, never just on test results alone.*

Signs of Low Estrogen
- Dry eyes (may be present with intermittent tearing)
- Begin to develop vertical lines round the lips
- Difficulty wearing contact lenses
- Dry mouth
- Dry vagina
- Hot flashes (possibly with cold flashes in between). Hot flashes probably occur because of relative drops in estrogen, so you can have normal blood levels but still have "heavy duty" hot flashes.
- Blood cholesterol levels start to rise, while good cholesterol—high-density lipoprotein (HDL)—may begin to lower.

Signs of Low Testosterone
- Low libido
- Fatigue

- Loss of muscle mass
- Bone loss

Testosterone is one hormone that usually wanes more slowly than the others, but not in all women.

For signs of other low hormones, see *Perimenopause*.

For low estrogen, try either estrogenic herbs (see *Menopause*) or natural estrogens (estriol with estradiol). Many doctors avoid using estrone since some studies link it to breast cancer, but not all agree. Check testosterone with a blood test. Testosterone replacement comes in creams. Do not use methyltestosterone, which has been shown to cause prostate cancer. Even though women don't have prostates, a known carcinogen isn't good for ladies, either.

If you choose to take any form of estrogen, it is best if you get an ultrasound before starting any hormonal program, synthetic or natural; then get another ultrasound six to eight weeks after starting your program to see what is happening to the lining of your uterus. If your uterus increases 5 mm or more, this greatly increases your risk of cancer, and your hormone replacement needs to be changed. Even though progestins reduce the risk of endometrial cancer, they don't prevent it 100 percent.

Standard Hormone Replacement Therapy

Initially women were put on estrogens, and this therapy was called estrogen replacement therapy. However, many women began to develop uterine cancer. Since progesterone opposes or balances the action of estrogen, progesterone was then added to the formula to minimize the risk of *uterine* cancer, although the recent use of cyclical progestins doesn't seem to protect against endometrial cancer as much as continual use. However, progesterone was added in synthetic form, called progestins; the most common progestin now being used is called Provera. The combination was called hormone replacement therapy, or HRT.

Approximately one-third of women between the ages of forty-five and sixty-five are on HRT, making female hormones the number-one-selling drug in the United States, as well as in the world. In America, more than 20 million prescriptions for Premarin are dispensed annually. The most commonly prescribed hormone replacement therapy is a low-dose synthetic estrogen like Premarin, made from horses' urine, along with Provera.

Despite the incredible volume of hormones being prescribed and taken, there are still real questions about hormone supplementation. The answers must come from each individual woman, taking into account her family and personal health history. With traditional HRT, giving only one or two hormones can actually unbalance a woman's complex hormonal system.

HRT and Heart Disease

HRT is officially approved only for the treatment of menopausal symptoms and to protect bones, but most doctors have earnestly believed that it helps women live longer and better by protecting against bone loss and heart disease. At least that was the story until July 24, 2001—the day the American Heart Association announced that women who have heart disease should *not* go on HRT, and other women shouldn't count on HRT to protect against heart disease.

Years ago, the National Heart, Lung, and Blood Institute launched a study, called the Women's Health Initiative, to figure out what HRT was actually doing for women (by randomly assigning 27,000 women to either HRT or placebo and watching what happened). In July 2001, four years into the eight-and-a-half-year study, they found the HRT group had more heart attacks, strokes, and blood clots than women on placebo. Both life-threatening clots in deep veins (thromboembolism) and clots in the lungs (pulmonary embolism) increased with HRT. These findings confirmed the preliminary results of the PEPI study

---

In human blood the estrogen ratios are estriol, 60–80 percent; estrone, 10–20 percent; and estradiol, 10–20 percent.

In Premarin the hormone ratios are estrone, 75–80 percent; equilin, 5–6 percent; and estradiol and others, 5–19 percent.

 Natural Hormone Replacement Therapy for Women Over 45,
by Jonathan V. Wright, M.D., and
John Morgenthaler (Smart Publications,1997)

(Postmenopausal Estrogen and Progestin Intervention trial done by the National Heart, Lung, and Blood Institute), which showed that healthy women on HRT had more heart problems, clots, and gallbladder disease than women on placebo (even though their cholesterol levels went down). Dr. Alan R. Gaby was one of the first doctors to publish warnings about this back in 1994.

Earlier studies on HRT are now recognized as biased: HRT was given to women generally known to be healthier, more compliant, with no histories of heart disease or estrogenic cancers, etc. The new test results don't make HRT look like the panacea it was once thought to be. Based on the latest information, the American College of Cardiologists said that *HRT should not be recommended to treat heart disease.* Other research also suggests that women who have any damage to their arteries (and most women in their forties, fifties, and sixties, if not younger, already have some vascular damage) may have this damage worsened by HRT. Why is that? One theory (based on a number of studies) shows that estrogen can sometimes promote inflammation, and heart disease is now thought to be partially, if not mostly, due to inflammation.

Dose: If you use oral conjugated estrogens, take 0.3 mg per day, as 0.625 mg or greater and in combination with progestin may increase your risk of stroke (*Annals of Internal Medicine* 133:933–41, 2000).

HRT and Breast Cancer

Synthetic progesterone, called *progestins* (specifically medroxyprogesterone acetate, or MPA), used in standard HRT has been shown to increase significantly the risk of breast cancer over and above the modest increase already recognized with prolonged use of HRT. But well-run studies have shown that Provera increases the risk of *breast* cancer by as much as 30 percent. This means that for every 1,000 women on traditional HRT (Premarin and Provera), 30 will eventually develop breast cancer from taking it. Some studies suggest that adding synthetic progestins to estrogen has also blocked some of the protective effects of estrogen—like protecting cognition (thinking and memory). *Research has not yet found similar problems with natural progesterone.*

It appears that progestins intensify the action of estrogen on breast estrogen receptors, causing a form of hormone disruption, and may also promote some adverse heart effects. Progestins are associated with a number of other adverse reactions, such as bleeding, loss of menstruation, bloating, feeling poorly, sleepiness, and altered glucose tolerance. Provera causes mammary tumors in dogs. Even though it has not been shown to do this in humans, this is a more than worrisome finding.

Women with hormonal cancers have historically been guided to avoid HRT. New studies suggest that taking hormones five years after diagnosis may not increase risk of recurrence or death. However, the National Toxicology Program clearly stated in 2001 that estrogens are carcinogens. Some new designer estrogens don't affect the breast, and estriol is thought to be gentler on breast tissue than estradiol in conventional HRT. This is a confusing issue that must be dealt with on an individual basis with much discussion with several doctors. Some doctors even suggest *natural* progesterone protects against breast cancer, while others disagree (*Molecular and Cellular Biochemistry* 202:53–61, 1999).

Nonhormonal treatments for hot flashes for breast cancer patients could be herbs, diet (see *Menopause*), or nonestrogenic drugs.

HRT and Longevity

Doctors have been led to believe that HRT increases longevity because some studies show that women on HRT live longer. This turns out to be mostly in women on HRT with heart disease who die less often from heart attacks but who get *more* heart attacks (at least during the first year of being on HRT, along with increased risk of stroke and dangerous clots). The improved longevity for most women diminishes over time (about ten years) as more women start to die of breast cancer. But when women on HRT get breast cancer, they appear to get kinder forms and have better survival rates. Then again, who wants *any* kind of breast cancer? As a population, women on HRT are often healthier, followed more closely, and take better care of themselves. So is it the HRT or these other factors that are promoting longevity? Studies clearly show that a daily multivitamin/mineral reduces heart disease by 25 percent (and adding extra vitamin E improves this to a 40 percent reduction), so why take synthetic HRT for the heart when it puts our hearts, breasts, and gallbladders at such risk?

HRT and Thyroid Medication

L-thyroxine, in dosages that are too high, *suppresses* the pituitary and negates the benefits of HRT on bones. If you are taking both HRT and thyroid medication, get yearly thyroid and TSH (thyroid-stimulating hormone) tests. Weight gain on estrogens suggests a sluggish thyroid.

HRT and Osteoporosis, see *Osteoporosis*.

DES Daughters

Tell your doctor you are a DES (diethylstilbestrol) daughter before you are given HRT. Studies suggest 67 percent of pregnant women were not told they were given DES. Call DES Action (800-DES-9288) for more information. See *DES Daughters*.

Common Side Effects of Standard HRT
- Resumption of menstrual cycle
- Spotting
- Stomach upset and nausea
- Fluid retention
- Swollen breasts, mastitis (breast infections), nipple sensitivity, cyst formation, and denser breast hard to read on mammograms
- Vaginal pain
- Skin pigmentation changes
- Leg and uterine cramps
- Harder-to-read mammograms
- Weight gain
- Asthma
- Gallbladder problems

Words of Warning: The Benefits of HRT Are Not What Many Doctors Think!

Sally McNagny, M.D., former associate professor of medicine, Emory University, says: "Estrogen has been removed by the FDA as treatment for osteoporosis, even though most doctors aren't aware of this. The American Association of Clinical Endocrinologists' Guidelines no longer lists estrogen as a first-priority medication to prevent bone loss. The Women's Health Initiative found a small but significant increased risk of cardiovascular disease (stroke and heart disease) after patients were on HRT for two years. A *randomized* trial shows HRT increases urinary incontinence." (Grady, D., et al., *Obstetrics and Gynecology* 97:116–20, 2001; Manson, J., et al. *New England Journal of Medicine* 345:34–40, 2001)

The bottom line is that the *only* uses for HRT are: 1) for symptom relief, to be taken *no longer than five years;* and 2) prevention of bone loss when other medications aren't tolerated. *All* other women should avoid HRT because it may make them prone to blood clots, possible breast cancer, increased urinary incontinence, heart problems, possible uterine bleeding, headaches, and possible increases in asthma symptoms—not to mention the high cost of the regimen. *Findings about risks of HRT are recent, so many physicians are unaware of them.*

Dr. John A. Blakely, cardiologist at Women's College Health Sciences Center in Toronto, Ontario, adds: "There's risk that women *without* coronary heart disease might experience even greater net harm from HRT." (*Archives of Internal Medicine* 160:2897–2900, 2000).

Appropriate individualized choices must be made. Ask about customized therapies; tri-estrogens—natural compounded estrogens often combined with hormones such as progesterone, DHEA (dehydroepiandrosterone), and testosterone; or try herbs and diet, or request Premarin with *natural* progesterone. Ask!

Natural Hormone Replacement Therapy (NHRT)

Menopause is not just a time of lowered levels of estrogen. Other hormone levels—such as those of progesterone, DHEA, and sometimes testosterone—may drop at this time. NHRT (also called bio-identical replacement therapy) involves supplementing with compounds that have the *exact* molecular structure of our body's own natural hormones, unlike synthetic hormones, which can be patented because they have been altered in some way. The sensible approach to hormone supplementation is to test for *all* the hormones and keep a balance among them all, making sure to supply the gentler hormone estriol. NHRT uses the three major estrogens (tri-estrogens) along with natural progesterone (first popularized by John R. Lee, M.D.) and other hormones if needed. In 1982, Jonathan V. Wright, M.D., started the first clinical treatments with triple estrogen and DHEA (which couldn't even be found in the United States at the time), and sometimes testosterone.

Studies are showing that these natural hormones, while weaker, have protective actions similar to those of traditional HRT. One study of sixty-eight postmenopausal women showed that estriol (2 mg per day continuously) effectively reduced hot flashes, night sweats, and insomnia without risking the harmful effects of estradiol (*Maturitas* 34:169–77, 2000). Therapy with natural progesterone has been effective for contraception, maintaining pregnancy, premenopausal bleeding disorders, endometriosis, mood disorders and premenstrual syndrome (PMS), and in HRT. In studies so far, natural progesterone does not seem to create adverse effects on heart and breasts. Dr. Wright reminds us that these hormones need more testing and research on humans. As 50 million women in America reach menopause in the next few years, there will be the impetus to do so. Read *Natural Hormone Replacement for Women Over 45,* by Jonathan V. Wright, M.D., and John Morgenthaler (Smart Publications, 1997).

To Find a Doctor Who Will Prescribe Natural Hormones: These natural hormones need to be prescribed by a doctor or nurse practitioner and ordered from compounding pharmacies. The beauty of compounding hormone replacement therapies is that the doctor can take a detailed history and order the pharmacist to make a customized program for you. Look for medical or osteopathic doctors who are members of the American College for Advancement in Medicine (ACAM). Call 800-532-3688 for a doctor in your area. In some states, nurse practitioners may also prescribe hormones. If you insist on getting insurance reimbursement, you may have to choose traditional hormonal pharmaceuticals, although more insurance companies are covering natural compounded hormones these days.

How Some Holistic Doctors Treat Hot Flashes: Before starting on a maintenance topical program: ¼ to ½ tsp. progesterone cream (containing 3 percent progesterone) daily, four times in the hour immediately following a hot flash.

Hormones That Help Hot Flashes: Progesterone, testosterone, estrogen, DHEA, and pregnanolone. Often doctors will give one or several of these hormones to treat menopausal symptoms.

Oral Versus Topical Hormone Replacement

If you have a history of any kind of liver disease or heightened risk of hormonal cancers, you may opt to use creams. Oral (ingested) progesterone has to go through digestion. Therefore, oral doses must be ten times greater than those of topicals to create the same amount of blood and saliva progesterone after digestion. A typical dose of oral progesterone is 200 mg, while that of a topical is around 20 mg. Oral administration of any hormone produces a mild but real stress on the liver, compared to that of skin application. However, some women just can't adjust to dermal application versus popping a capsule.

According to Dr. John Lee, researcher and author on progesterone, the oral form may be better than the topical form in some cases of PMS and postpartum depression. This is because the oral form produces more of a metabolite called *allopregnanolone*—a brain-calming substance. If too much oral progesterone is used, mental sluggishness can occur.

HORMONES

All life is about communication. In the body's Internet system, hormones deliver the e-mail information that coordinates major bodily functions and activities. These messages are received mostly by proteins called receptors. The endocrine system is made up of a group of glands that produce and secrete hormones directly into the bloodstream. The endocrine glands are the hypothalamus, pituitary, thyroid, parathyroid, the islets of the pancreas, the adrenals, and the gonads (testes and ovaries). During pregnancy, the placenta also acts as an endocrine gland.

The hormones that are discussed in this book are primarily those that regulate sexual function—the sex steroids (estrogens, progesterone, testosterone, and dehydroepiandrosterone)—but also included are the thyroid and adrenal hormones. However, scientists now understand that hormones, even sexual ones, regulate numerous and varied functions. For example, the female and male hormones—estrogens and androgens—affect various functions, such as determining what gender the fetus will become and how well our short- and long-term memories work.

Hormones connect the dots of many of our body's internal systems, thus their effects and dynamics are highly individual, depending on many facets of our body's unique makeup. For example, the number of hormone receptors we have varies from person to person, as well as from organ to organ. So when using therapies containing any kind of hormone, no treatment can be completely standardized or generalized. Each woman must be tested and monitored.

See appendix A for information on hormone testing and supplementation.

Adrenal Hormones

The adrenal glands sit on top of the kidneys. The inner adrenal gland (*medulla*) produces and secretes epinephrine and norepinephrine, known as *adrenaline* and *noradrenaline*, the "fight or flight" hormones. The outer portion *(cortex)* produces and secretes *hydrocortisone* and *cortisol*, the body's natural cortisone-like steroids. Cortisol is important when the body is dealing with inflammation, stress, metabolism of carbohydrates, healing, and maintaining blood pressure. Another adrenal hormone, *aldosterone*, influences the blood pressure by maintaining the body's potassium and sodium balance. The adrenal glands also produce sex hormones like testosterone and dehydroepiandrosterone (DHEA). See *Adrenal Insufficiency and Adrenal Fatigue*.

Adrenal "burnout" or fatigue, a common condition found in today's stressful society, is not an outright organic condition frequently recognized by most physicians, but it does exist. Symptoms

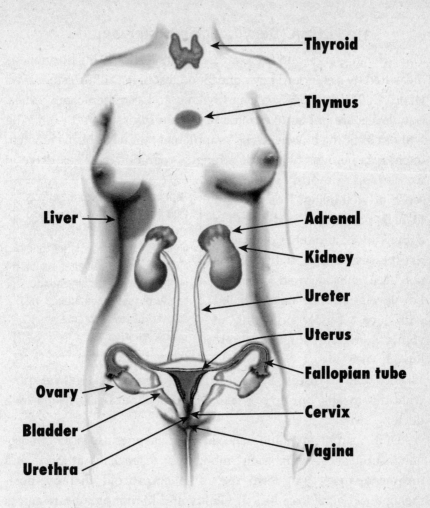

include: fatigue, especially in the morning, after exercise, or after orgasm; using sugar and caffeine to pull you out of "low-energy slumps"; insomnia; inability to lose weight; craving junk food; urinating several times a night; irritability, anxiety, depression, hopelessness, or loss of passion and creativity; common female problems like premenstrual syndrome (PMS); and dependence on antidepressants. Get your adrenal hormone levels tested (see *Adrenal Insufficiency and Adrenal Fatigue*), work with a holistic physician to identify your solutions, and read *Tired of Being Tired,* by Jesse Hanley, M.D. (Putnam, 2001).

DHEA (Dehydroepiandrosterone)

The adrenal glands and the ovaries secrete DHEA. This hormone is measured by a standard hormone blood test of its sulfate ester called DHEA-S. DHEA has weak androgenic and estrogenic properties. Low levels are linked to aging and certain diseases, and exercising without building muscle. DHEA supplementation has been shown to increase bone density, muscle strength, cognition, and sex drive in women and to improve a woman's sense of well-being. It is thought to help protect the body against aging, cancer, and other degenerative processes, although this has not been substantiated clinically. Low levels of DHEA are associated with breast cancer occurring in young women, and high levels are linked with breast and ovarian cancer and heart disease in older women. Researchers don't yet know what this means, but do not take DHEA without being tested by a doctor.

> Remember that hormone effects vary from woman to woman, so always get a baseline test before you start supplementation and always then repeat after six to eight weeks to carefully monitor results of supplementation. Oral contraceptives suppress DHEA levels.

DHEA supplementation should be considered in cases of adrenal insufficiency, depression, moodiness (especially at peri- and postmenopause), long-term use of glucocorticoid therapy, postmenopausal bone loss, loss of vitality and libido, premature aging, lupus, and chronic stress. Under stress, levels of the adrenal hormone cortisol rise while DHEA levels go down, both of which can have adverse health effects. Supplementation with DHEA lowers cortisol levels, which is a good thing since chronically high cortisol levels are associated with various health risks such as cancer, depression, and insomnia. It may improve mood and fatigue in patients with human immunodeficiency virus (HIV) infection. DHEA doses for women start at 5 mg per day and gradually build to 15 mg per day, taken three to seven days per week.

DHEA may be contraindicated in patients with hypertension. Very large doses have been associated with masculinizing side effects, such as increased body hair growth. Conflicting studies show both increased and lowered incidence of breast and ovarian cancer with high amounts of DHEA. One woman taking 150 mg per day developed liver problems. Play it safe and don't take large doses. DHEA most often is contraindicated for those with a history of hormonally responsive cancers.

DHEA used to be thought to increase estrogen. Several studies as of the writing of this book demonstrate that DHEA may lower estrogen and elevate testosterone in some women, while doing the opposite in men.

Estrogen

"Estrogen" is an umbrella term for various forms of this family of female sex hormones. The three most well-known and studied are *estrone, estradiol,* and *estriol,* named for the number of hydroxyl groups (pairs of hydrogen and oxygen atoms) attached to the main body of the hormone. Estr*o*ne has one, estra*d*iol two, and es*t*riol three. Men and women both have estrogens, just in different quantities. Since hormones are active in tiny amounts, even minuscule imbalances make a difference. Natalie Angier explains in her book *Woman: An Intimate Geography* (Anchor, 1999) that if we drained the blood of a quarter of a million premenopausal women we'd only get 1 tsp. of estradiol. What a powerful spoonful that is! Men depend on estrogen (as well as on male hormones) for the development of their maleness as much as women depend on estrogen for their femaleness.

Elevated levels of estrogen is a risk factor for various hormonally driven diseases, such as breast and uterine cancer and fibroids. See *Estrogen Dominance.* Estrogens were named as a carcinogen in 2001 by the National Toxicology Program. Take this into consideration when planning any synthetic hormone treatment. Estrogen is metabolized in the liver to various metabolites, some of which may be protective against cancer (2-hydroxyestrone estrogen) and some of which may promote cancer (4- and 16-alpha-hydroxyestrone estrogens). Exercise, protein, cruciferous veggies (high in indole-3-carbinol), and soy appear to increase the protective estrogen metabolites. This is an area of new research.

Plant hormones, such as those in soy and flaxseed, are called *phytoestrogens*.

Melatonin

This hormone is released from the brain's pineal gland during nighttime hours. Its production does not decline with age as it does with most hormones. Studies are associating abnormally low levels of melatonin with numerous health conditions from cancers to heart disease and depression. In the future we will probably test melatonin levels to see if replacement therapy is needed. Melatonin has a host of functions, including being a very potent antioxidant, enhancing thought processes, and regulating brain cell activity and the body's internal clock. It also has anticonvulsive properties.

If we spend hours at night in front of big screen TVs, computer screens, or with reading lights on, there is less time for the body to produce melatonin. Decreased melatonin results in overproduction of hormones like estrogen, which can promote hormonally associated diseases. Prolonged use of certain drugs, such as aspirin, ibuprofen, and beta-blockers, inhibits melatonin release. To increase melatonin levels, sleep in a completely darkened room. Pregnant or nursing mothers should avoid using melatonin. Melatonin supplementation may worsen rheumatoid arthritis.

Progesterone

Progesterone is formed in the ovaries, adrenal glands, placenta, and glial cells in the central nervous system, but it is present in its highest concentrations in the ovarian corpus luteum (the scar on the ovary where an egg was released). It gets the lining of the uterus ready to host the fertilized egg. The cessation of progesterone is crucial for the onset of menstruation. During pregnancy, the placenta makes progesterone, which maintains the pregnancy.

Progesterone needs to be in proper ratio with estrogen during the reproductive years for optimal effects of both hormones, and to offset health problems from estrogen dominance. Dr. John Lee says the balance between estradiol and progesterone is more important than levels of either hormone alone. Progesterone helps make other hormones, usually protects breasts from abnormal changes, is a natural diuretic, helps burn fat for energy, is a natural antidepressant, normalizes blood clotting, and enhances libido, blood sugar, and zinc and copper levels.

Signs of inadequate progesterone levels are: fibrocystic breasts, ovarian cysts, premenstrual syndrome (PMS), dry skin, high blood pressure, infertility, miscarriages, low thyroid, water retention, midcycle pains, osteoporosis, and some hot flashes. Supplementing progesterone takes two to three months for full effectiveness. Stress lowers progesterone levels.

Too much progesterone *may* cause: depression, sleep disorders, loose ligaments, chin acne, hair loss, and thigh pain. Test levels with saliva or twenty-four-hour urine tests.

Exposure to environmental estrogens in utero may damage follicle cells (cells that make eggs) in the ovaries. When a child becomes a menstruating woman, the damaged follicle may produce the necessary progesterone for only two to three days, rather than twelve to fourteen days of the second half of the cycle, as well as not making enough during the first six to eight weeks of pregnancy. This may be a leading cause of estrogen-driven problems, such as early miscarriages, fibroids, endometriosis, PMS, and others.

Prolactin

This pituitary hormone is controlled by *dopamine,* a substance formed in the hypothalamus. In pregnancy, prolactin levels rise and, once the baby is born, suckling produces a rapid increase in prolactin. The main function of prolactin is to stimulate the production of milk in the breasts, but it also acts on the ovaries. Elevated levels of unopposed estrogen or tumors in the pituitary gland may increase a woman's level of prolactin. Elevated levels of prolactin contribute to the symptoms of PMS and the risk of breast cancer and may possibly worsen the symptoms of menopause. Studies suggest that women exposed to the powerful estrogen drug diethylstilbestrol (DES) in the womb may make more prolactin. Whether other environmental hormone disruptors do this or not remains a question.

Testosterone

This sex hormone is found in both men and women, although women have much smaller amounts. Despite its small presence, it is an important hormone for women. There are receptors for testosterone all over the body, even in the brain and heart. Testosterone helps regulate cholesterol, improve surveillance of the immune system, keep sturdy bones, make muscle and red blood cells, and promotes a healthy sex drive. Women in peri- and postmenopausal years who lose their sex drive may be experiencing a deficiency of testosterone. This may be particularly true for women who have had their ovaries surgically removed. Have a doctor test your testosterone blood levels. Your body can make its own testosterone from DHEA, so many holistic doctors first recommend giving menopausal women DHEA if their levels of testosterone are low. If it is still too low after several weeks, consider supplemental testosterone. Women usually need from 5–25 mg per day of DHEA to see results. If you have had a hormonal disease like estrogen-receptor-positive breast cancer, *do not* take DHEA without a doctor's supervision.

Thyroid, see *Thyroid*

HYSTERECTOMY

Removal of the uterus. One of the most frequently performed operations in the United States, it's used most often to treat fibroids and cancer of the uterus or cervix; to relieve excessive bleeding or endometriosis; or to remove a severely prolapsed uterus. A *simple hysterectomy* removes the uterus and cervix; a *subtotal* removes the uterus and leaves the cervix. A *total hysterectomy* in medical terms is removal of the uterus, but in the lay community it has come to mean removing the uterus along with the fallopian tubes and ovaries. A *radical hysterectomy* also removes the pelvic lymph nodes in cases of advanced cancer. If your cervix and ovaries are left in, this may help with sexual lubrication and also avoiding urinary incontinence in the future. Hysterectomies increase the risk of urinary incontinence in women over sixty years of age. There are alternatives now to hysterectomy for large and multiple fibroids. Additionally, ask your doctor about a new in-patient treatment—called NovaSure (FDA-approved)—to prevent a hysterectomy from heavy bleeding. See *Fibroids* and *Adhesions.*

I

IMMUNE ENHANCEMENT

The immune system is responsible for protecting us against the foreign substances, such as bacteria and viruses, that we encounter in our environment. The lymphatic system filters, attacks, and destroys harmful organisms that cause infections. The thymus, tonsils, liver, spleen, appendix, bone marrow, and intestinal tract also help the body fight infection. Defects in the immune system cause autoimmune disorders (see *Autoimmune Disorders*), recurrent infections, allergies, inflammation, chemical sensitivities, and cancer.

The immune system includes the skin, which acts as a protective barrier; mucus membranes in the mouth, throat, eyes, intestines, and vagina; and antibodies and other immune system factors. If infectious organisms get past the outer protections, the *inflammatory response* is the second line of defense. Chemicals like histamine are released, causing the area involved to become red, painful, swollen, and hot. The *adaptive immune system* kicks in next. The major cells of the adaptive immune system are the white blood cells, which attack invading organisms and cancer cells. T cells are comprised of helper, suppressor, and killer cells, which help to fight viruses, bacteria, and some types of fungi.

Symptoms: When the immune system is not working up to par, there can be chronic or continuing infections, colds, respiratory problems, candida yeast overgrowth, chronic fatigue, or chronic allergies.

Causes: Any chronic recurring infection, such as middle ear infections in children and recurrent bronchitis or cystitis in adults, may signal hidden food, inhalant, or chemical sensitivities. Genetic predisposition, poor diet and nutrition, or environmental pollutants and chemicals can cause the immune system to malfunction. Prolonged use of antibiotics, emotional stress, and work or family pressures can overload the system. Depression can suppress the immune system, as can an underactive thyroid. Chemotherapy and/or radiation, diabetes, AIDS, alcoholism, lupus, and a host of bacterial and fungal infections can cause immune system dysfunction.

In 1996, Drs. Robert Repetto and Sanjay Baliga conducted an exhaustive review of the scientific literature and found that certain pesticides clearly impair immune system function, sometimes severely. Dr. Repetto commented: "New research may well show that the most widespread public health threat from pesticides is immunosuppression that weakens the body's resistance to infectious diseases and to cancers." Much of this immune suppression from pesticides is through the mechanism of hormone disruption (see *Hormone Disruptors*).

Uniquely Female: Dr. Allen Silverstone at SUNY Health Science Center in New York has found that exposure in utero to higher than normal levels of estrogen, synthetic estrogens (such as diethylstilbestrol, or DES), or dioxin hampers proper development of T cells, which are made in the thymus and are an important part of the immune system. When T cells get damaged, the immune system can become its own enemy, as well as having trouble fighting off foreign invaders. Silverstone says, "We should be looking for immune problems, definitely, from environmental estrogens." With modern women exposed to more es-trogen (see *Estrogen Dominance*), we may be seeing an increase in immune problems and cancer.

What to Do
- Don't smoke. It depresses the immune system.
- Get enough rest.
- Regular daily exercise keeps oxygen levels high, although excessive exercising can stress the immune system. Walk out-

side in fresh air, visit green parks. Exposure to city traffic can lower immune function in women.

- Laugh a lot.
- Learn relaxation techniques, including visualization and meditation (pages 52–58).
- Eat organic foods.
- Identify and avoid allergens.
- Don't use recreational drugs and reduce your dependence on prescription drugs, especially antibiotics and corticosteroids.
- Tap your thymus gland (behind your breastbone) every morning to stimulate it.
- Have a hair analysis performed to evaluate heavy-metal poisoning. Mercury amalgam dental fillings have been linked to a weakened immune system in some individuals.
- Reduce your toxic exposure, especially in the home (see my book *Hormone Deception*, Contemporary/McGraw-Hill, 2000).
- Rule out thyroid problems (see *Thyroid*).
- Have your cortisol and DHEA (dehydroepiandrosterone) levels tested.

Diet: Fresh fruits and veggies, including a green salad every day, are rich in the enzymes that are basic to immune response. Especially high in enzymes are garlic, papaya, and sea vegetables. Try a daily Green Drink (page 465) with optional 1 tsp. whey protein concentrate. Olives and olive oil are beneficial. Consume yogurt.

Avoid: Processed foods, processed oils, and saturated fat; they suppress immunity. Reduce dairy and sugar (including honey). Studies show that consuming large amounts of refined sugar and alcohol reduce the immune system's ability to destroy bacteria. On the other hand, reducing overall dietary fat improves immune functioning. Thus, nutritionally oriented practitioners often recommend reducing sugar, alcohol, and fat during acute infections or serious illness and for preventing recurrences of a wide variety of diseases.

Nutrients
** Antioxidants: alpha-lipoic acid, 50–100 mg once or twice a day with biotin, 2–3 mg per day

** Vitamin A, 25,000 IU twice a day for four weeks, then once a day, then 10,000 IU per day
** Vitamin C with bioflavonoids, 1,000 mg three times a day
** Thymus polypeptides, 500–1,000 mg once or twice a day
** Zinc picolinate, 30–60 mg per day, balanced with copper, 2–3 mg per day and multiminerals
** Proteolytic enzymes, 1–2 g between meals for one to two months
** Selenium, 100–200 mcg per day
** Beta-glucan, 50 mg per day
• Colostrum, powdered, 1 heaping tsp. one to three times a day
• Melatonin 1–2 mg at night. (DHEA, melatonin, and vitamin C help lower harmful elevated cortisol levels, which stress the immune system.)
• Vitamin E, 400 IU per day
• L-glutathione, 400 mg per day
• Transfer factor, 2 capsules twice a day (available from 4Life Research, 310-914-5191)

Herbs: Shiitake and maitake mushrooms (numerous kinds) included in the diet and/or several capsules or more per day. Echinacea, astragalus, and goldenseal are the immune system's Three Musketeers. Only mushrooms and astragalus can be taken for prolonged periods of time, goldenseal just for three weeks at a time.

INFERTILITY

The inability of a couple to conceive after a year of regular intercourse without contraception. Conception depends on the man's healthy sperm mating with a woman's healthy eggs. The fertilized egg must be able to become implanted in the uterus, and the hormonal environment must be adequate for the development of the embryo. As many as one in five or six couples are infertile. A woman's fertility begins to decline in her thirties. The number of women starting families at that age has increased enormously in recent years, perhaps leading to the high amount of infertility being experienced.

Causes: In women, the failure to ovulate due to hormonal imbalance is the most common cause of infertility. Blocked fallopian tubes (frequent after pelvic inflammatory disease), fibroids, disorders of the pelvic cavity (such as endometriosis), or cervical mucus that is hostile to sperm are other causes of infertility. Low thyroid or celiac disease can also lead to infertility. The birth control pill does not cause infertility; fewer than 1 percent of women experience problems with ovulation after going off the Pill. Stress can cause infertility.

What to Do

 ** Don't smoke (tobacco or marijuana) or drink alcohol.
 ** The test for male infertility is much easier than the one for women. Have your male partner checked first.
 ** Have your thyroid function checked.
 ** Get screened for celiac disease (have a blood test for antigliadin antibody).
 ** Have your spouse avoid wearing jockey briefs and tight jeans, and get tested for mercury toxicity linked to infertility in men.
 ** Don't have intercourse more than three times a week to help increase number of viable sperm in each ejaculation.
 ** Time intercourse to coincide with ovulation. Buy an over-the-counter test kit to know when you're ovulating.
 ** Don't stand up for fifteen minutes following intercourse to allow the sperm time to reach the egg, or lie on your back with your legs up against the wall.
 • Acupuncture and Chinese herbs may enhance conventional therapies. Call Dr. Roger Hirsch for consultations at 310-550-8186.
 • Exercise moderately but regularly.
 • Know that a very low fat diet for weight reduction can impair fertility.
 • Learn relaxation techniques. Infertility can be stressful, and stress can cause infertility.
 • Get checked for undiagnosed sexually transmitted diseases. Chlamydia is a leading cause of infertility, yet most infected women don't know they have it.

- Have your doctor test your DHEA (dehydroepiandrosterone) level. Supplementation with DHEA can improve ovarian response to fertility stimulation programs.
- Avoid hot tubs and saunas; they can change your ovulation patterns.
- Avoid pesticide- and heavy-metal-contaminated sport fish (*Epidemiology* 11:388-93, 2000).

Diet: Emphasize organic foods. Take a Protein Green Drink in the morning (page 465).

Avoid: Both partners should avoid alcohol and reduce their intake of refined sugar, processed foods, food additives, red meat (unless organic), and chemical-laced foods while trying to conceive. Caffeine consumption (in coffee, black and green teas, some sodas, chocolate, and many over-the-counter medications) has been linked to decreased fertility. Studies show anywhere from one to three cups of coffee per day can delay conception or reduce fertility. Other studies cite the tannic acid in coffee and tea as well as caffeine as culprits.

Nutrients

For Both Partners
- ** High-potency multivitamin/mineral supplement
- ** Vitamin C, 1,000 mg twice a day
- ** Manganese, 20 mg a day
- ** Vitamin B complex, 25–50 mg once a day
- ** Evaluate your need for digestive enzymes (page 468).
- • PABA (para-aminobenzoic acid), 100 mg two to three times a day

For Women
- ** Vitamin B_6, 50–200 mg per day, may increase fertility in women with a history of moderate to severe premenstrual syndrome. Take with vitamin B complex.
- ** Folic acid, 400 mcg twice a day
- ** Vitamin E, 400–800 IU per day

** Rule out iron deficiency.
- Essential fatty acids, 500–1,000 mg two to three times a day
- Selenium, 200 mcg per day
- If in-vitro fertilization attempts have been unsuccessful, take L-arginine (10 g per day) for a month prior, along with backup whole amino acid blends twice a day. L-arginine has been found to improve pregnancy rates, the number of eggs harvested, and embryos transferred when used in conjunction with hormonal treatments. Refer your doctor to *Human Reproduction* 14 (7):1690, 1999. Don't take these high doses without supervision or for extended periods of time. If you get herpes from arginine (which is a possibility), see *Canker Sores*. High arginine can cause flare-ups in some folks. If so, take 2–5 g lysine away from arginine and eat lots of yogurt.

Herbs: Vitex, 40 drops of concentrated extract in a glass of water in the morning.

For Men
- Vitamin B_{12}, 100–500 mcg per day
- L-arginine, 2 g twice a day
- L-carnitine, 500 mg three times a day with meals
- Vitamin E, 200–400 IU per day
- Zinc, 30 mg once or twice a day (balance with 2–3 mg per day of copper) for men with low blood levels of testosterone.
- SAMe (S-adenosyl-methionine), 200–800 mg per day

INSOMNIA

Insomnia isn't a disease, although you wouldn't know it from the million and a half pounds of tranquilizers consumed annually by Americans. Trouble sleeping—either falling asleep or staying asleep—is a common problem that affects everyone at some time. There is no "normal" amount of sleep. Some people need ten hours a night, while others do well on as little as four hours of sleep.

Symptoms: Lack of sleep creates daytime fatigue, irritability, and difficulty coping. It is one of the major causes of auto accidents.

Causes: Insomnia is a symptom with many different causes— sleep phase disorders (such as sleep apnea), restless legs (common after age fifty), too much noise or light, and lifestyle factors (lack of exercise, erratic hours, too many supplements before bed, or misuse of drugs). Common causes are plain old worry, depression, too much caffeine, and menopause. Also, as people grow older, they generally need less sleep and wake more frequently during the night. Chronic stress elevates the stress hormone cortisol, which can cause insomnia.

Uniquely Female: Hormonal changes during the premenstrual phase of menstruation, perimenopause, and menopause alter sleep patterns or can bring night sweats and hot flashes, which disrupt sleep off and on, sometimes for several years. Awakening between 3:00 and 4:00 A.M. is classic during menopause. For pregnant or nursing women, avoid all sedatives, especially during the first trimester of pregnancy. Women with sleep apnea who experience chronic snoring, frequent morning headaches, and debilitating daytime fatigue are at increased risk for heart attacks, stroke, and other cardiovascular events, and have twice the risk of heart failure. See your doctor about treating the apnea.

What to Do

- Acupressure can help. Apply gentle pressure on the feet at the big toes, tips of toes, and up the sides and the middle of the lower legs. Hold for ten seconds at a time, then rub gently.
- Make sure your mattress and pillow are comfortable. Wear loose-fitting sleepwear. Turn bright-light digital clocks away from the bed. Make sure the room is completely dark and isn't too hot or too cold.
- Sleep on 100 percent cotton sheets. Poly/cotton sheets or any new bedding treated with formaldehyde can cause insomnia. Wash new bedding three times with baking soda and air outside for a week before using it.
- If you are sensitive to electromagnetic fields, move all electrical appliances at least six feet from the head of your bed.

- Try a relaxing fifteen-minute hot bath with 2 cups of Epsom salts or baking soda before bed.
- Don't use your bedroom for anything other than sleeping and sex.
- Avoid stimulants (coffee, tea, cola, and amphetamine-type drugs) for two to three hours (six to eight hours for sensitive folks) before bed.
- Avoid large meals before bed. However, do eat a light snack of healthy food prior to bedtime if you are hungry.
- Develop regular sleeping habits, including a quiet activity, such as reading, before bed.
- Learn deep breathing and muscle relaxation techniques (see pages 52–58).
- Don't nap during the day.
- Don't use tranquilizers or alcohol to help with insomnia.
- Take medication for underactive thyroid first thing in the morning, not in the evening. Other medications, such as decongestants, appetite suppressants, blood pressure or seizure medication, and beta-blockers, can interfere with sleep if taken too late in the day, as can certain supplements (except melatonin).
- Consider a "white noise" machine.
- Nicotine is a stimulant. Don't smoke, especially before bed.
- Get regular daily exercise. Exercise in the mornings, except for a "constitutional" walk before bed; vigorous exercise in the evening can keep you awake.
- Don't fall asleep in front of the TV; the flickering light affects your nervous system.
- If yours or your partner's snoring keeps waking you up, have the snorer try the following suggestions: use nasal strips; encourage the snorer to sleep on his or her back; elevate the head of the bed; lose weight; cut back on alcohol at night; or try nasal douching if stuffiness is from allergies (buy a "neti pot" from your alternative practitioner—fill with a solution of ¼ tsp. sea salt and ¼ tsp. baking soda in spring or distilled water and alternate pouring through each nostril. It works incredibly well).

Diet: Increase calcium- and magnesium-rich foods such as leafy green vegetables, salmon, soy products, raw seeds and nuts. Eat foods high in tryptophan at dinner or bedtime: bananas, figs, dates, yogurt, cottage cheese, fish, peanuts, and turkey. Sometimes 1 tsp. honey in a warm glass of milk before bed helps.

Avoid: The major culprits—coffee, chocolate, sugar, and alcohol. Sometimes fruits and starchy foods consumed after midafternoon may be troublesome. Strong spices and MSG (monosodium glutamate) may affect sleep. Avoid taking too many of your regular supplements before bed, including vitamin C.

Nutrients

- ** Melatonin, 0.5–3 mg, especially if you're over age forty-five, one to one and a half hours before bed, or chew and let dissolve under your tongue twenty minutes before bed. For those who work at night, taking 10 mg of melatonin when going to bed in the daytime may improve daytime sleep; however, doses this high, if taken for several months in a row, may create early menopausal symptoms.
- ** Pantothenic acid, 200 mg with dinner, if melatonin doesn't work
- ** Magnesium, 250 mg one hour before bed
- • Vitamin E, 400 IU before bed, and folic acid, 800 mcg per day, for insomnia caused by restless legs
- • Choline, 200 mg with dinner
- • Vitamin B_1, 500 mg at night to reduce nightmares
- • Take vitamin B_{12} and B complex in the morning so they don't keep you awake at night.

Herbs: One cup of tea at bedtime made from equal amounts of any or all of the following: chamomile, passionflower, catnip, and valerian. Steep for ten minutes and drink one half hour before bed. Try valerian, 300–500 mg concentrated root extract one hour before bed. Valerian does not have an adverse impact the next day on reaction time, alertness, or concentration, as do drugs like benzodiazepines, and it can be taken by pregnant or lactating women. Try lavender oil on your temples, pillow, and the bottoms of your feet.

Note: If nutrients and herbs don't help, try sleeping pills (especially less addictive ones like Ambien), taken at the lowest dose for several nights followed by several nights off to avoid dependency. Long-term use can cause liver stress in some women, which can then cause hormonal imbalance. Going off long-term use of sleeping pills can produce withdrawal symptoms, particularly insomnia, which can last for weeks.

INSULIN RESISTANCE (Syndrome X)

A combination of conditions that results in cells becoming less able to utilize insulin for nutrient uptake into the cells. The pancreas tries to overcome the resistance by pumping out more insulin. If the resistance continues, diabetes can result. See *Diabetes Mellitus*. Our body cells use glucose (blood sugar) for nourishment. When the cells become resistant to insulin, sugar gets stored in other inappropriate tissues while the cells miss out on using it as their proper fuel. Degeneration and faulty functioning of numerous tissues occur over time. Insulin resistance may also play a role in many health problems such as heart disease, hypertension, and certain cancers, such as breast and colon cancer.

There is growing evidence that classic type 2 diabetes is caused by obesity-related insulin resistance in conjunction with a pancreas that is unable to compensate for this problem. Impaired insulin secretion and insulin resistance are universal in all obese women with type 2 diabetes, and probably in many who are not overweight.

Symptoms: Carrying too much weight over the belt (the "apple") as opposed to weight around the hips (the "pear") is a visible sign of higher risk. People who have a hard time losing weight, are prone to elevated blood fats like cholesterol and triglycerides, have a history of low blood sugar problems, and have numerous skin tags on their torso, neck, and armpits are at risk. Higher readings on glucose and insulin tests and elevated blood pressure all indicate a growing inability to utilize sugar properly. Insulin resistance syndrome is linked to double or triple the risk of heart disease and increased risk of breast cancer.

Causes: Runs in families, and the predisposition may be genetic. *If any member of your family has type 2 diabetes, take a test to determine your insulin resistance.* Insulin resistance may cause diabetes and, once a person is a diabetic, the disease and treatments increase potential loss of minerals, which worsens insulin resistance and the diabetes. Overconsuming refined sugars, overeating, nutritional deficiencies, and major depression (high cortisol levels) all contribute to developing insulin resistance.

Uniquely Female: An apple shape (fat around the middle) as well as fatty thighs, with unhealthy muscle that is marbled with fat (from a sedentary lifestyle), is associated with increased insulin resistance. These women may be more prone to conditions caused by unopposed estrogen, since fat cells make estrogen. Also, apple-shaped women may make less of the healthy proteins that bind or neutralize circulating estrogen, resulting in higher levels of active estrogen.

What to Do

- Regular exercise combined with weight loss and an improved diet is the best way to beat insulin resistance. Read *The Zone* by Barry Sears, M.D. (Regan Books, 1995) and *Protein Power* by Eades and Eades (Bantam Books, 1996).
- Thirty minutes of moderate physical activity each day decreases fasting insulin by 6.6 percent in African Americans, Native Americans, and white women.
- Keep your waistline down—it's not just for cosmetic reasons!
- Removal of ten pounds or more by liposuction has been shown to decrease insulin resistance and the subsequent risk of diabetes.

Diet: High-fiber foods lower insulin levels. Salt-restrictive diets can actually aggravate insulin resistance. Diets higher in protein (in relation to carbohydrates) reduce insulin resistance and associated risks. Avoid processed fats and switch to good fats. See *Fats and Essential Fatty Acids.* Beans are excellent. Good glycemic diets are strongly related to beneficial levels of good cholesterol.

Avoid: Greatly reduce simple carbohydrates like refined breads and pasta, sweet foods, and fruit juices, and when you do eat them, eat them early in the day. Don't overeat potatoes, including chips and fries.

Nutrients

Certain nutrients in the blood are inversely related to insulin resistance; the most important ones are listed below:

** High-dose multivitamin/mineral supplements

** Magnesium, 250–800 mg per day

** Potassium, 99 mg per day

** Calcium, 500–1,000 mg per day

** Chromium, 500–1,000 mcg per day, improves glucose intolerance and lowers elevated insulin.

** Vitamin K, 5 mg per day

• CLA (conjugated linoleic acid), 1,000 mg twice a day

J

JOINT PAIN

Soreness or severe pain in the joints, the points at which two bones meet.

Causes: Common joint injuries such as sprains, ligament tears, cartilage damage and tears, subluxations, muscle spasms, arthritis, bunions, and bursitis can cause joint pain. Infections like Lyme disease, secondary syphilis, intestinal parasites, bacteria, and yeast can cause chronic joint pain. Conditions associated with joint pain and/or aching include the common flu as well as chronic fatigue syndrome, fibromyalgia, and various types of arthritis (there are two hundred arthritic diseases). Joint pain can also be caused by hidden food allergies, toxic exposures to chemicals such as paints, inflammatory processes from acid-producing diets (high in protein but devoid of fruits and veggies), and from emotional states. Joint pain in feet can be caused by years of wearing high heels or tight-fitting shoes.

Uniquely Female: In women, joint pain is usually due to one of the many forms of arthritis (see *Arthritis*), autoimmune disease, allergies, or traumatic joint injury. Joint problems can be aggravated two weeks before the period or at menopause and by hormonal imbalances, especially low progesterone. Women are more often affected by TMJ (temporomandibular joint) disorders of the jaw than men.

What to Do

- When a joint feels hot to the touch, try applying ice packs, ten minutes on, ten minutes off. After the heat is gone and if the swelling is not acute, try ten minutes of ice followed by ten minutes of heat.

- Apply moist heat—hot baths, hot water bottles—for chronic pain.
- Regular rest is especially important.
- Regular exercise, especially stretching exercises and swimming in a heated pool, can help.
- Test for allergies.
- Test for mercury toxicity (find a dental specialist to check for a reaction to the mercury in amalgam fillings).
- For TMJ, avoid chewing on hard foods, gum, or ice or avoid cradling a phone receiver on one shoulder. Talk to your dentist about getting a protective appliance to wear at night. Consult a chiropractor or osteopath for treatment.
- Recurrent or chronically inflamed joints can come from feeling "held back" in life.
- Check for low nutrient levels (pages 35–39).

Diet: Emphasize vegetables and fruits and some seeds and grains like pumpkin seeds and lentils. Make a Green Drink (page 465) and sip throughout the day.

Avoid: Food, inhalant, or chemical allergens; excessive meat consumption; excessive refined sugars; caffeine; alcohol.

Nutrients: See the section on osteoarthritis under *Arthritis*.

K

KIDNEY INFECTIONS (Pyelonephritis)

The kidneys are the organs responsible for filtering the blood and excreting waste products and excess water in the form of urine. They also produce several hormones that regulate the production and release of red blood cells from the bone marrow. Only one normal kidney is needed for good health.

Symptoms: In acute infections, symptoms come on very fast—fever, shaking chills, burning and/or frequent urination, cloudy or bloody urine, lower back pain on one or both sides, abdominal pain, marked fatigue, nausea, and vomiting. Chronic infections develop slowly, grow steadily worse, and can lead to kidney failure. Symptoms include anemia, weakness, loss of appetite, hypertension, lower back pain, and protein and blood in the urine.

Uniquely Female: Kidney infections are far more common in women than in men. Vigorous sexual activity is one way that bacteria can enter the urethra and bladder; the bacteria can then travel up to the kidneys and infect one or both of them. Risk may increase with diabetes, chronic urinary tract infections, not emptying the bladder often enough, wearing synthetic panties and panty hose, and with pregnancy.

What to Do
- Take antibiotics and be monitored by a doctor.
- Drink lots of water and urinate immediately when you feel the need.

- See the section on urinary tract infections under *Urinary Problems* for more information.
- If you have recurrent or chronic infections, test for food allergies (especially to dairy products and wheat), other allergies, and hidden intestinal yeast infections or intestinal bacterial imbalance.
- Take a brisk walk or exercise daily to maintain kidney function.

Diet: Low protein. Eat several small meals a day rather than three large meals. Drink six to eight large glasses of liquid a day, including three glasses of unsweetened cranberry juice. Consume 75 percent raw foods. Eat plenty of celery, cucumber, parsley, watercress, potatoes, garlic, asparagus, and raw pumpkin seeds. Cultured dairy products, such as yogurt and buttermilk, are okay, as is goat's milk. Drink a Green Drink, three to seven times a week (see page 465).

Avoid: Reduce refined, fried, spicy, and sugary foods. Reduce animal protein and eliminate uncultured cow dairy products. Limit caffeinated beverages, such as coffee, tea, and soda, and full-strength fruit juices other than cranberry. Cranberry juice has a moderately high concentration of oxalate. Consume good fats. See *Fats and Essential Fatty Acids.*

Nutrients
- ** Vitamin C plus bioflavonoids, 2–4 g per day
- ** Lactose-free acidophilus, two to three times a day
- ** Vitamin B_6, 20 mg twice a day
- ** Vitamin A emulsion, 100,000 IU for three days; reduce to 50,000 IU for five days; then 25,000 IU per day; and be supervised by a medical doctor.
- ** Vitamin B complex, 50 mg twice a day
- ** Calcium, 400 mg twice a day with meals, and magnesium, 250 mg per day, taken as citrates. Does not increase the risk of calcium stones in most postmenopausal women.
- ** Multimineral once or twice a day
- Have your DHEA (dehydroepiandrosterone) level tested and supplement if low or very low.

Kidney Stones

Kidney stones are mineral salts combined with calcium that can lodge anywhere in the urinary tract. The most common kidney stone is made of calcium oxalate, and the following recommendations are for this type of stone. Recurrence rate after a first kidney stone is 27–50 percent at five years. To reduce recurrence, take vitamin B_6, 25–50 mg per day; magnesium, 250–600 mg per day; and vitamin E, 200 IU per day. Restriction of vitamin C is not warranted, except in high doses. Take vitamin A, 5,000–10,000 IU per day if deficient. Ask your doctor about potassium citrate and a low-purine diet, and *significantly increase your fluid intake*, especially in hot weather and after exercise. Reduce consumption of meat (a third of the kidney stone formers secrete oxalates after eating meat), sugar, salt, and colas, but do not restrict low-fat dairy and high-calcium foods and fiber. Low-calcium diets actually *worsen* recurrence rates. However, if you take calcium supplements, take only *with* food so they bind oxalates. Avoid excessive protein, which pulls calcium out of the bones; consume meat moderately. Citrus fruits, especially lemons, are good, but restrict excessive grapefruit juice, which studies have linked to kidney stones. Coffee and tea drinking are linked to less stone formation. Avoid chocolate, spinach, rhubarb, and other foods that contain oxalic acid. Reduce animal fat to increase urinary excretion of oxalates. Rice bran, 10 g twice a day after meals, is said to reduce recurrence rate. Talk with your doctor.

Herbs: Siberian ginseng extract, 100 mg in the morning, can improve kidney function in acute infections. Kidney flushing teas, 4–6 cups a day for ten days, from any combination of parsley, watercress, watermelon seeds, uva-ursi, and juniper can help. Burdock root tea can be used to detoxify kidneys. One quart of marshmallow tea per day for ten days three times a year strengthens the bladder and cleanses kidneys. Horsetail, 2 g two to three times a day for two weeks, can increase urine volume and decrease stone formation.

L

LEAD TOXICITY

Lead is a toxic mineral and hormone disruptor. Low levels of vita-min C, calcium, and zinc result in the body retaining the lead to which it is exposed. This in turn translates into higher blood levels of lead and more chance for toxicity problems. Acute lead poisoning is easy to avoid, but low-grade lead toxicity is not.

Symptoms: Headaches, personality changes, cognitive changes, metallic taste in your mouth, loss of appetite, fatigue, abdominal pain, constipation, and bone problems.

Causes: Lead can come from storing acidic foods and beverages (fruits, fruit juices or cola drinks, tomatoes or tomato juice, wine or cider) in lead-glazed ceramic ware. Other sources include leaded crystal, some calcium supplements (see page 352), and exposure to lead dust at work or in the home from the peeling of lead-based paints or carried in on the bottom of shoes, especially if there is new home construction happening in your area.

Uniquely Female: Lead competes for calcium in the bony matrix and results in bone loss, contributing to osteoporosis. Some bone meals have been found to contain lead.

What to Do
- Hair analysis is a valid test for lead toxicity in the body.
- Once the source of contamination has been identified and removed, discuss with your doctor chelation therapy—a

TOXIC METALS

Lead is not the only toxic metal. Women can have problems with cadmium, mercury, aluminum, and others. The best tests for metal toxicity are hair analysis or a urine test after a "chelation challenge"—a substance is taken that

 pulls toxins out of the tissues and dumps them in the urine for removal. Testing the urine then shows how much metal is in the body.

method of removing toxic substances from the body. For mild cases, oral chelation is available. Intravenous chelation is available for more difficult cases.

- Take vitamin C, 1–5 g per day; calcium, 500–1,000 mg per day; and zinc, 20–40 mg per day, and eat whole foods high in these nutrients.
- Wipe feet twice on a mat before entering home or have everyone take off their shoes.

LIVER HEALTH

The liver is an industrious and vital organ. It absorbs oxygen and nutrients from the blood, regulates blood sugar and amino acid levels, breaks down drugs and various toxins so they can be removed from the body, and manufactures important proteins. It also produces bile, which removes waste products and helps process fats during digestion, and is responsible for breaking down 80–90 percent of the hormones in the body. Since the liver is so vital to general health and well-being, it should be treated with respect.

Symptoms Suggestive of Liver Malfunction: General depression and melancholy, chronic anger, unexplained weight gain, extreme tiredness, poor digestion, food sensitivities and allergies, premenstrual syndrome, constipation, congestion, nausea, dry tongue and mouth, jaundice, and itchy skin.

Causes: The liver may be affected by vitamin B deficiencies, toxic chemical exposure, bacterial and parasitic infection, circulatory disturbance, metabolic disorders, or autoimmune disease. The most common cause of liver disease in the United States is excessive alcohol consumption. Overeating, as well as acute or chronic exposure to toxic chemicals, such as pesticides, solvents, preservatives, and other petrochemicals, and long-term use of various drugs (over-the-counter, prescription, or recreational) strain the liver. The liver also works harder if you are chronically constipated or taking oral birth control pills, fertility drugs, or hormone replacement therapy.

Uniquely Female: The liver is the primary site for the metabolism and excretion of estrogen as well as estrogen mimickers in the environment. It secretes metabolites of estrogen through the bile into the large intestine. If the breakdown of estrogen is impaired, it can result in local liver damage, continual recycling of estrogens, and alterations in immune function. If liver function is sluggish and estrogen metabolism is compromised, it can lead to conditions of estrogen dominance (see *Estrogen Dominance*). Women with chronic active hepatitis and those with cirrhosis often have trouble getting pregnant and are more likely to miscarry or deliver premature babies.

What to Do
- Eat smaller meals. Don't eat late at night.
- Eat quality protein with good fats. See *Fats and Essential Fatty Acids*.
- Get enough sleep.
- Exercise every day.
- Use coffee enemas to help detoxify your liver (appendix E).
- Take dry saunas to help detoxify your liver.
- Avoid toxic chemical exposures.
- Try topical treatments: Dissolve one pound of Epsom salts in a basin of very hot water. Soak a bath towel in the water and place it over a plastic bag or thin washrag placed over the liver to avoid burning the skin. Leave on until the towel cools; repeat several times. Or soak the towel in castor oil and place it over your liver with a heating pad on top, set to low, for fifteen minutes. Don't burn yourself.

Diet: Liver-friendly foods include whole grains, carrots, kale, brussels sprouts, broccoli, cauliflower, and cabbage. Liver-cleansing

LIVER-CLEANSING PROGRAM
(ONE TO TWO TIMES A YEAR)

For two weeks, once or twice a year, take:

- Milk thistle, 70–210 mg three times a day, or phyllanthus, 1 capsule two to three times a day with meals
- Cysteine/methionine, 700 mg per day
- Vitamin B complex, 50 mg once a day
- N-acetyl-cysteine, several hundred mg per day to be taken under a doctor's supervision (avoid if you have a history of active liver disease) or reduced L-glutathione, 400 mg per day
- Bioflavonoids, 1,000 mg twice a day
- Probiotics, two to three times a day
- Vitamin C, 500 mg two to six times a day
- Start and end each day with 2 Tbsp. olive oil mixed with the juice of one lemon.
- Each day, consume 2–3 Tbsp. shredded beets, at least two foods of the cabbage family, and plenty of raw seeds, nuts, beans, eggs, fish, and yogurt. Sauté grated burdock root along with other veggies.
- Consider doing a coffee enema during the first few days and the last several days (unless you have active intestinal disease).
- Get at least twenty minutes of exercise each day, drink plenty of filtered water, and get sufficient rest.
- Start and end each day with skin brushing. Purchase a skin brush at a health food store. Gently brush your arms and legs from the torso outward with long strokes to activate your lymph system.
- Extend the benefit of the cleanse by taking nettle and yellow dock teas, steeped fifteen minutes, two to three times a day for two weeks.

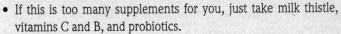

- If this is too many supplements for you, just take milk thistle, vitamins C and B, and probiotics.

foods include beets, artichokes, lemons, dandelion greens, watercress, and burdock root. Onions, garlic, and leeks are helpful, as are vegetable proteins, soy, almond and other nut butters, salmon, turmeric, ginger, and flaxseeds. Ghee (clarified butter) is easy for the liver to digest and helps restore enzymatic function. Increase foods high in potassium, including kelp, blackstrap molasses, brewer's yeast, rice and wheat bran, almonds, raisins, prunes, bananas, and seeds.

Avoid: Saturated fats, sugars, excessive caffeine, alcohol, and junk foods, which all interfere with the liver's ability to metabolize estrogen and other hormones and interfere with the metabolism of B vitamins, which the liver needs to regulate estrogen and other hormone levels. Avoid animal protein, fried foods, and too much salt until the liver is functioning properly. Don't use foods with saccharin or drugs containing acetaminophen (Tylenol) over extended periods of time.

Moderate drinking (one drink a day) is considered safer these days. However, two studies suggest that it is beneficial on the liver for some people but not others. Everything is individual. Be careful. Don't overdo alcohol (*Gastroenterology* 119 (5):1399–1401, 2000).

Nutrients
- Lecithin, 1 Tbsp. before meals, twice a day
- Inositol, 200–500 mg once or twice a day—especially if taking oral contraceptives
- Caution: Niacin, 100 mg twice a day, can trigger or aggravate liver disease in alcoholics, and high doses of niacin should not be taken if you have a history of liver disease. Higher doses of niacin (over several hundred milligrams per day) should be monitored even in healthy persons through liver enzyme blood tests.
- Ask your doctor about vitamin B_{12} plus liver injections.

Herbs: Milk thistle regenerates injured liver cells. Take 420 mg per day of milk thistle extract for three to four months, then reduce to 280 mg. Phyllanthus (available from Tahoma Clinic dispensary, 888-893-6878). Dandelion root, 2–5 g two to three times a day in divided doses for two to four weeks. Liver-rebuilding tonic: 4 oz. hawthorn berries, 2 oz. red sage, 1 oz. cardamom; steep for twenty-four hours in 2 qt. water. Add honey. Take 2 cups per day for two to four weeks. Schisandra tincture, 2–4 ml three times a day, helps reduce elevated liver enzymes. Ayurvedic combinations sold as Livit or Livotrit can help.

For severe liver damage, work with a naturopathic doctor and take mistletoe, which has been shown to help patients with hepatitis C.

LUPUS (Systemic Lupus Erythematosus, SLE)

A chronic autoimmune disease that causes inflammation of the connective tissue, which affects many systems of the body, including the joints and the kidneys. Discoid lupus erythematosus (DLE) is a skin disorder and is not discussed here.

Symptoms: Most sufferers have a characteristic butterfly-shaped rash on the face, with chronic inflammation of the connective tissue that can affect various joints throughout the body as well as the kidneys and blood vessels. Lupus can come on suddenly with great fatigue, infection, and fever or develop slowly over time with episodes of fever, fatigue, headaches, epilepsy, and psychosis. Symptoms can include recurrent mouth ulcers, especially on the hard palate, loss of appetite, red palms and hands, swelling of the lymph glands, nausea, joint pain, and weight loss. Intolerance to sun develops in 40 percent of women. There may be anemia, kidney failure, personality changes, inflammation of the lining of the lungs (pleurisy), inflammation of the membrane surrounding the heart (pericarditis), and many joints affected by arthritis.

Causes: Unknown. Suspected causes include low immunity, genetic predisposition, and viral infections, as well as nutrient deficiencies (such as antioxidants, vitamins A and E, and beta-carotene), food allergies, emotional stress, and reactions to environmental pollution and industrial emissions. Immunizations and some drugs (especially penicillin) may cause relapses or worsen symptoms, and lupus may be linked to some childhood vaccines and adult immunizations. People with this disease (and their relatives) have been shown to have more of a particular estrogen metabolite. Unopposed estrogen could contribute to SLE. In the Nurses Health Study, the risk of SLE was slightly increased in women who had ever used oral contraceptives (older forms with higher amounts of estrogen and progestins than what is used today), and there was a suspicion that fertility drugs also increased risk. The authors of this study say that estrogenic hormone disruptors should be investigated as a cause of lupus. Menstrual irregularities, menstruation starting at fifteen or older, and a history of other collagen diseases and asthma increase the risk. Several drugs can cause lupus-like symptoms, including procainamide, hydral-azine, methyldopa, and chlorpromazine.

Uniquely Female: Ninety percent of SLE cases occur in women between the ages of thirty and fifty. The incidence of lupus is increasing worldwide. Birth control pills or hormone replacement therapy may cause flare-ups of lupus. Risk increases with strep infections, abnormal estrogen metabolism, pregnancy, and stress.

What to Do

Natural therapies are helpful, especially for mild cases of lupus, but require many months of treatment.

- ** Rule out candida-related complex and treat with antifungals.
- Flare-ups may be triggered by exposure to sunlight, so symptoms may get worse in spring and summer. Wear protective clothing if you go out in the sun, but avoid commercial sunscreens.
- Use only hypoallergenic makeup and body products.
- Avoid overmedication, especially of corticosteroid drugs, which eventually suppress the immune system.
- Check for and treat food and chemical allergies, especially to dairy, beef, wheat, and chocolate.
- Take a rest period every day.
- Do gentle daily exercise like yoga, stretching, and t'ai chi.
- Learn stress-reduction techniques (page 52).
- Avoid environmental pollutants, including secondhand smoke, air fresheners, perfumes, pesticides, toxic fumes from paints and glues, etc.
- Avoid the amino acid L-canavanine found in raw alfalfa sprouts.
- Take ⅛ tsp. of ground flaxseeds per day; this has been shown to protect against lupus nephritis (*Journal of the American College of Nutrition* 20 (2):143–48 2001).

Diet: Eat a low-calorie diet, specifically a diet low in sugar, saturated fat, and protein and high in good fats (see *Fats and Essential Fatty Acids*) with many raw and steamed vegetables, especially broccoli, kale, arugula, artichokes, and beet and collard greens. Use olive oil and flaxseed oil and eat fish generously.

Avoid: Raw alfalfa sprouts, alfalfa, and possibly nightshade plants (eggplant, potato, peppers, tomato, tobacco).

Nutrients

See recommendations under *Liver Health*.

** Assess your need for digestive enzymes (page 468).

** Take a high-potency multivitamin/mineral supplement with extra zinc, 20 mg per day, and copper, 2–3 mg per day.

** Flaxseed, 1 Tbsp. per day for one month, then add a second dose, or fish oil, 6–10 g per day, with vitamin E, 800 IU per day. Flaxseed may be especially helpful with lupus nephritis.

** Have your DHEA (dehydroepiandrosterone) hormone level tested. In one study, women with lupus were given 100 mg per day, which decreased symptoms and improved overall condition, but doses this high can cause acne and body hair growth and must be monitored by a doctor. Recommended dosages are much smaller, more in the range of 20–25 mg per day. Avoid DHEA if you have a history of breast or ovarian cancer unless you are working with a specialist.

• Pantothenic acid, 10 g per day in divided doses for nineteen months (work with your doctor)

• Beta-carotene, 15,000 IU per day

Herbs: Tripterygium, 30–60 g per day for two to four weeks, but you must use under the direction of an expert in Chinese herbal treatments.

LYMPHEDEMA

An abnormal accumulation of lymphatic fluid in the tissues. The skin becomes puffy or swollen and is often painful.

Lymphedema can occur at birth in an infant but often develops from blocked or damaged lymphatic vessels from infection, trauma, or after the surgical removal of the lymph nodes, causing poor drainage of lymph. It is particularly common after surgical removal of lymph nodes in the armpits associated with breast cancer surgery, when it can cause swelling in the arm. It usually occurs within three to six months after surgery, but can happen at any time. Today, women with breast cancer should be given the option of sentinel node removal or doing chemotherapy without testing nodes. Many women have suffered too many disabilities from outdated lymph node surgery.

For postcancer lymphedema, see a lymphedema drainage expert for wrapping and lymph massage. Exercise regularly, using light weights. Take bilberry, 80 mg two to four times a day, and homeopathic lymph formulas, which may require several months to make a difference but eventually help to bring down the swelling in the arm. Once normal size is reached, take bilberry, 80 mg once or twice a day for six months to a year, and keep on a moderate exercise program. See *Bloating* for food suggestions. Lymph fluid can be thinned with iodine to help improve flow. Try kelp tablets or ask your doctor for an iodine prescription (5–6 drops per day). Avoid IVs, blood pressure readings, or having blood drawn from the affected arm. Lymphodiruril (a homeopathic rub-in), just released in the United States, has been used in Europe extensively for years.

M

MASTURBATION

Self-stimulation of the clitoris or vaginal opening (or the penis in men) to reach orgasm. This is healthy. It teaches women what their bodies need to reach orgasm and what to tell their partners to do to help them achieve orgasm. Research suggests that regular masturbation increases circulation and thus retards aging of the vagina, lengthens and strengthens sexual enjoyment, and may even produce hormonal stimulation that may protect against illnesses like breast cancer.

Masturbation does *not* lead to impotence, heavy menstrual bleeding, blindness, or premature senility. Try vibrators and/or massagers available at places like local drug stores (you don't have to go to sex shops) or www.goodvibs.com.

MELATONIN, see *Hormones*

MEMORY

The ability to remember what has happened in the past. There are three main stages:

- *Registration*—Information is perceived, understood, and retained for a limited time in short-term memory;
- *Long-term memory*—Storage involves associations with words or meaning, with visual imagery, or smell or sound; and
- *Recall*—Retrieval of information stored at an unconscious level.

Symptoms: Memory ability increases from birth to around the age of thirty, when a very gradual decline begins. About 5 percent of people over age seventy suffer some degree of impaired memory, reduced clarity of thinking, and ability to concentrate, and another 5 percent suffer from severe irreversible mental impairment, or *dementia* (sometimes called *senile dementia*). Dementia is usually the result of stroke or a brain disease such as Alzheimer's. *Delirium,* caused by illnesses, chronic alcoholism, or drug reactions, results in mental confusion and memory loss that is reversible.

Causes: Certain drugs, such as antihistamines, caffeine, marijuana, diet pills, and daytime sedatives can affect memory, as can vitamin and mineral deficiencies, anxiety, and depression. Certain medical conditions can adversely affect memory, such as allergies, chemical sensitivities, head injury, toxic-metal buildup, candidiasis-related complex, stress, thyroid disorders, and hypoglycemia. People regularly exposed to pesticides, like farmers and gardeners, are at higher risk for cognitive dysfunction. It is presently theorized that a diet low in fish, or baby formulas low in "good" fats, may contribute to low levels of a beneficial fat (phosphatidylserine) in brain membranes that help memory.

Uniquely Female: What did I come into the kitchen for? What was the name of the movie I saw yesterday? There are specific changes in cognition that happen when estrogen drops rapidly, commonly resulting in short-term memory loss, especially in verbal or recall memory. It is common during menopause, after childbirth, or after the removal of one or both ovaries. Hormone replacement therapy, natural hormones, and certain nutrients seem to improve both memory and cognitive function. Alzheimer's disease, the most common cause of dementia, affects almost three times as many women as men.

What to Do

- Get a physical to rule out disease, liver damage, thyroid problems, etc.
- Reduce distractions, like TV.
- Pay attention, as when hearing a person's name for the first time.
- Focus on what is happening and find devices that will help you remember, such as pretending to take a photo of where you're putting your keys.
- Go ahead—put a colorful ribbon on your car antenna so you can find it in the parking lot.
- Get more organized. Write lists, set aside a box for bills, leave yourself notes on the refrigerator or front door, have a special spot for your purse, keys, or briefcase.
- Have your doctor evaluate you for allergies or chemical sensitivities, which can cause "brain fog."
- Alzheimer's may be related to aluminum and other heavy metals. Avoid aluminum in deodorants, pots and pans, dandruff shampoos, antidiarrhea compounds, canned foods, etc.
- Women at high risk for Alzheimer's may benefit from a daily low dose of aspirin (80–100 mg) or low dose nonsteroidal anti-inflammatory drugs (less than 500 mg per day). These anti-inflammatories may protect the brain. Or try herbal anti-inflammatories such as cat's claw and turmeric.
- Mild aerobic exercise (such as a twenty-minute walk) increases oxygen to the brain.
- Learn deep breathing and other relaxation techniques (page 52).
- Remember, memory doesn't have to be perfect to still be okay.

SEE A DOCTOR ABOUT MEMORY LOSS IF:

- You are losing contact with reality, lose track of where you are, can't remember if it's morning or evening, can't remember your spouse's name.
  - You are uncomfortable and anxious about memory lapses.
  - You are not able to take care of day-to-day business and activities.

Diet: High fiber with lots of raw vegetables, whole grains, and lean protein (fish and chicken). Fish contains choline, which the brain converts to acetylcholine, a neurotransmitter that plays a big role in memory. Fish also contains DHA (docosahexaenoic acid), a brain essential fatty acid. Eat frequent, small, high-protein, low-carb meals. Drink eight 8-oz. glasses of pure water each day. Foods that help reduce oxidative stress that leads to age-related declines in cognition include strawberries, spinach, and blueberries.

Avoid: Overeating, processed foods, refined sugars, excess caffeine, and alcohol. Junk food diets adversely affect memory and the ability to learn.

Nutrients

** Phosphatidylserine, 100 mg per day with a fatty meal. It's a naturally occurring compound in the brain that assists neurotransmitters. It's not a guaranteed cure, but numerous studies show that it improves mental function, even in Alzheimer's patients (take three times a day for Alzheimer's). Take it daily until memory returns, and then reduce to three to six times a week, depending on response. It usually works within one to two weeks. If it doesn't help within four weeks, try several of the following:

- PABA (para-aminobenzoic acid), 100 mg three times a day for four weeks
- High-potency multivitamin/mineral supplement (should contain vitamin E)
- Evaluate your need for digestive enzymes (page 468).
- B complex, 25–50 mg once a day, plus 500 mcg of vitamin B_{12} and 800 mcg of folic acid
- L-tyrosine, 500 mg first thing in the morning for one to two months (don't take this if you're already on a monoamine oxidase inhibitor)
- Essential fatty acids, 250 mg twice a day (especially DHA), or ½–1 Tbsp. flaxseed oil once a day, balanced with vitamin E, 400 IU per day
- Free-form amino acids, once or twice a day on an empty stomach

- After age thirty-five, melatonin, 500 mcg–3 mg at night to enhance neurologic and cognitive functioning. After age fifty, increase to 6 mg per night. However, some women's levels of estrogen lower radically with more than 2 mg per night, so watch for hot flashes or other signs of low estrogen.
- Ask your doctor about vitamin B_{12} intramuscular injections.
- Have all hormones tested, especially DHEA (dehydroepiandrosterone) and testosterone. These may help peri- and postmenopausal women think better. Estrogen-only therapy does not protect against age-related cognitive decline.

Herbs: Ginkgo biloba extract, 60 mg twice a day (some supplements combine phosphatidylserine and ginkgo); gotu kola, 200 mg two to three times a day for up to six weeks; Siberian ginseng, 100 mg twice a day. Ginkgo helps if problems are mild, and 80–120 mg per day reduces side effects of antidepressants (selective serotonin-reuptake inhibitor type). Do not take with blood thinners.

MENOPAUSE (Climacteric, Change of Life)

A woman reaches menopause once her period has stopped completely for one year, usually between the ages of forty-five and fifty-five. It is a natural part of life and not a disorder. The end of menstrual cycles is a result of reduced production of several hormones: estrogen, progesterone, prolactin, and DHEA (dehydroepiandrosterone). Testosterone wanes more slowly than the other hormones at first. By the year 2015, 50 percent of adult U.S. women will be menopausal. Many women will spend a third of their lives or more beyond the age of menopause.

Too many menopausal women become embarrassed, feel invisible, and get depressed about this sign of aging because American society worships youth. We need to break through this stifling collective paradigm. In other cultures, older women are honored for their wisdom and maturity. We can start a positive groundswell by choosing to be joyously alive rather than depressed at not being young anymore.

We can nurture our relationship with ourselves (our bodies, lives, and purpose) as well as with those around us. See *Aging*.

Symptoms are varied, and some women experience nothing more than the ending of menstruation. Most common symptoms are hot flashes (experienced by 50–80 percent of women) and night sweats of varying frequency and severity. Hot flashes usually stop two to five years after menopause but may go on longer. Sleep disturbances are common.

Other symptoms include moodiness (who wouldn't be this way if they aren't sleeping well?), vaginal dryness, dry and thinning skin, acne, head hair loss, facial hair growth, poor circulation, cold "spells," painful intercourse, urinary symptoms, weight gain, and poor short-term memory. Changes in metabolism may lead to osteoporosis, rise in blood pressure, increased fats in the blood, atherosclerosis, and increased incidence of coronary heart disease and stroke. Depression, irritability, and anxiety can plague normally well-adjusted women. Symptoms may be more pronounced in women who are hypoglycemic, very stressed, particularly low in certain nutrients such as magnesium and vitamin B complex, and/or low in digestive enzymes. As hormone levels drop, tissues thin, including the lining of the gastrointestinal tract where certain digestive enzymes are made (page 468). The gums and teeth can develop problems during menopause. See *Gingivitis*.

Causes: Menopause occurs naturally when periods stop. However, it may occur earlier in life as a result of illness, chemotherapy, surgical removal of the uterus and/or ovaries, cigarette smoking, eating disorders, or long-term, intense physical activity.

Note: It is possible to get pregnant while going through menopause. You are not free from possible pregnancy until you have gone a year (some say two) without a menstrual period.

What to Do

- Have your thyroid levels checked.
- Have a hormone panel done for estrogen, progesterone, DHEA, and testosterone. Consult with a doctor about various forms of replacement therapies as well as herbs and nutrients.

There are lots of alternatives. See *Hormone Replacement Therapy*.

- The average woman gains eight pounds in the first two years of menopause, and the weight distributes itself in new places (bummer). This can be somewhat modified by eating fewer carbohydrates, eating fewer calories in general, and exercising more. You just have to decide that the effort is worth it. It may also be due to low DHEA, testosterone, and to a lesser degree, estrogen levels.
- Exercise becomes very important to prevent osteoporosis and heart disease. The more healthy muscle you have (not marbled with fat), the younger you remain, no matter what your biological age. Weight training four to five times a week along with aerobic exercise keeps tissue and skin from sagging and keeps muscles strong; three times a week maintains the level of fitness you already have. Exercise early in the day if you are prone to insomnia.
- Stretch. Keeping flexible physically also keeps you flexible emotionally.
- Quit smoking. It contributes to breast cancer, emphysema, osteoporosis, wrinkles, and early menopause.
- Try acupuncture and/or biofeedback.

When trying any treatment, conventional or alternative, for menopausal symptoms, see how it affects your digestion, energy level, mood, appetite, and sleep. If the treatment improves all of these, it's a good one for you. If it relieves hot flashes but gives you insomnia, for example, consider something else.

Diet: Consume more soy products (tofu, soy milk, tempeh, soy cheese, miso soup) if you have not had an estrogen-dependent cancer or other estrogen-dominant problems (page 226). Ground flaxseeds are another good source of phytoestrogens. Try goat's milk products, as they have less cholesterol than cow's and cause less allergies. Eat lots of dark green leafy vegetables (kale, collard greens, romaine lettuce, spinach, Swiss chard) for good sources of calcium. Cold-water fish (salmon, tuna, mackerel, herring, sardines, and halibut) are good sources of the omega-3 fatty acids that help prevent heart disease. Eat smaller meals, graze, and, in general, realize that it is time to start eating less.

Avoid: Reduce refined sugars, red meat, chocolate, alcohol, most sodas, and caffeine. They may make menopausal symptoms worse, and a diet excessive in these foods and/or with too much protein increases bone loss, as does chronic stress.

Nutrients

Try one or two under each section.

For Menopause in General

* ** Multivitamin/mineral formula
* ** Calcium, 800–1,500 mg per day; magnesium, 300–400 mg per day; vitamin D, 400–800 IU per day; and trace mineral supplement
* ** Vitamin E, 400–800 IU per day
* ** Evaluate your need for digestive enzymes (page 468)
* ** Fish oil, 1,500–3,000 mg per day in two or three divided doses
* Folic acid, 400 mcg per day
* Bioflavonoids, 500 mg three times a day
* Vitamin C, 500 mg three times a day
* Boron, 1–2 mg per day
* Vitamin B_6, 50–200 mg per day, and vitamin B_{12}, 250 mcg per day

Herbs: Black cohosh extract, 1–2 capsules twice a day. Angelica, dong quai, vitex, fenugreek, ginseng, and licorice root often help.

DHEA and Progesterone—Various Alternatives for Hot Flashes

* ** Hormone potentiators—various formulas that contain PABA (para-aminobenzoic acid), 100 mg two to three times a day. PABA safely slows the breakdown of your body's own hormones and is one of the only substances associated with increased libido (aside from testosterone, L-arginine, some herbs, and sometimes DHEA and/or progesterone. Estrogen

does *not* improve libido). Do not take without supervision of a doctor if you have a history of liver disease or elevated liver enzymes.

** Black cohosh, 20–40 mg of concentrated extract twice a day

** Hesperidin (a bioflavonoid), 500–1,500 mg per day in divided doses

- Vitamin E, 1,000–2,000 IU per day
- Vitamin C, 1,000–2,000 mg per day
- Pantothenic acid, 250 mg twice a day for a week to see if it works
- Garlic, 500 mg twice a day
- Gamma-oryzanol, 100 mg three times a day
- Flaxseed oil, 1 Tbsp. per day (balance with 400 IU vitamin E)
- Sage (for severe sweating with hot flashes), 3–5 g per day, or tea from 2–3 tsp. steeped fifteen minutes, 3 cups per day, or 4 ml tincture three times a day
- Some women with hot flashes and associated anxiety and stress have been found to have a higher ratio of cortisol to DHEA. Ginseng, vitamin C, and phosphatidylserine appear to improve this ratio.
- One study on soy did not find it more effective than placebo for controlling hot flashes, and another did, but many women feel it helps (*American Journal of Epidemiology* 153:790–93, 2001).
- Progesterone, DHEA, and testosterone have all been shown to be helpful for hot flashes.

For Heavy Menstrual Flow

** Bioflavonoids, 1,000 mg per hour until bleeding reduces (should take three to four hours to give it a chance to work) and then take 1,000 mg two to four times a day for one to two more days as needed

** Vitamin A, 25,000–50,000 IU per day, and vitamin A–rich food for several months

- Have your blood ferritin and iron levels tested.
- Have your thyroid levels tested.
- Vitamin C–rich foods and/or vitamin C supplementation

For Breakthrough Bleeding
- Citrus bioflavonoids or rutin, 600–1,000 mg per day

For Fatigue
- ** PABA, 100 mg one to four times a day
- ** Pantothenic acid, 500–1,000 mg one to three times a day
- Siberian ginseng, 300–500 mg once or twice a day
- Magnesium/potassium aspartate (up to 2 g per day of combined formula)
- Herbs—valerian root, passionflower, hops, chamomile, and scullcap—soothe and aid in sleeping. Do breath and relaxation exercises.

For Hair Loss and Thinning
- ** Progesterone (most hormones except testosterone can act at follicles on scalp as an anti-androgen and help some women); dose customized for patient by doctor after testing
- ** Pregnanolone; dose customized for patient by doctor after testing
- Biotin, 3 mg per day

For Insomnia
- Melatonin, 1–2 mg, chewed and held under tongue for one to thirty seconds before bed
- Alive Calm herb, 1–6 capsules before bed. It can be ordered from Inventive Biomedical (415-464-1347).

For Breast Tenderness
- ** Eliminate or reduce caffeinated products.
- ** Vitamin E, 800 IU per day
- ** Magnesium, 250–400 IU per day
- ** Vitamin B$_6$, 25–50 mg per day
- ** Iodine (prescription)
- Essential oils such as evening primrose, flaxseed, and fish oils, 2–8 g per day; or ground flaxseeds, ⅛ tsp. per day
- DIM (diindolylmethane) metabolite of indole-3-carbinol *theoretically* helps.
- Testosterone and/or progesterone decrease breast pain in some women.

- Eliminate or reduce estrogen supplements.
- Eat organically as much as possible.

For Depression and Anxiety (Midlife Dysthymia)

- ** Vitamin B$_6$, 50–100 mg once or twice a day for up to three weeks, along with vitamin B complex, 50 mg per day
- ** St. John's wort for depression
- ** Ask your doctor about DHEA (5–20 mg per day has reduced loss of energy, motivation, emotional "numbness," sadness, inability to cope, and worry, and improves cognitive function and memory). Avoid if you have a history of hormonal cancer, or work with a doctor. DHEA levels have been found to be inversely related to depressed mood in postmenopausal women. Transdermal DHEA patches have been shown to increase bone density.
- PABA, 300 mg three times a day
- SAMe (S-adenosyl-methionine), 200–900 mg per day (aids mind, joints, liver)
- Magnesium, 250–500 mg per day
- Scullcap, valerian, and passionflower are botanical relaxants.

For Vaginal Atrophy

See vaginal atrophy under *Vaginal Problems.*

For Food Allergies/Intolerances and Maldigestion at This Time

- ** Evaluate your need for digestive enzymes (page 468).
- ** Rotate your foods as much as possible.
- ** Glutamine, 500 mg two to four times a day (builds up thinning gastrointestinal lining)
- ** Vitamin A, 5,000–10,000 IU per day
- ** Zinc picolinate, 30 mg per day
- Vitamin B$_1$, 50 mg once a day
- Balancing and supplementing with hormones can often reduce allergies.
- Consider a detox and rebuilding gastrointestinal program (read my book *Healthy Digestion the Natural Way*, John Wiley, 2000) and test for intestinal infections.

For Urinary Problems

For disorders such as incontinence and prolapse, see *Urinary Problems*.

For Loss of Libido

- PABA, 500–2,000 mg per day in divided doses to begin, building up to a level that improves your libido. After several days, see if you can reduce the dose while maintaining the benefit.
- Identify and treat progesterone/testosterone and/or DHEA deficiencies. Also rule out hypothyroidism.
- Thirty minutes of exercise four times a week increases energy and sex drive.
- Testosterone (2 percent) creams, applied to the clitoris and surrounding area, may increase sexual desire. Try a small amount daily for one week, then two to three times a week as needed.

Early Menopause

Menopause usually occurs between the ages of forty-five and fifty-five, but it can start much earlier. Spontaneous cessation of the menstrual period before age forty is called *premature menopause* or *premature ovarian failure*. It is not known why some women enter menopause early. Possible causes include smoking, genetic abnormalities, disorders of the ovaries, excess exposure to ionizing radiation, chemotherapy drugs, surgical procedures that remove the ovaries or impair their blood supply, and severe infections or tumors of the ovary. Some type of hormone replacement therapy is the primary treatment. Early menopause increases the risk of a form of glaucoma (open-angle).

MENSTRUAL CALENDAR

Mark on your calendar when you get your period. Also mark down *any* symptoms (pelvic pain, fatigue, back pain, infections), anything you are feeling. Keep the calendar for two to three months, noting if any of the symptoms are cyclical, usually for the two weeks out of the month between ovulation and your period.

Recurrent cyclical symptoms are often due to a hormonal imbalance. In this case, treating the imbalance, such as a progesterone deficiency, is what is needed to get rid of the health problem. Also, we all have weak links in our bodies, which can be a result of an old severe illness or accident. For example, if a few years ago you had severe bronchitis or had an injury to your knee, these old symptoms can recur cyclically due to hormonal imbalance.

Not all cyclical pain has its origin in hormones. The problem may be aggravated by hormones but not caused by them. However, it is always important to rule out this hormonal link.

MENSTRUATION

The cyclical shedding of the lining of the uterus (endometrium), accompanied by bleeding. Menstrual periods begin at puberty and continue until menopause. The menstrual cycle usually lasts from twenty-four to thirty-five days, with day one being the day bleeding starts and counting until the day before the next period. *Ovulation,* the release of an egg from the ovaries, occurs around midcycle and is accompanied by the production of progesterone and some DHEA (dehydroepiandrosterone). If the egg is fertilized, a pregnancy results; if not, the uterus sheds its lining and the unfertilized egg about fourteen days after ovulation. A period usually lasts two to seven days, and a woman normally loses up to four tablespoons of blood. If the flow is heavier, the blood will clot. Menstruation usually takes place every four weeks, but exposure (both in utero and throughout life) to plant and environmental estrogens may be shortening this cycle in certain women, thus laying the groundwork for hormonal and fertility problems and cancers. Short and irregular cycles do start to happen from the mid-thirties on, with the beginning of the perimenopause.

The delicate balance of estrogen and progesterone hormones is easily upset, making abnormal menstruation a common disorder of women. Any change in a woman's periods can indicate a problem in the pelvic area, including fibroids, endometriosis, or pelvic inflammatory disease. Tell your doctor.

Amenorrhea (Absence of Menstrual Periods)

This symptom can come from any number of complex causes. *Ruling out pregnancy and disease is vital before trying any treatment.*

Primary amenorrhea is the failure to start menstruating by the age of eighteen as a result of delayed puberty, usually from a hormonal disorder such as an underactive thyroid or an adrenal tumor. *Secondary amenorrhea* is the temporary or permanent cessation of periods in a woman who has menstruated regularly in the past. The most natural cause is pregnancy. Amenorrhea occurs permanently after menopause or after a hysterectomy. Periods that occur four months or more apart may be caused by hormone imbalances related to stressful situations, such as emotional problems, crash diets, extreme low-fat diets, extreme weight loss, or extreme exercise; due to the effects of drugs, including tranquilizers and antidepressants; or the result of an ovarian cyst or tumor.

What to Do: Have your doctor perform a complete hormone evaluation and an essential fatty acid blood screen. Balancing essential fatty acids or adding quality fats like flaxseed to the diet while avoiding all hydrogenated fats can be surprisingly helpful. Eat a diet high in vegetables, especially yellow ones. Rule out hypothyroidism. Consider ovarian and pituitary glandulars. Vitex (40 drops of concentrated extract to a glass of water in the morning) is an herb that increases the production of progesterone, balances prolactin, and helps regulate the menstrual cycle naturally and safely. Work with a naturopathic doctor.

Polycystic Ovary Syndrome (POS)

POS is a hormone imbalance caused by lack of ovulation due to excessive stimulation of the ovaries by some hormones and a deficiency of others, characterized by scanty or absent menstruation and sometimes excessive hairiness and obesity. Often, multiple ovarian cysts are present. Women with this problem usually have their periods very irregularly with variable flow patterns, such as intervals from every six weeks to every six months, and tend to have problems with infertility, insulin resistance, and more classic risk factors for heart disease. Close female relatives are at risk.

What to Do: Vitamin D (ergocalciferol-type, 50,000 IU per day) and calcium therapy (1,500 mg per day) help normalize menstrual cycles and stop dysfunctional bleeding. D-chiro-inositol, 1,200 mg per day, helps you resume ovulation. Electro-acupuncture and some Chinese herbs induce regular ovulation in some women with POS. Ask an acupuncturist. Prevention includes maintaining adequate levels of calories and fat in the diet; regular eating habits; avoiding underweight or obesity; avoiding excessive exercise; and learning stress-reduction techniques. See *Insulin Resistance.* For depression, try amino acid blends and up to 12 g per day of inositol. You must work with a doctor.

Dysfunctional Uterine Bleeding (DUB)

Most abnormal uterine bleeding is a benign condition. It can take many forms, including heavy and/or prolonged bleeding *(menorrhagia)*, frequent bleeding *(polymenorrhea)*, infrequent bleeding *(oligo-menorrhea)*, anovulatory bleeding *(menometrorrhagia)*, intermenstrual bleeding (bleeding between menstrual cycles), or postmenopausal bleeding. Half of DUB cases are in perimenopausal women due to changing ovarian function and/or underactive thyroid (most commonly associated with abnormal bleeding problems) and unopposed or excess estrogen/progesterone deficiency. *Nonovulatory cycles* cause progesterone deficiency and promote estrogen excess. Lack of or imbalance of vitamin B_6, magnesium, and essential fatty acids can contribute to progesterone inadequacy problems.

Another 20 percent of DUB cases happen in adolescents before their hormones "even out," and the remaining 30 percent occur among women aged twenty to forty as a result of polycystic ovarian syndrome, elevated prolactin levels, emotional stress, obesity, weight loss from anorexia, or intense athletic training.

Differentiate benign DUB from premalignant, malignant, or other diseases. If a woman saturates a super tampon or heavy pad more than every hour for six to eight hours, she requires prescriptive hormones. Bleeding more often than this may require surgical intervention, such as a D&C, in which the lining of the uterus is scraped to stop the bleeding. Ask your doctor about natural hormones, including natural progesterone (especially suppositories). Reduce stress, which elevates cortisol and prolactin and, in turn, can imbalance hormones.

Any bleeding that occurs between periods may indicate cancer of the cervix or uterus, particularly if you are over forty and have not had a period for more than six months, or if the bleeding follows intercourse. See a doctor right away. However, midcycle bleeding is also a sign of hormonal imbalance and has been anecdotally reported to occur in a number of DES daughters. It may suggest low progesterone and/or thyroid hormone. Have your doctor evaluate your hormone levels.

For all DUB, take ⅛ tsp. ground flaxseeds or 1 Tbsp. flaxseed oil daily (balance with vitamin E, 400 IU per day).

For *menorrhagia* (excessive bleeding and clotting), which may be caused by hormonal imbalance, have your doctor check for pelvic infection, fibroids, or polyps, or consider removal of your intrauterine device (IUD) if you've been using this method of contraception.

What to Do

- Have your doctor check for endometriosis or uterine fibroids.
- Have your doctor check thyroid and all other hormones, especially progesterone.
- Try castor oil packs on your abdomen, or use a hot compress of chopped cabbage.
- Place a ginger tea pack over your sacrum or lower abdomen.
- Vitex is helpful for many menstrual disorders. Take for oligomenorrhea (infrequent bleeding) or for irregular periods in general, and for four to six months for polymenorrhea (frequent bleeding). Work with your doctor.

Nutrients (For Heavy Bleeding)

** Bioflavonoids, 1,000 mg per hour until bleeding slows down, then reduce dosage to two to three times a day for several days

** Iron—Heavy bleeding causes iron loss, and iron deficiency causes more heavy bleeding. Only supplement with iron if blood tests (iron and ferritin) are low.

** Vitamin A, 50,000–75,000 IU per day for two to four weeks, then 10,000–25,000 IU per day for several months, especially for women in their twenties and thirties. You must see a doctor.

• Bromelain, 500–1,000 mg per day, and magnesium, 250 mg several times a day on an empty stomach, to reduce the inflammation often associated with heavy bleeding.

Herbs: Vitex, 40 drops of concentrated liquid herb in a glass of water in the morning for four to six months, is the herb of choice, but it's slow-acting. While taking this, use false unicorn root tincture, 2–5 ml three times a day for one to two months. Herbal products with astringents and uterine tonics (equal parts of yarrow, greater periwinkle, shepherd's purse, and life root), 20–30 drops every two to three hours. If you have heavy cramps accompanying heavy bleeding, try butiao, 500 mg three times a day for two weeks before your period. Herbal bath: 1 qt. strong chamomile tea and 1 qt. ginger tea each in a warm-to-hot bath. Use vitex only under a doctor's supervision.

For Metrorrhagia (Bleeding Between Periods)
** Have your doctor rule out disease.
** Citrus bioflavonoids, 1,000–3,000 mg per day or every hour for several hours when bleeding
• Evaluate and treat overt or subclinical hypothyroidism and inadequate progesterone.
• Vitamin C, 1,000 mg one to three times a day
• Some DES (diethylstilbestrol) daughters have abnormal bleeding, which may be due to in utero preprogramming. They should have an essential fatty acid blood test and get a customized therapy program as well as consider melatonin, 1 mg per night during bleeding, along with vitamin B_6, vitamin B complex, and magnesium; and test hormones, especially progesterone.

Dysmenorrhea (Painful Periods, Cramps)

Almost 50 percent of menstruating women are affected by menstrual cramps, with 10 percent having severe pain, mostly between twenty and twenty-four years of age. Cramping occurs only in menstrual cycles during which ovulation has taken place; anovulatory cycles are usually painless. Generally, the cramps are caused by muscles tightening in the uterus. Also, the cervix needs to stretch when large blood clots are passed, which contributes to menstrual pain. The tendency to suffer from cramps runs in families.

Primary dysmenorrhea usually lasts for one or two years in women who have just begun to menstruate. Hormone imbalance is normal during adolescence. Childbirth dramatically relieves this form of dysmenorrhea.

Secondary dysmenorrhea is due to an underlying disorder, such as endometriosis, fibroids, unopposed estrogen in relation to progesterone, underactive thyroid, or pelvic inflammatory disease. Either type can be accompanied by premenstrual syndrome (PMS). A doctor needs to evaluate any woman with painful cramps to rule out disease.

Symptoms: Cramps and pain in the lower abdomen, which may come and go in waves; dull lower backache; diarrhea and possibly nausea and vomiting. In severe cases, the woman may be dizzy and/or faint. Some have pelvic congestion and bloating.

Causes: Lack of blood flow (and oxygen) to the uterus; imbalance in uterine prostaglandins (related to excess estrogen and low progesterone levels or possibly an imbalance in the ratio of estrogen metabolites), hypothyroid, and possibly estrogenic pollutants. The high-stress lifestyle and low-nutrient diets of contemporary women have also been implicated in dysmenorrhea.

What to Do
- Don't smoke. Even passive smoke makes cramps last longer.
- Carrying excess weight doubles the odds of having long, painful periods.
- Don't use an IUD.

- Use a heating pad set on low or a warm water bottle on the abdomen, or take a warm bath for ten to fifteen minutes to relieve pain.
- Try NPRx™, a new natural topical alternative to NSAIDs (aspirin, ibuprofen, and prescription medications), for the relief of pain related to cramps.
- Constipation makes cramps worse. Eat a high-fiber diet.
- Take Epsom salts baths two days before and on first day of your period.
- Try using pads instead of tampons.
- Spinal malalignment can contribute to cramps. Get evaluated by a chiropractor or osteopathic doctor and practice regular exercise along with good posture.

Avoid: Identify and avoid food allergies, which can cause water retention and increase cramps. Avoid foods that increase inflammatory prostaglandins—dairy, beef, pork, lamb, and poultry. Limit salt and sugar. Avoid alcohol the week before your period as it may prevent your liver from metabolizing hormones. Avoid caffeine.

Nutrients

Long-term treatment with magnesium, vitamin B_6, and essential fatty acids gradually decreases cramps in most women as long as they also reduce the processed fats in their diets.

- ** Magnesium (as citrate/aspartate combination), 100 mg two to three times a day one week before the onset of your period; on the day before, take 100 mg three times a day; on the first day, take 100 mg four to five times a day. Reduce the dosage if diarrhea occurs.
- ** Vitamin B_6, 50 mg twice a day five days before your period, three to four times a day on the first day, and a lower dose throughout the month. Do not take more than 200 mg per day.
- ** Iron deficiency can cause cramps. Take if blood tests show your iron is low.
- Niacin, 100 mg once a day one week before your period and 100 mg every two to three hours while you have cramps

- Gamma-linolenic acid (from borage, evening primrose, flaxseed, or fish oils) balances out prostaglandins. Take 2,000 mg two to three times a day for two to six months.
- Vitamin E, 100–200 IU per day
- Calcium (as citrate/aspartate combination), 800–1,000 mg throughout the month and 250 mg three times a day with cramps
- Rutin, 200 mg during your cycle and 500 mg two to three times a day while cramping (rutin with vitamin C, 300–1,000 mg per day helps the effectiveness of niacin)
- Melatonin, 2 mg for the five nights before your period, may help.
- If nothing helps, ask your doctor for intravenous magnesium, vitamin B_6, and B complex at the onset of cramps (see Myer's Cocktail on page 471) or try nonsteroidal anti-infammatory drugs (NSAIDs) such as Anaprox while waiting for natural therapies to take effect.

Herbs: Valerian tincture, 1 tsp. every three to four hours as needed; cramp bark, 4–8 ml of tincture three times a day as needed. Black cohosh, 250 mg three times a day or 2–4 ml three times a day (do not take if allergic to aspirin or take for longer than six months). Also try turmeric, 250 mg three to four times a day between meals while having cramps, or yarrow, 3–4 ml three times a day—both act like natural anti-inflammatory agents (don't take them with NSAIDs).

Mittelschmerz ("Middle Pain")

Lower abdominal pain or discomfort during ovulation, about halfway between menstrual periods. The pain is felt on one or the other side of the abdomen, depending on which ovary is releasing an egg.

MISCARRIAGE (Spontaneous Abortion)

The loss of a pregnancy before the baby is born, usually within the first two to three months of pregnancy. Occurs in 10–15 percent of pregnancies with obvious cramping and bleeding, but the true rate of miscarriage is closer to 40 percent, since many occur early and may be confused with a heavy or late period. Most miscarriages are random events and don't have any bearing on a woman's ability to bear a child later on.

Symptoms: Spotting or bleeding, strong abdominal pain, lower back pain, heavy cramps.

Causes: More than half of all miscarriages are caused by damaged or abnormal chromosomes in the sperm or egg. Sometimes it is a result of a fetus not growing normally. Increased risk factors include high levels of homocysteine in the mother, excess caffeine intake during pregnancy, fibroids, diabetes, exposure to X rays or toxic chemicals, the mother being over the age of thirty-five, smoking, pollutants in the environment (such as solvents in the workplace), drinking alcohol, very poor nutrition, or drug abuse. Having sex, exercising, working, suffering a minor fall, or using birth control pills before pregnancy do *not* cause miscarriage.

What to Do
- Get checked for fibroids. If you have them, consider non-adhesion-forming surgery (page 74).
- Use sanitary pads rather than tampons to prevent infection.
- Wait two or three normal periods before trying to get pregnant again.
- Recurrent early miscarriages have been linked to high levels of homocysteine during pregnancy. Have your doctor test your homocysteine levels.
- Get tested for celiac disease. Hidden problems with gluten increase the risk of miscarriage.
- Start exercising slowly. It will take your body six to eight weeks to return to normal.
- Feelings of loss and grief are normal. Don't blame yourself for the miscarriage. In most cases, nothing could have prevented it.
- Don't smoke. Smokers are twice as likely to miscarry and have low birthweight babies.

FOR A THREATENED MISCARRIAGE

If it's early in your pregnancy and you begin spotting or light bleeding with mild or no cramps, lie very still and drink a cup of false unicorn tea every half hour. As bleeding decreases, drink the tea every hour, then every two hours. Add lo-belia extract (6 drops) to the last cup. Other options: Steep 1 tsp. wild yam root in 2 cups hot water for fifteen minutes; take 2–4 oz. every half hour (don't use the tincture, as it may induce nausea). Try comfrey/wild yam/cranesbill tea every hour until bleeding stops, or hawthorn extract, ½ dropperful, and bee pollen, 2 tsp., every hour until bleeding stops. Obviously, contact your doctor when spotting begins.

- Some women are affected by the benzene in gasoline, which can shorten pregnancy. Avoid pumping gas, or stand upwind from the fumes.

Foods: The more green vegetables, fruit, milk, cheese, and eggs you consume, the less risk you will have of a miscarriage.

To Lessen Your Chances of Miscarriage
- ** Vitex, 40 drops in a glass of water in the morning for women in their thirties with inadequate progesterone
- ** Multivitamin/mineral supplement daily
- ** Zinc, 20 mg per day
- ** Vitamin E, 400 IU per day
- ** Manganese, 20 mg per day
- ** Fish oils, 2–6 g per day for six to twelve months
- • Bioflavonoids, 200 mg three times a day, help chronic aborters.
- • False unicorn root, 3 drops of tincture four to five times a day throughout the first trimester (especially for chronic aborters, but you must work with a specialist)
- • If traveling in a foreign country and you are pregnant and begin to spot, do not let a doctor give you a shot of DES!

MOOD DISORDERS

When your mood or emotions go out of control, leaving you overly happy or sad for prolonged periods, you're said to have a mood disorder (also called an *affective disorder*). Moods are often associated with menstruation. Keep a menstrual calendar (page 328). See *Depression* or *Premenstrual Syndrome*.

MULTIPLE CHEMICAL SENSITIVITIES (MCS)

A medical condition characterized by debilitating chemical sensitivities, which can affect any organ in the body. It is becoming a widespread problem. People with MCS react to chemicals at levels that ordinarily do not affect others. It's sometimes called "chemical allergy," although the mechanism is not the same as in more traditional allergies. Examples of MCS include sick-building syndrome, Gulf War syndrome, and latex and insecticide allergies. There are undoubtedly more to come.

Symptoms: Can be mild to life-threatening. Includes headache, trouble concentrating, nausea, fatigue, muscle and joint pain, dizziness, difficulty breathing, irregular heartbeat, and seizures. Also mood disturbances, panic attacks, depression, memory loss, low energy despite enough sleep, abnormal metabolism, learning and behavior disabilities, skin rashes, chronic respiratory inflammation, ringing in the ears, diarrhea, low immune response, and chronic infections. Reactions may last from a few seconds to weeks or months. People with MCS often react to foods, drugs, molds, and pollen as well as chemicals.

Causes: Repeated exposure to low-level toxic chemicals or acute high-level exposure and a genetic predisposition to slow detoxification processes. Some of the chemicals known to cause reactions are found in many common products such as pesticides, perfumes, tobacco smoke, new carpets, air fresheners, new paint and building materials, and many cleaning and laundry products. Our immune systems can be affected by the chemicals in the water we drink and

DON'T BE BUG-FREE OBSESSIVE

Many women are swayed by advertising into thinking we should use anti-bacterial formulas in soaps, shampoos, toothpaste, moisturizers, dish detergents, etc. Avoid ones that contain triclosan and use simpler cleaning mixes such as baking soda and vinegar and water (cheaper and safer), and purchase products at health food stores. Excessive antibacterial products are triggering genetic changes in bacteria that make them super-resistant.

the food we eat, as well as by toxic metals in our environment. There are more than 70,000 chemicals in production in the United States. More than 2,000 new chemicals have been added *each year* since the end of World War II.

Uniquely Female: The majority of people affected are women. In general, women and children are more affected by toxic chemicals and environmental pollutants than men. Women work in the home more often than men, which has been proven by Environmental Protection Agency studies to have the highest exposure to pollution. And when women are exposed to pollutants, they don't clear them from their bodies as efficiently as do men, and they have more fat cells, which can store more toxins than men.

What to Do
- Ventilate, especially near the washer and dryer and in the kitchen.
- Use exhaust fans in bathrooms while showering.
- Use air filters, especially in the bedroom and office.
- Wipe your feet on a good-quality doormat several times before entering your home, or remove your shoes when you step inside.
- Use "greener" cleaning products or baking soda and vinegar rather than commercial cleansers with numerous chemicals.
- Dust and vacuum frequently, preferably with a vacuum that has a HEPA (high-efficiency particulate air) filter.

- Air out dry-cleaned clothes for several days before putting them inside your house.
- Leave garage door open for fifteen minutes after pulling your car into an attached garage.
- Avoid most commercial air fresheners, avoid fabric softeners, use unscented detergents.
- Read my book *Hormone Deception* (Contemporary/McGraw-Hill, 2000) for a full discussion of how to reduce your exposure.
- When remodeling, use less toxic materials.
- The liver and kidneys need to be working well to clear out toxins.
- Work with a physician who is trained in environmental medicine to learn how to reduce chemical exposure and which nutrients to take.

MULTIPLE SCLEROSIS (MS)

A progressive disease of the central nervous system in which the protective covering (myelin) of nerve fibers in the brain and spinal cord are destroyed. This results in multiple and varied neurological symptoms that usually wax and wane. Age of onset is usually between twenty and forty.

Symptoms: Most common are numbness, weakness, and clumsiness of a hand or leg, painful muscle spasms, impaired vision, loss of balance, weakness, bladder dysfunction, and psychological changes. May also have urinary tract infections and skin ulceration. Some people have only mild attacks and long, symptom-free periods and few permanent effects; others have a series of flare-ups that leave them with gradual deterioration and disability.

Causes: MS is thought to be an autoimmune disease with a strong genetic factor. A virus in the first fifteen years of life may be responsible for the disease's later development in susceptible people. It is also much more common in cold and temperate climates. There are theories that some cases are related to mercury toxicity, food allergies, chemical sensitivities, and/or candidiasis-related complex.

__Uniquely Female:__ The disease affects more women than men, especially white women.

What to Do

- Check for food allergies (especially dairy) and toxic chemical exposures. Avoiding allergy-causing foods may completely resolve symptoms for some people early in the disease.
- Acupressure and massage are helpful.
- Tobacco smoke makes symptoms worse.
- Get enough rest.
- Moderate exercise can help maintain mobility.
- Learn stress-reduction techniques (pages 52–58).
- Extremely hot baths, showers, or any overly warm environment may trigger an attack.
- Test for Lyme disease. The symptoms often mimic MS.
- Test for *Chlamydia pneumoniae*, as it is now linked to some cases.
- Mineral baths are helpful.
- Excess dental cavities have been found in MS patients, and whether this is cause or effect is not known. Consider having mercury amalgam fillings removed (while having an intravenous vitamin C drip, followed by an oral chelation program). Order a copy of the *60 Minutes* TV show on MS and dental amalgams ("Is There a Poison in Your Mouth?," Patti Hassler, producer; order from BBC: P.O. Box 7, London, England, W36XJ; send check for £3.50); talk to dentists and doctors. Refer to *British Dental Journal* 187 (5):261, 1999.
- Evaluate for candida infection and consider antifungal medications.

__Diet:__ Try the Swank Diet—restrict saturated fats (animal fat, including red meat and cow's dairy products) to less than 20 g per day. Reduce all processed fats like hydrogenated and partially hydrogenated oils and margarines, and avoid refined sugars. Supplement with cod liver oil, 1 Tbsp. per day; sunflower oil, 2–8 tsp. per day; and vitamin E, 400 IU per day. Include regular rest periods and stress-reduction sessions. Read *The Multiple Sclerosis Diet Book* by Dr. Roy L. Swank and Barbara Brewer Dugan, R.N., Doubleday, 1987. Use olive oil liberally.

Avoid: Avoiding gluten foods (gluten is a protein found in wheat, rye, and barley) is controversial. Try it for a month and see if your symptoms improve. Alcohol and caffeine may aggravate symptoms.

Nutrients

- ** Cod liver oil, 15–20 g per day (build up to this amount and balance with vitamin E, 800 IU per day), or 1 Tbsp. of flaxseed oil per day
- ** Calcium, 1,000 mg per day, and magnesium, 500 mg per day in divided doses
- ** Vitamin B complex, 50–100 mg per day with extra vitamins B_1 and B_3
- ** Antioxidants of all kinds are helpful.
- ** Evaluate your need for digestive enzymes (page 468).
- ** Ask your doctor about Procarin patches. These are histamine patches from compounding pharmacies developed by Elaine DeLack, R.N., who put her own MS symptoms into remission with them. They are tremendously helpful, not widely known, and need to be closely monitored (especially in redheads and blondes). MS patients who are very heat sensitive tend not to respond as well as others. Procarin action is blocked by histamine-blocking antacid medication but not by the antihistamines found in cold remedies.
- • Thymus glandular extract, 500 mg three times a day for two months, then 250 mg per day
- • Multivitamin/mineral supplement
- • Ask your doctor about vitamin B_{12} injections (1,000 mcg intramuscularly) once a week or as needed, and adenosine monophosphate (AMP) injections (25 mg per ml), 3 ml intramuscularly one to three times a week. Or liver extract injections, 20 mcg once a week.
- • Have a doctor evaluate your DHEA (dehydroepiandrosterone) hormone level. Supplement if borderline low or below.
- • Ask your doctor about antifungals like Diflucan and nystatin.

Herbs: Padma 28, two to three times a day (call PADMA AG at 877-877-2362 to order the commercial preparation), helps half of the chronic cases when taken for one year. The cannabinoids in marijuana have been shown to control tremors and muscle spasticity (in animal studies). Ask your doctor about a prescription for medical marijuana.

N

NOSEBLEEDS (Epistaxis)

Loss of blood from the mucous membrane that lines the nose, most often from only one nostril. Common in childhood, nosebleeds in old age are more serious. If you lose a large amount of blood, you may get dizzy. If you swallow blood, your stools may turn black.

Causes: Most nosebleeds are caused by accidents, putting something in your nose, or just blowing your nose too hard. Inflammation from a cold, allergies, high altitudes, or dry winter air can cause nosebleeds. Occasionally, recurrent nosebleeds are a sign of hypertension, an infection, a bleeding disorder, exposure to mold, a tumor of the nose or sinuses, or fumes from chemicals like formaldehyde. If a nosebleed starts after a heavy blow to the head, it could indicate a fractured skull.

Uniquely Female: Estrogen influences mucus production. Anything that changes the level of estrogen can make a woman more prone to nosebleeds. Tell your doctor if you are prone to nosebleeds before starting any hormonal treatment, especially oral contraceptives.

What to Do

When Your Nose Starts to Bleed

- Sit calmly in an upright position with your head tilted forward. Blow out all blood clots from both nostrils, breathe through your mouth, and pinch the fleshy lower part of your nose for twenty minutes. Slowly release the pressure and avoid any subsequent contact with or pressure on the nose.

- If bleeding continues after the first twenty minutes of applying pressure, pack your nose with gauze or use cotton dampened with white vinegar (the acid cauterizes the nose) and apply wrapped crushed ice against the nose and cheek. Sit up straight so you won't swallow any blood. If bleeding still continues after twenty more minutes, notify a doctor.
- When bleeding stops, lie back and rest for a few hours.

<u>After the Bleeding Has Stopped</u>

- Squeeze the contents of a vitamin E and vitamin A capsule into the lining of your nose. You may also use zinc oxide, K-Y jelly, aloe vera gel, comfrey or calendula ointment in your nose and then place a small piece of gauze against the gel.
- Blood thinners such as Coumadin, aspirin, or excessive vitamin E may cause nosebleeds; if this happens, notify your doctor.
- Use a humidifier filled with distilled water if your room is too dry.
- Smoking dries out your nasal cavity. Don't smoke.
- Avoid decongestant nasal sprays. They constrict blood vessels.

Diet: Vitamin K is essential for blood clotting and is found in dark green leafy vegetables such as watercress and kale and in green tea.

Avoid: Foods high in salicylates (page 112).

Nutrients: Bioflavonoids, 500–1,000 mg at the start of bleeding and every hour if bleeding continues for four to six hours. Vitamin K, 5 mg per day may help intermittent and chronic cases.

Herbs: Try 1 tsp. aloe vera gel dropped into each nostril or a comfrey ointment to keep nasal membranes from drying out. One cup of nettle-leaf tea several times a week can be taken as a preventative (stop if nettle upsets your stomach).

O

OSTEOPOROSIS

Loss of bone mass, causing bone to become brittle and easily fractured. Osteoporosis affects more than 25 million Americans, causing 1.5 million fractures annually, including 300,000 hip fractures. About a third of these women end up in nursing homes, and 25 percent never get better. Most women don't know that osteoporosis is often preventable and usually treatable.

Symptoms: Wrist fractures in women often occur fifteen years before osteoporosis has become severe. If your wrist fractures, even in your thirties, get a bone density test. Chronic backache from bone loss occurs after 50 percent of bone mass is lost. Other indicators are chronic leg pain, unusual dental problems, or facial tics. Falls that would not cause a fracture in a young adult may produce fractures in older women, particularly in the hip and spine. Small fractures in one or several vertebrae cause bones to be compressed, leading to a progressive loss of height and possibly to a "dowager's hump" and pain due to spinal neck compression.

Causes: Inadequate calcium and/or vitamin D in the diet or factors that increase calcium loss, such as diets high in protein, sodas, caffeine, low levels of minerals that help keep calcium in the bony matrix, too much cadmium (test with hair analysis), inadequate stomach acid, chronic stress, certain hormonal disorders, or prolonged treatment with corticosteroid drugs. Low levels of vitamin D, or vitamin D resistance, may be the result of vitamin D receptors that are damaged by age or blocked by hormonal pollutants. Osteoporosis is more common in smokers and drinkers and is associated with chronic obstructive lung disorders such as bronchitis and emphysema. Celiac disease (intolerance to gluten foods) causes *osteopenia* (low bone mineral density).

Risk Factors
- Family history of osteoporosis or bone disease
- History of amenorrhea, infrequent periods, late menstrual onset, or anovulatory cycles
- Small bones, long thin bones, low skeletal mass
- History of anorexia, diabetes, hyperthyroidism
- Fair complexioned, blond, blue-eyed coloring
- Low percentage of body fat
- Over forty years old
- Had ovaries removed
- Never had children
- Early menopause
- Allergic to dairy products
- Celiac disease

<u>**Uniquely Female:**</u> Much more common in women (especially small-boned, lightweight white or Asian women) than in men, particularly after menopause or after the removal of the ovaries because of the reduction in estrogen. A woman's bone mass peaks around age thirty-five and rapidly decreases for several years right after menopause at the rate of 3–8 percent of bone mass per year. Approximately 50 percent of postmenopausal women over the age of sixty-five develop osteoporosis-related fractures. Women whose hair turns prematurely white may be at higher risk. Vitamin D supplementation in infant multivitamin formulas is linked to higher bone mass in adolescent girls. Young women on oral contraceptives lose less bone.

What to Do
- ** Have a baseline bone densitometry test *before* menopause and regular ones every several years after menopause to track bone loss over time. All women over sixty-five, regardless of

OSTEOPOROSIS AND HORMONE REPLACEMENT THERAPY

At this time, the exact role of all hormones in menopause is not known, but it is believed that natural progesterone (not progestins) may be the hormone responsible for building new bone, while estrogen (at the levels given in hormone replacement therapy) helps to prevent further loss. For women who do not respond to natural therapies, natural hormone therapy should be combined with vitamin D, calcitonin (a hormone that inhibits bone resorption), and new calcium-sparing medications like Fosamax (ask your doctor about the once-a-week pill). Some women can develop severe heartburn, even long after starting Fosamax, so trying natural treatments first makes sense.

Have your hormone levels checked for estrogen, progesterone, DHEA (dehydroepiandrosterone), and/or testosterone. Transdermal DHEA patches have been shown to increase bone density. Estrogen's bone-sparing effect is enhanced when vitamin D_3 is added to the diet. Estrogen alone is not the answer. Low levels of estradiol were *not* associated with spine fractures in the Rancho Bernardo Study (*Journal of Clinical Endocrinology and Metabolism* 85:219, 2000), meaning bone loss was due to other hormone deficiencies and factors.

risk, should have a bone scan. Urine tests can tell what is happening to bone in the moment, although they can sometimes give false alarms. Bone-specific alkaline phosphatase tests tell if bone is rebuilding (responding to a treatment program).

** Others who should be tested include women who have or have had anorexia nervosa; long-term users of Depo-Provera injections; and those with renal failure, hyperthyroidism, malabsorption, vitamin D deficiency, Cushing's syndrome, or rheumatoid arthritis. Chronic use of some medications may contribute to bone loss, and users should be tested.

** Have your stomach acidity evaluated. You need adequate stomach acid to absorb calcium and other minerals.

** Ask your doctor to test your homocysteine levels. High levels may cause bone loss (see *Homocysteine*).

** Weight-bearing exercise strengthens the bones and can actually increase bone mass. You're never too old to start exercising. Do thirty to sixty minutes four or more times per week.

Combine resistance training with light weights with cardio-vascular exercise, such as walking or running on a treadmill. Both impact and nonimpact exercises have been shown to increase spinal bone density in pre- and postmenopausal women.

- Each year about 250,000 osteoporosis-related hip fractures occur. To avoid falls:

  Keep your home well lit, including night-lights for the bathroom.

  Don't have throw rugs or scatter rugs in your home.

  Have room to maneuver around furniture.

  Use a cane if you are unsteady on your feet.

  Wear cushioned footwear to protect your feet and external hip pads worn under clothes to protect your hips.

- All women with osteoporosis should be tested for celiac disease (antigliadin antibody blood test).
- If relatives have celiac disease, get young girls tested; if high, have them consume a gluten-free diet to avoid poor calcium absorption.
- Sleep on a firm mattress if your back is affected.
- Don't smoke. It lowers estrogen levels. Over time, a pack a day results in a 10 percent loss in bone density.
- A Harvard study showed that hypnosis (plus standard care) lessened the need for pain medication, increased mobility and function, and provided easier rehabilitation and a more positive outlook for postmenopausal women with bone fractures from osteoporosis.
- If you have compression fractures, ask your doctor for a prescription for decompression water exercises with a physical therapist. For chronic severe pain, ask about vertebroplasty.
- Fluorescent lighting, electric blankets, aluminum cookware, and nonfiltered computer screens can all leach calcium from the body.
- Avoid fluoride toothpastes, especially during peri- and post-

menopause. It increases bone density, but with a poor-quality bone.

- Get a hair analysis to rule out cadmium and lead exposure.
- If osteoporosis runs in your family, avoid depo medroxypro-gesterone acetate for contraception.

Diet: Calcium, calcium, calcium. Good sources are low- or nonfat dairy products, especially yogurt. However, many people have trouble digesting dairy products. If you consume little or no dairy, it isn't easy to get the recommended dietary allowance (RDA) of this nutrient. High-calcium foods include dark green leafy veggies (except spinach), sea vegetables, nuts, salmon, and sardines (with bones). Vitamin K foods are excellent in helping to build bone mass: alfalfa, egg yolk, kelp, fish liver oils, leafy greens, and green tea. Soy prevents bone loss, but may be contraindicated in certain women (page 413).

Dairy and Bone

Yogurt elevates blood calcium longer and more effectively than milk, which only increases calcium levels for two hours, unless taken with calcium supplements. Cottage cheese and cheese actually rob the body of calcium due to their high acid content, high protein, and alteration of the calcium during processing.

Avoid: Too much protein depletes calcium, but the line between how much is too much versus too little is hard to say. Meat, poultry, and dairy (not yogurt) are all high in protein, and eating too much of these foods in proportion to veggies, fruits, and grains can weaken your bones.

Limit caffeine. If you drink two to three cups of coffee a day, consume at least 800 mg of calcium a day to avoid bone loss. Limit salt, which also increases calcium loss. High levels of phosphates, found in one or more colas a day, food additives, pesticides, and processed foods, deplete calcium. Excess alcohol reduces bone formation. Women should limit themselves to one alcoholic drink per day. Face it—women are just more sensitive to colas, caffeine, and alcohol than men. Also note that taking pharmaceutical antacids for one to two years has been associated with bone loss, and fluoride increases the risk of hip fractures in women. Don't eat too much chocolate (high in oxalic acid, which binds up calcium).

Between 40 and 60 percent of bone mass is accrued in adolescence. Teenage girls who consume carbonated beverages (especially colas with phosphoric acid) are three times more likely to break bones than girls who don't drink them. Natural colas use fruit acids and are a better choice.

Nutrients

Many of the minerals below come in multimineral formulas.

** *Calcium is the most important nutrient for bones.* Calcium absorption can vary from less than 10 percent to over 60 percent in healthy women, so these recommendations are approximate. You need to be tested and monitored to see that what you are taking is working.

Prevention: 800–1,000 mg per day added to a diet that contains 500–700 mg of calcium from food

To Stop Active Bone Loss: 1,000–1,500 mg per day. Natural hormone replacement therapy (HRT) plus calcium is much more effective than therapy without calcium.

Postmenopausal Women Not on HRT: 1,500 mg per day

Pregnant or Nursing Women over the Age of Eighteen: 1,000 mg per day

Pregnant or Nursing Women Under the Age of Eighteen: 1,300 mg per day

Take calcium with meals. Capsules and chewable tablets are more absorbable than compressed tablets (especially if you don't make enough stomach acid), and liquid is the most absorbable, especially for older women or those with digestive problems. There are a number of different types of calcium—citrate, lactate, malate, orotate, aspartate, or extracts of whole bone or compounds like hydroxyapatite calcium (a microcrystalline form of calcium with associated factors that is well absorbed). *Calcium citrate is the most absorbable.* Calcium carbonate (the calcium in some antacids) has been found to bind up thyroid hormone, which can cause thyroid problems in some women, and it is the form of calcium most often contaminated with lead. Look for labels that say "essentially lead free." Don't take calcium and iron together; each inhibits absorption of the other. The calcium in fortified soy milk is not as absorbable as the calcium in cow's milk.

Many bone formulas contain all the essential nutrients listed below.

** Magnesium, 250–650 mg per day or in a 2:1 (2 to 3 parts calcium to 1 part magnesium) ratio with calcium. Increase magnesium if you are prone to constipation and reduce if you are prone to loose stools. The most absorbable forms of magnesium are citrate, aspartate, or glycinate.

** Vitamins B_6, B_{12}, and folic acid, in amounts found in vitamin B complex supplements and multivitamins, reduce homocysteine levels and protect bones.

** Vitamin K, 150–500 mcg per day

** Zinc, 10–30 mg per day

• Manganese, 5–20 mg per day

• Silicon, 1–3 mg per day

• Strontium, 500 mcg–3 mg per day

• Vitamin D, 400–800 IU per day (low blood levels are associated with hip fractures, especially in winter and spring. Low levels are linked to bone loss. *If you have to be on corticosteroids for any reason, take vitamin D plus calcium to prevent bone loss.* Vitamin D reduces the number of falls and number of fractures by up to 50 percent.

• Copper, 500 mcg–3 mg per day

• Vitamin C, 500 mg per day or more; take with calcium

• Cod liver oil, 3–4 capsules twice a day

• Avoid boron if you have had hormonal cancers or estrogen-dominant health problems unless you are working with a doctor. Some postmenopausal women get fewer hot flashes with boron, while some get more.

• Ask your doctor about Ipriflavone, 300 mg three times a day. It's a synthetic phytoestrogen that acts like estrogen to protect bone, but, unlike estrogen, it may also enhance bone formation. Its safety for women with hormonal cancers is unclear.

• Have your thyroid checked. Women with too high or too low

thyroid levels and low DHEA (dehydroepiandrosterone) are at greater risk of bone loss.

- Calcitonin is a naturally occurring hormone involved in calcium regulation and bone metabolism. It reduces bone breakdown and appears to reduce pain. Currently it is available as an injection or nasal spray. Ask your doctor.

Herbs: Horsetail, 2 g three times a day; silica, 1–2 mg per day.

OVARIAN CYSTS

The ovaries are glands on either side of the uterus immediately below the opening of the fallopian tubes. Each ovary contains numerous follicles (sacs) in which egg cells develop. The ovaries also produce the female sex hormones estrogen and progesterone.

Ovarian cysts are abnormal, fluid-filled swellings in an ovary, benign in 95 percent of cases. The most common type is a *follicle cyst*, frequent in young women. They are usually small and go away by themselves. However, they can get large and cause problems, such as pain, rupture, bleeding, or scar tissue. Ovarian cysts are usually not a form of cancer. Cysts tend to appear when too much estrogen and inadequate progesterone are produced by the ovaries and tend to go away after menopause. *Chocolate cysts* are a type of ovarian endometriosis.

Symptoms: Most cysts are asymptomatic unless they rupture, twist, become infected, or bleed. Fever may indicate that a cyst has become twisted and needs surgical removal. Symptoms of cysts include late, irregular, or painful periods; abdominal pain that doesn't go away; enlarged or swollen abdomen; trouble emptying the bladder completely; pain during sexual intercourse; feelings of fullness, pressure, or discomfort in the abdomen; and weight loss for no apparent reason.

Causes: Unopposed estrogen or other hormonal imbalances, use of birth control pills, fertility drugs, or hormone replacement therapy. Inflammation of the ovary *(oophoritis)* may be caused by mumps or by other infections such as gonorrhea, pelvic chlamydia, or pelvic inflammatory disease.

What to Do

- If you are at high risk for ovarian cancer (you can get genetic testing to see if you carry the mutated genes), have a baseline vaginal ultrasound. Repeat yearly to monitor ovary size. Have a yearly blood CA-125 test to rule out ovarian cancer (although this does not pick up every type of ovarian cancer). Avoid bleached tampons, reduce or eliminate supplemental estrogen, and eat organic food as much as possible.

- *Ovarian cyst homeopathic formula:* 2 cc each from mother tinctures of phytolacca, byronia, gelsemium, and aconite. Put in an 8 oz. dark glass jar and fill with filtered water. Take 2 Tbsp. three times a day between meals. Pre- and postvaginal ultrasounds have found this to be effective in reducing large cysts within one to two weeks in a number of women. Do not continue after two weeks.

- Ask your doctor about iodine drops (6 drops per day of SSKI by prescription) for two to three months. While taking iodine, have your thyroid function monitored (based on clinical work by Jonathan V. Wright, M.D.).

Diet: Shred broccoli and cabbage into salads. Try broccoli sprouts.

Avoid: Caffeine, refined sugars, concentrated starches, hard liquor.

Nutrients

For recurrent cysts, take for a two-month trial:

- ** Alpha-lipoic acid, 50–100 mg once or twice a day
- ** B complex, 25–50 mg once or twice a day \
- ** Bromelain, 500–1,000 mg twice a day between meals
- ** Fish or evening primrose oil, 2–8 g per day in divided doses
- ** Vitamin B_6, 20–40 mg once or twice a day
- ** Magnesium citrate, 250–600 mg per day
- Melatonin, 1 mg for two to three days midcycle and for the last several days before your period, may *theoretically* work.
- Indole-3-carbinol, 200 mg twice a day if you weigh 120 pounds or less; or 300 mg twice a day (over 120 pounds);

or Indoplex by Tyler, 80 mg twice a day may *theoretically* work.

Herbs: Milk thistle, 300 mg two to three times a day. Vitex, 40 drops of concentrated herbal extract in a glass of water in the morning for up to six months. You must work with a doctor.

P

PELVIC INFLAMMATORY DISEASE (PID)

Severe or recurrent infection or inflammation of the upper genital tract. The disease starts in the vagina and moves into the uterus, up the tubes, and into the ovaries. Sometimes it spreads to other areas in the abdomen. It includes a variety of conditions, such as infection of the fallopian tubes (*salpingitis*) or ovaries (*oophoritis*), infection of the lining of the uterus (*endometritis*), and pelvic peritonitis. It is most common in women in their late teens or early twenties who have more than one sexual partner. More than 1 million women develop PID each year, which partially explains why the rates of infertility and tubal pregnancy have doubled in the last few decades. It is a common causes of pelvic pain in women. It seldom occurs after menopause.

Symptoms: Abdominal pain, tenderness, and rigidity; fever; an unpleasant-smelling vaginal discharge; and backache. The pain often occurs immediately after menstruation and may be worse during intercourse. There may be pain during urination, more frequent urination, and vaginal bleeding. Symptoms will depend on where the infection is and which organism has caused it. Repeated attacks may occur without reinfection.

Causes: Usually bacteria. Almost three quarters of all cases occur after a sexually transmitted disease (usually gonorrhea or chlamydia), while others occur after miscarriage, abortion, or childbirth. Women who use intrauterine devices have a three to five times greater risk of PID than those who use other methods of birth control.

What to Do
- Requires antibiotics immediately to prevent scarring of fallopian tubes and subsequent infertility.
- Don't put anything in your vagina until the infection is gone. Don't douche.
- Use sanitary pads if you have a period while taking your medication.
- Wait until your doctor tells you it's okay to have sex. Make sure your partner(s) have finished their antibiotic treatment before having sex with them. Use latex condoms.

Nutrients

Natural treatments can act as supportive and adjunct therapies for rebuilding pelvic health after medical treatment.
- After the infection is gone and the doctor says you can have sex, moisten a tampon with a vitamin A capsule and sprinkle it with a powdered probiotic culture. Insert and leave in place overnight. Remove in the morning. Repeat for five nights in a row.

For Two Weeks After Infection
- ** Consume live cultured yogurt, 4–8 oz. per day, to prevent yeast vaginitis that can accompany antibiotic treatment.
- ** Multivitamin/mineral supplement
- ** Vitamin C, 1,000–2,000 mg three times a day
- ** Vitamin A, 25,000 IU per day, then reduce to 5,000 IU per day
- ** Zinc, 20 mg per day (balanced with copper, 2 mg per day)
- Vitamin E, 400 IU per day

Herbs: Butiao (Chinese herbal) to reduce pain, 3 tablets twice a day; echinacea extract, ½ tsp. two to three times a day between meals; and goldenseal for lingering symptoms after antibiotic therapy. Drink nettle and yellow dock teas steeped fifteen minutes two to three times a day for several weeks after the infection has cleared.

PELVIC PAIN

Severe or chronic pelvic pain is a complicated problem because so many different abdominal organs can be the source of the pain. A doctor will want to know the following:

- Did the pain start suddenly or gradually?
- Is the pain in sharp intermittent waves; severe and steady; or a dull ache or pulling pain?
- Where is the pain located?
- Other symptoms associated with the pain, such as fever or chills
- Relationship of the pain to your menstrual cycle, diet and digestion, bladder function, and sexual intercourse

In Premenopausal Women, Pain Can Come From:
- Fibroids: Often produce chronic lower abdominal fullness and aching (some women get symptoms, most don't); the same pain can occur with moderate to severe premenstrual syndrome (PMS)
- Pelvic congestion: Poor circulation in the pelvis due to an imbalance of prostaglandins and inflammation, nutrient deficiencies, spinal malalignment, or PMS.
- Endometriosis: Episodes of pain (mild to severe) and fatigue that are often accompanied by pain on intercourse.
- Trigger points: Pinpoint areas that can mimic the pain of hernias and can occur in patterns of referred muscular pain that actually come from distressed abdominal organs. Can be treated by Dr. Janet Travell's trigger-point work. Read Travell and Simons' *Myofascial Pain and Dysfunction: The Trigger-Point Manual* (2-volume set), by Janet Travell, M.D., and David G. Simons, M.D., illustrated by Lois S. Simons (Lippincott, Williams & Wilkins, 1998).

In Postmenopausal Women: Abdominal fullness, pain, indigestion, and/or swelling may be a sign of ovarian cancer.

During Pregnancy: After the first trimester, pelvic pain is due mostly to pressure produced by the growing uterus. The pain may be sharp, dull, or stabbing and may radiate to the legs, hips, or vagina. In the second half of pregnancy, uterine contractions are the most common pains.

PERIMENOPAUSE

The years leading up to menopause when the menstrual cycle is likely to get shorter and irregular, and when other symptoms such as hot flashes begin to occur. Dr. Christine Green of Palo Alto, California, calls perimenopause "ovarian retirement."

Hormones stabilize multiple body systems as well as deliver the messages that act as directives for thousands of cellular tasks. When the hormonal environment starts to wax and wane during perimenopause, numerous systems become destabilized, and new health problems can manifest themselves. Women can suddenly experience confusing symptoms, all of which may be caused totally or in part by their new "crazy" hormonal environment.

You Are Probably in Perimenopause if:
- Your menstrual flow has changed (and you're in your forties)
- The timing of your cycles has changed
- You're starting to gain more weight around your middle
- Your muscles are less firm
- For the first time you are starting to have cramps or breast tenderness
- You get hot flashes (can recur during menopause)
- You get new health problems or old ones, such as headaches or allergies, go away

Symptoms
- *Mental*—Disorientation, depression, fear, apathy
- *Allergic*—Nasal congestion, recurrent respiratory infections, sneezing, fatigue
- *Neurologic*—Dizziness, headaches, memory loss, loss of balance

- *Rheumatologic*—Tingling, joint problems, arthritic aches and pains, numbness
- *Skin*—Gravity starts to win and old sun exposure begins to show

Signs of Excess Estrogen or Low Progesterone (see page 286)
- Breasts engorge before periods, enlarge, hurt
- Cramping with periods and midcycle pain
- Headaches before periods
- Bleeding problems, such as spotting or heavy periods

Signs of Low DHEA (Dehydroepiandrosterone) (see page 284)
- Fatigue
- Can't build muscle mass
- Lowered libido
- Weight gain around the tummy
- Wake up feeling groggy, need more sleep than you used to

Causes: Aging. During ovulation in the childbearing years, eggs burst through the ovary. This process leaves a scar, called the *corpus luteum*, which produces estrogen, progesterone, and DHEA. Women at twenty-eight generally ovulate twelve out of thirteen months and make lots of these hormones. By their late thirties and forties, women ovulate less often and make fewer hormones. By age fifty, women are ovulating maybe half the time—and no ovulation means no progesterone and much less DHEA. So many symptoms of peri- and postmenopause are caused by the waning of various hormones (though testosterone doesn't wane as much for quite some time). This process starts at about age thirty-five and up, with more irregular cycles, fewer hormones, bone loss, less energy, spotting; and *early onset is linked to a history of depression.*

Birth Control Pills and Perimenopause

Doctors frequently recommend birth control pills to women in their forties. Not good. This increases the risk of blood clots, stroke, diabetes, migraines, allergies, and gallbladder problems. Women are not told this, nor are they warned to take folic acid, which oral contraceptives deplete. Insufficient studies leave us not knowing if oral contraceptives at this age may increase the risk of breast cancer.

What to Do*

Whenever a woman in her mid-forties to fifties experiences a new set of symptoms that are confusing and not easily linked to causes, she and her doctor should consider hormonal imbalance or deficiencies. Have your doctor run hormone tests for the three estrogens, progesterone, DHEA, testosterone, and early-morning cortisol. If your hormones are low or out of balance, try hormonal supplementation for several months and see if your symptoms go away or greatly improve.

When women first start in the perimenopause, using natural progesterone in cream form is a good way to try to decrease symptoms, along with taking magnesium, 250–800 mg per day; calcium, 800–1,000 mg per day; B vitamins, 50 mg per day; and essential fatty acids like borage and fish oils, several grams a day.

Creams must be applied on a rotational basis to the torso, shoulder, sides, inner thighs, inner wrists, and soles of feet (if no calluses). *Never* use progesterone cream on the breasts. Your doctor should monitor your progress by how you "feel" and hormone tests. See if improving lifestyle habits helps. If you develop signs of low DHEA, have your blood levels tested and check to see if DHEA is needed. Oral forms of progesterone are available but not recommended if you have a history of liver disease.

Some women cannot handle progesterone, even the natural kind. They feel "odd" or get depressed. Some women are allergic to the peanut oil in Prometrium, and some women just can't handle creams. Some women do better and feel "safer" on herbs. The delivery system must work for your life.

---

* Co-authored with Christen Green, M.D.

PHLEBITIS (Thrombophlebitis)

Partial or total blockage of a vein by a blood clot *(thrombus). Superficial phlebitis* is the inflammation of part of a superficial vein, near the surface of the body, along with clot formation in the affected segment. *Deep vein thrombosis (DVT)* tends to occur in the leg or pelvis and is far more serious as it can lead to embolism (the sudden blocking of an artery by a clot). Pieces of the clot can break off and travel to one of the arteries supplying the heart muscle and cause a heart attack, or they can travel to arteries supplying the brain and cause a stroke. Deep vein thrombosis is a medical emergency!

Symptoms: In superficial phlebitis, there is obvious swelling and redness along the affected segment of vein, which is extremely tender to the touch and can feel warm and like a hard cord. The condition occurs most often in leg veins close to the skin. There may be limitation of movement or fever. There are more symptoms with superficial phlebitis than with DVT. In DVT, there may be dull aching pain and possibly swelling, or there may be no symptoms at all.

Causes: Can occur after minor injury to a vein and is common in intravenous drug users. Can come from varicose veins, sitting for extended periods on an airplane, especially with crossed legs, resting in bed for a long time, or wearing a cast. Other causes include side effects from oral contraception, smoking, clogged arteries, toxic blood from excess consumption of saturated fats and a sedentary lifestyle, inflammation, infection, obesity, stressed liver, poor circulation from constipation or a weak heart, high blood pressure, or starting a new medication or supplement. Risk increases with being over sixty years old and being overweight. Phlebitis in an upper extremity can come from physical trauma, extreme exercise workouts (especially abduction exercises), or after getting lymph nodes removed as part of breast cancer surgery.

Uniquely Female: During pregnancy there is a rise in the level of coagulation factors in the blood, which may lead to DVT. Women who take birth control pills have an increased tendency for blood to clot, get deep vein thromboses three to four times more often than nonusers, and have a higher risk of recurrence of superficial phlebitis.

Smoking while using birth control pills can lead to more than the usual amount of clotting. High levels of homocysteine may be connected. Women who have had lymph nodes removed during cancer surgery are at increased risk in the nearby limbs. Women on traditional hormone replacement therapy are more at risk.

What to Do

- For superficial phlebitis, keep the affected arm or leg elevated. If pain is severe, rest. Use towels, soaked in warm water, wrapped around your arm or leg to relieve the pain. You may use ginger tea instead of water.
- Don't sit or stand for long periods of time. Don't cross your legs when you sit.
- To keep from getting blood clots: Move your legs as soon as possible after surgery or during long periods of bed rest; exercise your legs every one to two hours while on long car or airplane trips.
- Avoid tight clothes, especially at the groin, where deep vein pressure may originate.
- Wear elastic stockings, support hose, or elastic bands on the arms to reduce pain, although they do not promote quicker healing.
- Exercise. Walk or move several times a day for twenty to thirty minutes.
- Stop smoking, especially if you are taking birth control pills.
- Ask your doctor to test your homocysteine levels, and take B vitamins if they are elevated.

Diet: Drink quality liquids such as Green Drink (page 465), filtered water, berry drinks (especially black cherry juice), or berry mixes once a day. Beneficial foods include garlic, ginger, onions, and hot peppers (which contain capsicum), which protect against heart attack and stroke. Use granulated garlic on food as a regular spice. Fish oils help to reduce clotting of blood. Increase consumption of cold-water fish to at least three times per week. Beets, especially grated raw beets, are a classic remedy for improving veins. Consume extra-virgin olive oil rather than refined, and eat nuts and seeds.

Avoid: Alcohol, caffeine, and excess refined sugars. Avoid all saturated and hydrogenated fats.

Nutrients

For an Acute Attack

- ** Cod liver oil, 2–3 Tbsp. per day until pain settles down, then taper down to 1 Tbsp. per day
- ** Bromelain, 1,000 mg two to three times a day, between meals
- ** Bioflavonoids, 500 mg of mixed three times a day, plus butcher's broom, 300–500 mg three times a day
- ** Aspirin or nonsteroidal anti-inflammatory drugs (NSAIDs) taken with meals. Discuss the dosage with your doctor, and avoid if you have ulcers.
- ** Vitamin E, 800 mg per day
- • Niacin, 50 mg once or twice a day

To Prevent an Attack (If You Have Had Two Recurrences)

- ** Bromelain, 500–1,000 mg twice a day between meals, plus butcher's broom, 200 mg once a day
- ** Bioflavonoids, 200 mg twice a day
- ** Cod liver oil, 1 Tbsp. per day (balance with vitamin E, 800 IU per day)
- • If you are prone to phlebitis, take one prophylactic enterically coated baby aspirin (81 mg) and/or several bromelain (1–3 g once or twice a day between meals) before prolonged periods of travel, bed rest, or surgical procedures.

Herbs: Drink green tea especially with high-fiber meals. Hawthorn extract, two to three times daily, improves circulation; horse chestnut extracts with 50–75 mg of aescin twice a day for two months, then reduce to once a day, to strengthen veins.

PREGNANCY

Getting pregnant, being pregnant, labor, and delivery are huge topics, with many available sources of excellent information. In this book we are just touching on some aspects of pregnancy that respond to natural treatments.

Some suggestions for a good pregnancy:

- Make sure your multivitamin contains choline, which is needed for normal development of your child's memory. Eggs are another good source.
- Opiates and barbiturates given in labor and delivery have been linked to drug abuse when these children grow up.
- Taking fish oil and/or eating fish promotes higher DHA (docosahexaenoic acid) fatty acid in blood of newborns, good for baby's brain. Taking cod liver oil during pregnancy leads to kids with a lower risk of diabetes.
- Prenatal perineal massage with warm olive oil reduces tearing during delivery, even for women with a previous episiotomy.
- Vitamin A and beta-carotene help with maternal night blindness. Ask your doctor about the correct dose.
- The way a mom eats during her pregnancy affects her child's bone density later in life.
- Women with celiac disease have a greater risk of miscarriage, unfavorable birth outcomes, and low birthweight babies. Get tested.
- Elevated levels of estriol, in one single saliva testing, is a useful marker for assessing women at risk of having premature birth, even before physical symptoms manifest, especially in women with known risk factors.
- If there is a family history of atopy, avoid peanuts during pregnancy (Committee on Toxicity of Chemicals in Food, United States government).
- Moms who take multivitamins greatly reduce the risk of heart abnormalities in their babies. Starting at end of first

month does not offer protection, so women of childbearing age should take multivitamins on a regular basis. They should also take folic acid, which prevents neural tube defects forming during the first two weeks of pregnancy, and B vitamins. Birth control pills and smoking deplete folic acid, and folic acid in food is not very well absorbed.

- Sexual intercourse during the last few weeks of pregnancy greatly increases the risk of preterm delivery, especially in women twenty-five to twenty-nine years of age.
- Don't go off vitamin C cold turkey. Take 70–100 mg of vitamin C per day. Don't take quercetin when pregnant.
- Eat tuna only once a week and avoid shark and swordfish, which are high in mercury.
- Vitamin K_3 stops nausea and vomiting, but it's not available in pharmaceutical form. Doctors should demand this.
- Magnesium, 250–300 mg per day, reduces uterine cramping.
- Limit caffeinated beverages; high consumption of these is linked to fetal loss.
- Prenatal multivitamins/multiminerals with lower levels of iron (27 mg) and more of vitamin C meet recommended iron levels (> 3 mg) and cause less tummy irritation and fewer problems with blocking zinc levels.
- Certain drugs block the action of folic acid and may increase the risk of neural tube defects even though you are taking folic acid. These pharmaceuticals are: aminopterin, carbamazepine, methotrexate, phenobarbital, phenytoin, primidone, sulfasalazine, triamterene, trimethoprim, and valproic acid.
- Take calcium (see page 352) to protect your bones, and to protect your baby's brain from lead (*Nutrition Reviews* 59 (5):152–55, 2001).
- Low zinc in blood or hair analysis has been linked to increased risk of neural tube defects.
- Avoid chemicals like wood varnish and perchlorethylene found in cleaners. Let someone else pick up your dry cleaning, and air it out in the garage for four days before wearing.

Symptoms

Here are some tips to discuss first with your doctor for controlling the many symptoms that accompany pregnancy:

Anemia: Have your doctor run iron and ferritin blood tests in early pregnancy to see if you require iron supplementation.

Back Pain: As the baby grows, it is common to experience back pain. Try squatting instead of bending over (which also helps develop those thigh muscles so important during labor). Try to maintain good posture by standing straight. Wear shoes with good support. Don't wear high heels. Do stretching exercises each day. Back rubs are helpful. Try soaking a towel in cider vinegar, squeezing out the excess, and lying down on your side with the towel spread across your back for fifteen to twenty minutes. Acupuncture helps reduce pain.

Bleeding Gums: Brushing and flossing during pregnancy will keep your gums and teeth healthy. Use liquid folic acid mouthwash and rinse for thirty seconds after flossing. Increase vitamin C foods, calcium, and protein. Be sure to tell your dentist that you are pregnant, and don't have any X rays taken.

Constipation: Drink plenty of liquids (six to eight 10-oz. glasses a day) and eat foods such as bran cereal, bran muffins, raisins, fruits (at least one fresh fruit a day), and raw vegetables. Daily exercise helps, especially walking. Check with your doctor before taking a laxative.

Edema: Toward the end of pregnancy, there may be six or more quarts of excess water in the mother (half of which is in the fetus, placenta, and surrounding the fetus). The mother's feet and legs swell because the uterus compresses the large veins that return blood from the legs to the heart. Also a rise in estrogen causes swelling of hands and feet. Be sure to remove your rings before they have to be cut off. Don't eliminate salt from your diet. Lying down two or three times a day and raising your legs above your heart for ten to fifteen minutes will reduce the swelling. Lie on your left side while sleeping to help prevent swelling. Drink plenty of liquids. Do not use diuretics. You may want to wear elastic support stockings.

Abnormal fluid retention during pregnancy may indicate

preeclampsia (see the discussion of preeclampsia later in this section). Consult with your doctor or midwife and consider adding more protein and magnesium in your diet. In pregnancy, generalized edema may be a sign of hypertension or high blood pressure, especially when there are headaches, blurred vision, or dizziness.

Frequent Urination: You will urinate more often as the growing uterus presses on your bladder. When lying down, the uterus no longer blocks the blood vessels in your legs, which is why you urinate frequently at night, as fluid from the legs becomes available for excretion. You could also pass urine when you cough, sneeze, or move. Don't cut down on liquids! Infections in the urinary tract are more common during pregnancy. Call your doctor if you have burning or pain when you urinate.

Hemorrhoids: See *Hemorrhoids.*

Heartburn: See *Digestive Disorders.*

Insomnia: Very common during last weeks of pregnancy when it is hard to find a comfortable sleeping position. Use a long body pillow or a number of smaller pillows behind or under your belly. Staying active during the day helps. Increase vitamin B foods like whole grains and fresh veggies. Try herb teas—chamomile, marjoram, and lemon balm. Scullcap and passionflower may also help.

Itching: Milk thistle, 200 mg per day, can help relieve itching skin due to poor gallbladder function during pregnancy.

Leg Cramps ("Charley Horse"): May result from varicose veins, from a deficiency of calcium, magnesium, or potassium or an excess of phosphorus in the diet, and the growing uterus can affect blood circulation to and from the legs. Leg cramps can develop when you are tired. Try to rest often with your legs higher than your heart. Put a hot water bottle or heating pad on the cramped area and apply pressure with your hand.

Moodiness: Those crazy-making hormones! Your moods may change from joy to sadness or mild depression in rapid succession. Crying jags for no reason are not unusual.

Morning Sickness: Nausea and vomiting are especially common during the first half of pregnancy. Although unpleasant, it is usually not serious. Hormone changes and a sluggish digestive system may contribute to morning sickness. Nausea is sometimes relieved by lying down immediately after meals, which should be frequent and small. Eating saltines or dry toast before getting out of bed in the morning may help. Avoid greasy, fried, or spicy foods. Stress can worsen nausea. Women with severe nausea have higher rates of birthing girls.

Take vitamin B_6, 10–25 mg once a day, for mild nausea. Do not go over 25 mg, as higher levels can inhibit future milk production. When morning sickness is severe, swallow vitamin C, 100 mg, plus vitamin K, 5 mg, in the same mouthful every three to four hours. If this doesn't work, try adding ginger, 1 g a day (*Obstetrical Gynecology* 97:577–82, 2001). Teas from red raspberry leaf, basil, ginger, and peppermint help relieve nausea. Don't smoke, and ask others not to smoke around you. Acupuncture can help stop vomiting.

Sciatica: Irritation of the large nerve that runs through the hip joint and down the back of the thigh is common during pregnancy. A chiropractor or physical therapist can help.

Sore Breasts and Nipples: Breasts will get larger, heavier, and possibly sore during pregnancy. Get a good support bra and wear it around the clock if necessary. Toward the end of pregnancy, clear or milk-like liquid may come from your nipples, which is perfectly normal. Wash them only with water. If the nipples are sore, apply lanolin or calendula ointment.

Stretch Marks (Striae): These fine, wavy, pinkish marks on the lower abdomen or upper thighs may not be due only to stretching, but also to the increased amount of a hormone in the tissues which "fragments" the elastic fibers in the skin, as well as zinc deficiencies. They often fade after pregnancy.

For prevention, apply the following recipe to the areas in which stretch marks usually appear: Mix in a blender ½ cup virgin olive oil, ¼ cup aloe vera gel, the oil from 6 capsules of nonsynthetic vitamin E, and some essential *fun* oil. Refrigerate in a jar and apply some each day. (You can also apply this ointment daily with stretching massaging motions around the vaginal opening to reduce the need for episiotomies during delivery. Or have your partner apply.) Make sure you're on a multivitamin/mineral supplement that contains zinc.

Round Ligament Pain (a "Stitch" in the Side): On each side of your uterus are bands of tissue called ligaments that hold the uterus in place. As the uterus grows, these ligaments are pulled and may cause abdominal pain. This is normal. Lying on your sore side may help the pain, as may deep breathing. Daily exercise helps.

Skin: Apply lotion if your skin feels dry and itchy. *Chloasma* (mask of pregnancy) is a darkening of the skin on your face, around the nipples, and below the belly button. It results from an increase in pigmentation and affects more than 50 percent of pregnant women, particularly brunettes.

Sweating: Dress in loose, comfortable clothing. Don't soak in hot tubs during pregnancy.

Tiredness: You may need more sleep than usual. If you can, try taking a few ten- to fifteen-minute rest breaks during the day.

Vaginal Discharge: You may have thicker and heavier vaginal discharge, possibly with an odor. Check with your doctor if the discharge is accompanied by burning or itching.

Varicose Veins: The growing baby and long periods of standing can put pressure on the veins in your lower body, often the legs, where blood moves slowly. You are more likely to get varicose veins if other members of your family have them. Rest often with your legs raised higher than your heart. Wear support panty hose. If you have varicose veins in the genital area, rest often with a small pillow under your bottom. Varicose veins should improve or disappear after delivery. Heat and massage may help. Try vitamin C, 500 mg, with bioflavonoids and rutin twice a day.

The Centers for Disease Control reported in 2000 that the chemical called dibutyl phthalate (DBP) has been found in the highest levels in the urine of women of childbearing age. Although the Food and Drug Administration and the cosmetic industry regard DBP as safe, studies have shown it to cause birth defects in lab animals, and various phthalates have been linked to reproductive problems in boys. Women who are thinking of becoming pregnant or are pregnant should avoid colognes, perfumes, and nail polishes that contain phthalates.

TOP TEN WARNING SIGNS IN PREGNANCY

Tell your doctor immediately if you have:

1. Any vaginal bleeding or spotting

2. Severe, persistent headaches

3. Prolonged vomiting (over one to two days, preventing adequate intake of liquids)

4. Blurring of vision; spots before the eyes

5. Fever (over 100°F) and chills not accompanied by symptoms of a cold

6. Sudden intense or continual abdominal pains

7. Sudden gush of fluid from the vagina

8. Sudden swelling of hands, feet, and ankles

9. Frequent, burning urination

10. Pronounced decrease in fetal movement

(from *The Complete Guide to Women's Health*, by Bruce D. Shephard, M.D., and Carroll A. Shephard, R.N., Ph.D., Plume, 1997, p. 115)

Herbs for Pregnancy: Red raspberry leaf tea (the best uterine tonic), peppermint, ginger root, bilberry, burdock root, yellow dock root, and chamomile. Shepherd's purse is helpful for good strong uterine contractions during birth. In the case of all herbs, check with your doctor.

For more information, see *Women's Encyclopedia of Natural Medicine* (Hudson/Keats, page 234, 1999).

Serious Problems of Pregnancy

Before or during pregnancy, have your blood homocysteine levels tested. Elevated levels of homocysteine may be risk factors for pregnancy complications (preeclampsia, spontaneous abortion, placental abruption) and adverse pregnancy outcomes. These events are linked to nearly 30,000 infant deaths before age one in the United States as well as to birth defects. If homocysteine levels are high, ask your doctor for supplemental levels of folic acid, vitamins B_{12} and B_6, and B complex.

After one month, rerun blood test. Do not go higher than 25 mg per day of vitamin B_6.

AIDS

Although AIDS (acquired immunodeficiency syndrome) began as an epidemic among gay males, women currently account for 13 percent of all U.S. AIDS cases. Women are two to five times more likely than men to acquire HIV (human immunodeficiency virus) from heterosexual sex. Only blood, semen, vaginal discharge, and breast milk contain enough of the virus to infect others, so it can only be transmitted by sexual contact, sharing contaminated needles, and by an infected woman transmitting the disease to her fetus or through breast-feeding her newborn. If a pregnant woman has HIV, cesarean birth may offer the best protection to her child since there is a 20 percent risk of the infant's contracting the virus before or during delivery. Breast-feeding transmits the virus roughly 14 percent of the time; using milk substitutes reduces transmission of HIV from an infected mother to her infant by 44 percent.

Various perinatal antiretroviral regimens now available help to prevent transmission of HIV from mothers to babies, although the benefit of perinatal treatment is diminished in breast-fed infants. Women who receive effective antiretroviral therapy as a matter of routine care have a relatively low risk of transmitting the virus to their babies.

Gestational Diabetes

Vitamin B_6, 25 mg used one time a day, is the most important nutrient for warding off this disorder. Chromium supplementation improves glucose intolerance and lowers elevated insulin. Refined carbohydrate restriction improves the condition and reduces the mother's need for insulin. Have your blood glucose, urine ketones, appetite, and weight gain monitored and develop an appropriate treatment program with your doctor. Diets higher in vegetable and fish oils compared to animal fats appear to be protective against blood sugar abnormalities. Be careful about iron supplementation, as there is a link between increased iron stores in moms and this condition in offspring (*Diabetes Medicine* 18:218–23, 2001).

Toxoplasmosis

Eating raw meat or being around cat litter can cause an infection from this organism that can result in birth defects and other pregnancy problems. Wash your hands after touching raw meat and make sure it is well cooked before you eat it. Let someone else clean the cat's litter box. Do not garden in soil that cats use as a bathroom.

Preeclampsia (Pregnancy-Induced Hypertension)

Also known as *toxemia of pregnancy*, this is a serious condition in which high blood pressure, edema, and protein in the urine develop in a woman in the second half of pregnancy. Other symptoms can include headache, nausea and vomiting, abdominal pain, fluid retention, and visual disturbances. It affects about 7 percent of pregnancies and is more common in first pregnancies and in women under twenty-five or over thirty-five. There is less than a 5 percent chance of preeclampsia in a second pregnancy.

The rise in blood pressure usually occurs after the twentieth week, unless diabetes, hypertension, or kidney disease already exist. After delivery, the mother's blood pressure usually returns to normal. Untreated, preeclampsia may lead to eclampsia (convulsions and coma). Bed rest improves the flow of blood through the uterus. Ask your doctor about magnesium sulfate, which appears to be more effective than phenytoin sodium in preventing recurrence of seizure in eclampsia. Preeclampsia and eclampsia are the most common causes of maternal death and increase the risk of infant mortality even in industrialized countries.

Tom Brewer, M.D., is credited with encouraging the consumption of high-quality protein to combat this disorder, while John Ellis, M.D., pioneered the use of vitamin B_6 in preeclampsia. Intravenous (IV) magnesium has been standard care for years in the later stages of preeclampsia. Vitamin B_6, magnesium, and protein in the early stages can entirely prevent this condition. Even in later, more serious stages, intravenous amino acids or human albumin, vitamin B_6, and magnesium sulfate reduce or eliminate the problem. Inadequate levels of vitamins E and C increase risk, as does a low level of calcium.

To Prevent Preeclampsia

Eat high-protein foods like eggs, turkey, or nuts along with whole grains, fruits, vegetables, and legumes. Avoid sugar and white flour. Take calcium, 1,200–1,500 mg per day, and magnesium, 400–600 mg per day. High-risk women should take 1,500–2,000 mg per day of calcium. Take a high-potency multivitamin/mineral supplement that includes 10–20 mg of vitamin B_6 and vitamin B_2; vitamins C and E; and evening primrose oil.

Miscarriage, see *Miscarriage*

Postpartum Depression

Depression in a woman after childbirth, ranging from an extremely common and short-lived attack ("baby blues") four to five days after giving birth, to a severe depression that may last for weeks, with a constant feeling of tiredness, difficulty sleeping, loss of appetite, and restlessness. You may feel sad, nervous, irritated, moody, or cry a lot. It affects 10–15 percent of women and can occur with any birth, the first or the sixth. A small number of women may develop a severe depressive psychosis two to three weeks after childbirth. Some women can develop transient underactive thyroid within one to six months after delivery, which may coincide with postpartum depression. Post-traumatic stress disorder is common after stillbirths. See a therapist.

What to Do
- Rest whenever possible. Nap when the baby naps.
- Don't try to do everything yourself. Do only what is needed and let everything else go. Ask others to help.
- Talk to other mothers about how you are feeling.
- Take care of yourself as well as the baby. Shower and dress each day. Don't forget to eat. Try to get out of the house each day.
- Request a complete hormonal workup.
- If you cannot take care of the baby or feel negative toward the baby, it is okay and normal; get help in taking care of the child for the first weeks. This is part of the depression and is *not* a part of your ability as a mother.

PREMENSTRUAL SYNDROME (PMS)

A common group of symptoms that occur one or two weeks before a woman starts her period and go away when her period begins or several days into it. In severe cases, symptoms can occur for three weeks out of each month. At some time in their lives, around 90 percent of women experience PMS. In 15–25 percent of women, these symptoms are severe enough to disturb life and relationships for a number of days each month. *Premenstrual dysphoric disorder* is an aggravated form of PMS with extreme moodiness and depression that interfere with functioning.

Symptoms are many, all the way from retaining fluid and getting irritable to having a recurrence of a common ailment (like bronchitis or a rash) or feeling exhausted. Most women can reduce PMS symptoms through general lifestyle and nutritional improvement.

PMS symptoms can be divided into four categories that may further help treatment (though these aren't set in stone):

1. *Anxiety (PMS-A)*—Includes anxiety, irritability, irrational anger, short temper, aggressiveness, and nervous tension. Usually from too much estrogen and inadequate progesterone.
2. *Cravings (PMS-C)*—Eating disturbances, such as increased appetite, craving for sweets, and binge eating. Fatigue, faintness and/or dizziness, and possibly heart palpitations can occur. Comes from low levels of prostaglandins and changes in carbohydrate metabolism.
3. *Depression (PMS-D)*—Crying fits, confusion, absentmindedness, depression, and insomnia. Comes from low levels of estrogen and high levels of progesterone, high levels of prolactin, possibly low levels of DHEA (dehydroepiandrosterone), plus elevated adrenal hormones.
4. *Hyperhydration (PMS-H)*—Fluid retention, abdominal bloating, breast pain/tenderness, and weight gain. Comes from inadequate vitamin B_6, possibly low thyroid, low progesterone levels, or excess aldosterone (adrenal hormone).

Other physical symptoms include headache, backache, acne flare-ups, and constipation or diarrhea. You can experience symptoms from all categories.

Causes: PMS is a syndrome with many possible causes, including hormone imbalance or deficiencies due to less frequent ovulation; essential fatty acid imbalance; nutrient deficiencies; and hypoglycemia. Stress can cause or worsen the problem. Most women develop PMS in their thirties and forties following an interruption of the hormonal cycle, such as after a pregnancy or after stopping birth control pills. In rare cases some women can be sensitive or allergic to some of their own hormones. It has been estimated that 10–40 percent of women with PMS may have subclinical or overt low thyroid.

What to Do

** Ask your doctor to run multiple hormone panels, especially progesterone, and check your thyroid to rule out over-low thyroid or subclinical hypothyroidism. If nutrients and lifestyle change don't help, check out progesterone therapy (from ovulation to beginning of menses) and in rare cases hormone "desensitization" (some women are allergic to their own hormones).

Note: Regarding commercial formulas touting progesterone from unprocessed wild yam—the body *cannot* make progesterone from wild yam; wild yam molecules need to be processed by a compounding pharmacist in order to turn into "natural" hormones.

- Keep a menstrual calendar for two or three periods (see *Menstrual Calendar*). Knowing when you are likely to have PMS symptoms will help you plan your activities and nutrients.

  When using progesterone cream, *never* use it on your breasts. Rotate on thin-skinned areas of body, such as wrists, shoulders, inner thighs, etc. Some thin-skinned women can't handle even natural progesterone and may get depressed or feel "off" when using it.

- Moderate exercise every day can help relieve symptoms.
- Remember to breathe deeply.

- Try a mineral bath. Add 1 cup sea salt and 1 cup baking soda to bathwater and soak for at least twenty minutes.
- Test for food allergies, and have a hair analysis done to rule out heavy-metal poisoning.
- Don't smoke, and avoid secondhand smoke. Nicotine inhibits hormone function.
- Try ice packs on the pelvic area, or fresh ginger root compresses covered with a hot water bottle.
- Massage, sauna, and shiatsu are helpful.
- Get at least twenty minutes of sunshine a day, preferably while taking a walk.
- Orgasm helps move blood and other fluids away from congested organs and can relieve the sluggish circulation that comes with PMS.
- In rare cases, candida-related complex may be causing or aggravating PMS.
- Progesterone helps some, even if not all studies agree. *Oral* progesterone is good for anxiety and mental symptoms.

Diet: High-protein snacks, especially sources like seeds and nuts, eaten between meals can prevent low blood sugar. Consume quality proteins such as legumes, soy, and fish. Eat lots of veggies and fresh fruit.

The Chocolate Connection: It's not your fault when you reach for that chocolate bar or knock off that pint of ice cream right before getting your period. Hormone disturbances seem to affect the area of the brain responsible for carbohydrate cravings. And chocolate has the amino acids the brain needs at that point, along with magnesium. Try eating fruit when the cravings hit, or consume chocolate in tiny amounts.

Avoid: Head off constipation by reducing your intake of red meat and alcohol. Avoid drinking three or more alcoholic drinks a day, which can reduce your level of progesterone. Constipation promotes the absorption/recycling of estrogens from the intestines and can lead to hormone imbalances. Avoid or limit sugar, refined carbohydrates, caffeine, and identify and avoid food allergies. Avoid hydrogenated oils carefully. Some women may need to go off dairy. Eat moderate amounts of cabbage, cauliflower, and brussels sprouts, especially raw, which are good if you have high estrogen/low progesterone. Don't overconsume these foods if you have underactive thyroid.

Some women do well on an anti-candida or antifungal program (no refined sugars, fruit juice, processed foods, or dairy) and when taking an antifungal medication or oil of oregano. Women with a history of recurrent vaginal yeast infections and those who took glucocorticoid medications, birth control pills, or multiple antibiotics might try this approach.

Nutrients: Try nutrients and diet change first. If these don't help, ask your doctor about progesterone therapy.

- ** Vitamin B$_6$, 50 mg one to three times a day. Studies show that doses of vitamin B$_6$ up to 100 mg per day most often help PMS and associated depression, mood changes, and anxiety. Women with acne, bloat, and headache before their period do well with B$_6$.
- ** Vitamin B complex, 50 mg per day
- ** Magnesium (citrate and others), 200–600 mg per day in divided doses
- ** Essential fatty acids like black currant seed oil, borage oil, evening primrose oil, flaxseed oil, or fish oils. Example: 2,000 mg twice a day of gamma-linolenic acid (GLA), 1 Tbsp. per day flaxseed oil, or 500–1,500 mg evening primrose oil twice a day. (There are conflicting studies about evening primrose oil, but many women feel it helps.)
- ** Calcium (citrate and other forms), 800–1,200 mg per day in divided doses with meals and before bed (less if you consume high-calcium foods). Calcium supplementation has been consistently shown to be effective when taken for at least three months.
- ** Vitamin E, 400–800 IU per day
- ** Evaluate your need for digestive enzymes (page 468).
- • Acidophilus decreases the reabsorption of estrogens from the intestines.
- • Zinc picolinate, 15 mg once or twice a day, and backup trace minerals in a multimineral formula

- Tryptophan, 1,000–1,500 mg per day. Tryptophan and St. John's wort help most with depression, sweet cravings, and trouble sleeping.

Herbs: Vitex (herbal support to increase production of progesterone), 40 drops of tincture with a glass of water in the morning for two weeks before your period, is especially good for acne associated with PMS, as well as reducing irritability, mood swings, anger, headache, and breast fullness. Some doctors feel that vitex (which works at the level of the pituitary gland) is not safe for long-term use. Discuss with your doctor. *Do not use at the same time as progesterone.*

St. John's wort, 300 mg per day, can reduce symptoms by 50 percent. Dong quai, black haw tea for women between fifteen and thirty-eight, bupleurum and peony for women over age thirty (½–1 tsp. three times a day for two weeks before your period). False unicorn root, ¼–½ tsp. two to three times a day with meals one week before your period, but only with supervision.

If Diet, Nutrients, and Progesterone Therapy (Used Day 12 Through Day 25 of Cycle) Don't Help

Consider any of the following treatments and/or anti-candida therapy (page 444):

- *For PMS-A,* add mixed bioflavonoids, 500 mg twice a day; indole-3-carbinol, 200 mg twice per day; melatonin, 1 mg at bedtime for several days midcycle and several days before your period. Eat less animal products and some raw broccoli in salads.
- *For PMS-C,* add chromium, 100 mcg three times a day, and emphasize evening primrose oil, 500–1,000 mg twice a day, and bromelain, 250 mg three times a day between meals one week before your period. Cut down on carbohydrates in your diet in ratio to proteins. Eat often (every three to four hours) and consume lots of veggies.
- *For PMS-D,* tyrosine, 500–1,000 mg each morning the week before your period until your period is finished, and free-form amino acid blend every night before bed for several months. Take 1,500 mg tryptophan twice a day. Take folic

acid, 800 mcg per day. Two weeks before your period, take DLPA (D, L-phenylalanine) three times a day for extreme moodiness. Do not take tyrosine if you are taking an MAO (monoamine oxidase) inhibitor.

- *For PMS-H*, check thyroid hormone and progesterone levels. Take extra vitamin B_6. Avoid allergens.

> Some new drugs used for PMS are actually just antidepressants (like Prozac) with another name. Beware!

PROGESTERONE, see *Hormones*

PUBERTY

"Puberty" is the term used for the physical changes (development of secondary sex characteristics) that underlie the emotional changes of adolescence (the period between childhood and adulthood). Usually occurs between the ages of twelve and fifteen, and is initiated by the pituitary gland producing hormones that stimulate the ovaries to increase secretion of estrogen.

The first sign of puberty in girls is usually breast budding, although some girls develop pubic hair first. The development of a wider pelvis and fat distribution in the hips and buttocks may lead some girls to anorexia and/or bulimia. The circulating sex hormones initiate sexual fantasies and sexual arousal, resulting in vaginal lubrication, which in turn can lead to teenage pregnancy and sexually transmitted diseases.

Menarche (the First Menstrual Period)

Usually occurs a year or more after the beginning of puberty, by which time pubic and underarm hair are in a fully developed adult pattern. Girls who are overweight tend to start earlier than average, which may be related to the critical body weight-to-height ratio that a girl has to achieve before menstruation starts (although the essential change that triggers menstruation takes place in the brain). GnRH (gonadotrophin releasing hormone) is secreted steadily during childhood until a few years before menarche, when GnRH is released in pulses that stimulate the release of hormones from the pituitary gland which, in turn, stimulate the ovaries to make and release estrogen.

Precocious Puberty

Sexual development that begins very early (between the ages of five and ten) may be related to hormone disruption, or exposure in the womb from environmental and plant substances that can mimic the action of human hormones. The age at which menstruation begins has been getting younger for the past century. Studies on boys and girls suggest that those who go through puberty too early (and also too late) are at risk for lower IQ; more behavior problems, such as higher level of crime, unruly behavior in school, greater frequency of delinquent acts; and generally poor mental health when compared to children with normal age of puberty. Early puberty also puts young girls at higher risk of hormonal problems, including cancer, later on in life.

What to Do When Your Daughter Hits Puberty
  ** Hold on to your hat, and pray.
  ** A daily multivitamin/mineral supplement with B complex has been shown to consistently lower antisocial behavior, such as disrespect, disorderly conduct, defiance, obscenities, etc. in children and teenagers.
  • Encourage good nutrition, healthy exercise, and a positive body image.
  • Discourage smoking, drinking, and drug abuse.
  • Good communication skills are a must.
  • Talk openly about sex, sexually transmitted diseases, and contraception. If you are uncomfortable doing this, have a woman friend, relative, nurse, or counselor talk with your daughter.
  • Melatonin, 1–3 mg at night, helps adolescents with school phobia and sleep disturbances. Try for one week. If it helps, continue for one to two months, but it shouldn't be used on an ongoing basis.

R

RAPE

A sexual assault in which the woman is forced to have vaginal, oral, or anal intercourse against her will. It is also a sexual assault if she is forced to masturbate the man or to be masturbated by the man. In half the cases of rape, the woman knows her assailant.

In the event of rape, a woman should not bathe or shower, wash her genitals, or change her clothes until she has seen a doctor, and she should not drink any alcohol before talking to the police, as she may be accused of being drunk and submitting willingly to the rapist. Try to remember exactly what took place and in what sequence. Rape crisis centers help a woman come to terms with her pain and anger as well as shameful feelings of being "dirty" or "used." Get checked by a doctor for sexually transmitted diseases. Rape is not your fault, and not all men are bad. See the discussion of post-traumatic stress disorder, page 415.

RAYNAUD'S DISEASE

A disorder of the blood vessels in which fingers (or less commonly toes and face) turn bluish white or patchy red and blue from lack of blood when exposed to cold. When symptoms are secondary to some other condition, the disorder is termed *Raynaud's phenomenon*.

Symptoms: Spasm and contraction in the capillaries in fingers and toes that reduce the blood supply. There may be tingling, numbness, pain, or burning in the affected digits. Warming your hands or feet usually helps relieve these symptoms. In longstanding Raynaud's, the skin of fingers or toes may look smooth, shiny, and tight.

Causes: The immediate cause of symptoms is exposure to cold or emotional stress. It is often associated with migraine headaches, various anginas, and high blood pressure, so it is thought that all these disorders share common underlying problems with abnormal constriction of the blood vessels. Raynaud's disease has no known cause, whereas Raynaud's phenomenon is secondary to illnesses such as scleroderma, arthritis, and systemic lupus erythematosus, as well as nerve disorders, thyroid deficiency, and reaction to certain drugs (channel blockers, ergot, antihypertensives). A history of smoking is often linked to this illness. Like carpal tunnel syndrome, Raynaud's happens more often in those who use their fingers continually, such as pianists, computer operators, etc. Also, those working jobs with repetitive activities or vibrating tools may develop occupational Raynaud's.

Uniquely Female: Between 60 and 90 percent of cases occur in young women, especially those between the ages of twenty and forty. Linked to estrogen-driven autoimmune problems (see *Estrogen Dominance*).

What to Do
- Keep your whole body warm and dry. Dress in layers. Choose fabrics that wick away perspiration (such as cotton-blend socks instead of pure cotton). Wear a hat; the greatest loss of body heat is from your head.
- Don't let your hands or feet get cold. Always wear mittens or gloves in cold weather and when handling ice or frozen food. (Mittens are warmer than gloves because they trap more body heat.) Use holders for glasses or cans containing cold drinks. If possible, stay indoors during very cold weather.
- Stop smoking and stay away from secondhand smoke. It narrows the small blood vessels.
- Learn stress-reduction techniques (pages 52–58).

- Wear loose-fitting socks and comfortable, roomy shoes.
- Avoid using tools and machinery that vibrate.
- Have a hormonal evaluation of progesterone, DHEA (dehydroepiandrosterone), and thyroid. Rule out underactive or subclinical thyroid disease.

Diet: Drink plenty of fluids.

Avoid: Coffee and other caffeinated beverages that constrict blood vessels, and alcohol, which lowers body temperature. Identifying and avoiding food allergies helps some.

> **A SIMPLE WARM-UP EXERCISE**
>
> Swing your arm downward behind your body and then up in front at about eighty rotations per minute. This forces blood to the fingers.

Nutrients
- ** Inositol hexanicotinate, 500–1,000 mg two to four times a day (must be monitored with blood liver enzyme tests). Do not take if you have a history of liver disease. Or take vitamin B_3 (niacin), 100 mg two or three times a day. Start low and increase the dose until you feel flushing.
- ** Magnesium, 300–600 mg per day. Ask your doctor about intravenous magnesium.
- ** Multivitamin/mineral supplement with trace minerals
- ** Fish oil concentrate, 5–10 g per day
- ** L-carnitine, 1,000 mg two or three times a day
- ** Evaluate for digestive enzymes (page 468).
- Folic acid, 5 mg per day for one or two months (shown to relieve symptoms in clinical practice; see doctor)

Herbs: Padma 28 (call PADMA AG at 877-877-2362 to order), twice a day, or ginkgo biloba, 40 mg three times a day.

RESTLESS LEGS SYNDROME

A syndrome that features unpleasant tickling, burning, pricking, or aching sensations in the muscles of the legs, particularly at night in bed. Affects around 5 percent of the population. Tends to run in families, and is most common in people who consume a lot of caffeine, in smokers, and in people with rheumatoid arthritis or diabetes. Can be a warning sign of lung disease, kidney disease, Parkinson's, and many neurological disorders, so get checked out by a doctor.

Symptoms: Usually affects both lower legs and occasionally the thighs and arms. Symptoms are worst when trying to sit still, rest, or sleep.

Causes: Possibly related to a problem in the nervous system that originates in the brain or spinal cord. May be linked to mineral deficiency or genetics.

Uniquely Female: Most common in middle-aged women and during pregnancy.

What to Do
- Exercise regularly.
- Walk before going to bed.
- Change sleeping positions.
- Soak your feet in cool (not icy cold) water. Others may find a heating pad more soothing.
- Quit smoking.
- Rule out iron deficiency.

Diet: High-fiber diet with plenty of green vegetables.
Avoid: Refined sugar, caffeine.

Nutrients
- ** Folic acid, 5–30 mg per day. If it works, take with vitamin B complex, 50 mg twice a day, and zinc, 20 mg once a day, to balance.
- ** Vitamin E, 800 IU per day
- ** Multivitamin/mineral supplement twice a day (make sure it includes B vitamins)
- Calcium, 500 mg two to three times a day
- Magnesium citrate or malate, 200–300 mg two or three times a day
- Iron only if diagnosed iron deficient by a blood test

Herbs: Passionflower plus valerian, 150–250 mg of each (they often come together in herbal formulas) in the morning and evening or just in the evening.

RUBELLA (German Measles)

A viral infection that is serious only when it affects a woman in the early months of pregnancy and sometimes in children. If contracted during the first twelve weeks of pregnancy, one baby in three will be malformed, often severely (deafness, congenital heart disease, mental retardation, cerebral palsy, eye and bone disorders). In very early pregnancy, miscarriage may occur. Symptoms include a rash on the trunk and limbs, a slight fever, and enlargement of the lymph nodes at the back of the neck. Rubella vaccine provides long-lasting immunity.

S

SALPINGITIS,
see *Pelvic Inflammatory Disease*

SCIATICA

An inflammation of the sciatic nerve, which starts in the low back and runs across the buttocks and into the leg, calf, and foot.

Symptoms: Any or all of the following—nagging, aching, tingling, burning, or numbness that can start or remain in the buttocks, or travel the course of the sciatic nerve down the back of the thigh and the front of the foreleg. Pain is usually on one side. May be sensitive to temperature changes and touch and, in cases related to disc disorders, may radiate down to toes, affecting strength in the feet or walking gait. Disc causes are usually associated with low back pain, often worse on bending backward and better lying down.

Causes: Protruded disk pressing on a spinal root of the nerve, or pressure from a muscle that can surround the nerve like a clamp. In one third of people, the sciatica nerves go through the *piriformis muscle,* which can spasm down on the nerve. Any disorder that involves nerves (such as diabetes or alcohol dependence) may affect the sciatic nerve, as may arthritis of the vertebrae joints and spinal stenosis.

__Uniquely Female:__ There are documented cases of cyclical episodes of sciatica that are due to stray uterine tissue (endometriosis) wrapped around the nerve so that it swells and bleeds with the menses. Keep a menstrual calendar. If the pain is associated with or worsens from midmonth to several days into your period, try taking vitamin B_6 (25–50 mg per day) along with magnesium (250 mg per day) and evening primrose oil (several grams each day). Also, fluid shifts with premenstrual syndrome can cause surrounding tissues, including the piriformis muscle, to swell and increase pressure on the nerve, especially in women with a thick sciatic nerve passing right through this muscle.

What to Do

** A professional like a chiropractor must diagnose the cause of your pain. If piriformis syndrome is the cause, find a chiropractor or Rolfer who can do deep piriformis work. Chiropractic therapy often helps with unprotruded herniated discs if treated by an extension table (like the Cox table). Call around for chiropractors trained in Cox technique.

- Avoid activities that aggravate pain.
- Stretching rarely helps and may worsen the condition.
- If endometriosis is causing your problems, see _Endometriosis_. Try nutrients before surgery.
- Ice packs or wet heat may relieve pain.
- For prevention, exercise regularly.

__Diet:__ High fiber (constipation can make the pain of sciatica worse); drink six to eight glasses of bottled mineral water a day.

__Avoid:__ Caffeine, especially chocolate, and refined sugars.

Nutrients

** Bromelain, 300–500 mg three times a day between meals

** Magnesium, 500–600 mg twice a day

** Calcium, 500–600 mg twice a day

** Vitamin C, 500–1,000 mg twice a day

- B complex, 50 mg each day
- For prevention, take fish oils, 2–4 g per day in divided doses.
- If nothing helps, ask your doctor about vitamin B_{12} (1,000 mcg)

with vitamin B$_1$ (50 mg) injections, or intravenous magnesium injections given three to seven days during the first week, then tapering down (page 471).

Herbs: Boswellia, 400–800 mg three times a day, or turmeric, 500 mg four times a day, during acute symptoms as anti-inflammatory agents.

SEXUALITY

For those of us who don't choose to be celibate, sex can be an oasis of intimacy, pleasure, and a natural way to recharge our batteries. If sexual desire, sexual arousal, or the ability to have an orgasm is reduced or inhibited, self-esteem and relationships can suffer.

Some of the problems of sexual dysfunction include painful intercourse (*dyspareunia*) and failure to achieve orgasm (this used to be called frigidity, but now is called *inhibited sexual excitement* or *anorgasmia*). Only about 50 percent of women reach orgasm during intercourse, but more than 90 percent can climax through clitoral stimulation. More than 80 percent of women have masturbated (see *Masturbation*), and many obtain an orgasm this way that is even more intense than through intercourse or oral sex.

Sexual response and libido tend to change as we get older. As many as 85 percent of postmenopausal women experience some degree of reduced libido, related to a decrease in sex hormones.

Causes: When pain is felt deep in the pelvis during thrusting with the penis, it may be caused by pelvic infection or endometriosis. Some women experience temporary painful intercourse following stitches to treat perineal tears or episiotomies after childbirth. Failure to reach orgasm can stem from stress, poor diet, childhood abuse or rigid upbringing or other trauma, as well as insensitive partners. Vitamin deficiencies (especially vitamin A) can lower estrogen levels, resulting in vaginal dryness. Hormonal fluctuations greatly influence sexual desire.

What to Do
- Exercise, such as walking, swimming, or dancing, can increase your sex drive.

- Environmental estrogens from everyday foods and products can affect female hormone balance. Buy organic foods, especially meats and dairy products, whenever possible.
- Have your thyroid, testosterone, and DHEA (dehydroepi-androsterone) hormones tested, as low levels cause lower libido and enjoyment. Also test estrogens and progesterone.
- Anxiety and stress can be major factors in sexual responsiveness. Learn stress-reduction techniques (pages 52–58).
- Consider psychological therapies and/or couples counseling.
- Have your mate look at his issues. It is astonishing that during the first four months after the release of Viagra (March 27, 1998), 3.6 million prescriptions were filled. So part of your sexual problem may be your partner's problems.

Diet: Eating a healthy, whole-foods diet enhances vitality, including sexuality.

Avoid: Chronic abuse of sedatives or alcohol can result in a lack of sexual desire.

Nutrients
- ** PABA (para-aminobenzoic acid), 100 mg two to three times a day
- ** Niacin, 100 mg thirty minutes before sexual activity to intensify orgasm
- ** L-arginine, 1–3 g a day, in divided doses
- Amino acids (L-phenylalanine, 500 mg or more—start low first; and tyrosine, 1–3 g—start low first), taken on an empty stomach in the morning and 20 minutes before sex on day of intercourse
- Vitamin B_6, 50 mg once a day, and vitamin B complex, 25 mg once a day
- Zinc, 50 mg per day, with a multimineral that contains 2 mg of copper

Herbs: Siberian ginseng and/or gotu kola. Muira-puama, 250 mg three times a day, enhances erectile tissue and libido.

ArginMax is a product of herbs and arginine; a double-blind, placebo-controlled study showed statistically significant increase in sexual desire, satisfaction, and frequency of intercourse compared to those getting the placebo.

SEXUALLY TRANSMITTED DISEASES
(Venereal Disease)

A class of diseases that includes infections spread by having sex. Sexually transmitted diseases (STDs) are the most common type of infection in the United States today after the common cold. The growth in the rate of STDs has occurred because some sexually transmitted viral infections (such as herpes, human papilloma virus, hepatitis B, and AIDS—acquired immunodeficiency syndrome) cannot be cured, while other infections, such as chlamydia and gonorrhea (which can be cured), display few if any symptoms and may therefore go undetected. Many sexually transmitted diseases can be cured within a week or two with antibiotic treatment. If left untreated, some of these diseases can cause infertility, while others can be fatal.

> At some college orientations, students are told that one in every three will have had an STD by the time of graduation. Smarten up! Use condoms!

Symptoms: Often women have no early symptoms, or there may be slight vaginal irritation, itching, or discharge (can be smelly); burning with urination; or eyes can become red and irritated. There can be small wartlike growths around the genital area, painful ulcers in and around the genital area, painful urination, or painless ulcers around the genital area or mouth.

Causes: Most come from bacteria or viruses.

What to Do to Prevent STDs

- Use a latex condom to reduce your risk of being infected. Other kinds of birth control can help prevent pregnancy, but they do not stop infections.

WHAT IS SAFE SEX?

Hugging and body-to-body rubbing; masturbation alone or with someone else; massage; dry kissing; intercourse with the use of a condom. Unsafe practices include sharing sex toys; using saliva as a lubricant; and intercourse without the use of a condom.

- The more people you have sex with, the greater your chance of developing a sexually transmitted disease. The fewer your sexual partners the better.
- Practice safe sex, although this does not guarantee that you'll avoid infection. The only 100 percent safety is to never have sex, or to sleep with only one person who is completely faithful to you. However, if you do have sex with more than one person, practice safe sex *every time.*
- Condoms made from animal membranes are not safe because germs can get through them. Use latex condoms in conjunction with a sperm-killing gel (spermicide) that contains at least 5 percent nonoxynol-9. Some condoms are prelubricated with spermicide. Using just a spermicide alone is not a reliable way to kill all the germs.
- If you use a lubricant, choose a water-based brand such as K-Y jelly, Foreplay, or Wet. Vaseline, Crisco, baby oil, or cooking oil could make the condom break.
- If you have oral sex, use a dry condom. If you don't use a condom, don't brush or floss your teeth first. Small cuts in the gums make it easier for germs to get into your body. Don't let the person getting oral sex finish in your mouth.

The following are brief descriptions of the main STDs:

Chlamydia

These microorganisms cause various infectious diseases. The organism usually infects the cervix, although in some women it can infect the lining of the uterus or the fallopian tubes and cause infertility. Chlamydia is the most common STD in the United States; more than

10 percent of sexually active women have chlamydial infection of the cervix but don't know it because they have no symptoms. Some may have a vaginal discharge or pain on urination, or cervicitis. More than 4 million new cases are diagnosed each year, and 20 percent of American adolescents have had chlamydia. It is the leading cause of pelvic inflammatory disease in women. Using oral contraceptives can predispose a woman to chlamydial infection.

Gonorrhea ("The Clap")

Gonorrhea is the second most common STD, affecting 2 million people in the United States each year. Most prevalent among young adults (fifteen to twenty-nine years old) who have had multiple sexual partners. Caused by a bacteria, it has an incubation period of seven to twenty-one days and affects the sex organs and sometimes the throat and rectum. Untreated, in women it may spread to the fallopian tubes, causing pelvic inflammatory disease (in approximately 17 percent of women) and is a major cause of sterility. About 80 percent of infected women have no symptoms, or there may be a smelly vaginal discharge, a burning sensation when urinating, or pain during intercourse. Gonorrhea can be cured. If untreated, the infection can spread to the internal sex organs, joints, skin, eyes, and heart. Gonorrhea acquired early in pregnancy increases the risk of premature labor, stillbirth, and postpartum uterine infection. The newborn may develop a serious eye infection if gonorrhea is present in the birth canal during delivery.

Genital Herpes

Caused by the herpes simplex virus, this disease produces a painful rash on the genitals. An estimated 40 million Americans have genital herpes, with 500,000 new cases diagnosed each year. Women are more at risk than men because a woman's genital area is warmer and moister. People with herpes are believed to be at greater risk for acquiring AIDS. Intercourse and oral sex must be avoided when genital sores are present. Pregnant women with an active attack may need a cesarean section to prevent the baby from being infected during delivery. Women with genital herpes have a greater risk of cervical cancer and should have regular Pap smears. Ask your doctor about an ointment made from propolis (available from Ap-Remedica Industries, Winnipeg, Canada), which has been more effective in treating lesions than have pharmaceuticals (*Phytomedicine* 7 (1):1–6, 2000).

Symptoms: Itching, burning, soreness, and small blisters in the genital area that develop when you first get the virus (they are so small that most people see only red bumps with redness around them). The blisters burst, leaving small painful ulcers. The lymph nodes in the groin may be enlarged and painful, and there may be headache, fever, and very painful urination. Even after the sores begin to heal, *the virus remains in the body permanently* and can cause renewed symptoms at any time. Subsequent attacks tend to occur after sexual intercourse, after sunbathing, around menstruation, or when the person is run down or stressed. Without treatment, there is a greater risk of inflammation of the brain, spinal cord, or bone marrow, as well as nerve pain. Ask your doctor about taking lithium carbonate for a short period of time.

Human Papilloma Virus (HPV)

This highly contagious disease is caused by any of about seventy viruses of the human papilloma group. It is the fastest growing STD in the United States today. It usually manifests as venereal warts (*condylomata acuminata*). These warts—small, soft bumps that can be pink, red, white, or brown—vary in size from a pinhead to large cauliflower-like clusters. In women, they tend to grow in the warm, moist areas of the perineum, inside the labia, in the vagina or on the cervix, or in the urinary canal or rectum. Incubation may take up to three months, and it can be much longer until the warts appear.

HPV has been linked to precancerous changes and cancer of the cervix, vagina, and vulva and is believed to account for a majority of abnormal Pap smears. Many, if not most, of the 10 million or more women in the United States with HPV infections are never diag-

---

 To test if a man is infected with genital warts (which may not be visible to the naked eye), wrap his penis with a cloth soaked in vinegar for five minutes. If there are any white patches found on the cloth, be sure to use a condom.

nosed. The warts will not go away without repeated treatment. Do *not* try to treat the warts with medicine used for hand warts. Women with genital warts should have a Pap smear at least once a year. Using a condom doesn't necessarily prevent genital warts, because they can be anywhere in the pubic area and are spread by skin-to-skin contact.

Syphilis

This STD is caused by a corkscrew-shaped organism called *Treponema pallidum*. Incidence increased dramatically in the early 1990s in urban areas, and the infection is spreading faster among women than men. Approximately 20,000 cases are reported in women each year. Syphilis often goes hand in hand with AIDS.

The bacteria multiply rapidly and the first symptom—a highly infectious hard-edged ulcer (chancre)—appears twenty to thirty days after contact, usually located on the genitals (but may also be on the anus, mouth, rectum, or fingers). The soft center of the ulcer oozes fluid, which is alive with the syphilis bacteria. A woman will infect any man with whom she has sexual intercourse during this period. The ulcers usually heal in three to eight weeks, leaving scars. Although it may seem to go away without treatment, unless syphilis is cured with antibiotics it will return later, spread, and attack almost any part of the body, including the skin, heart, blood vessels, and brain. Antibiotics usually cure the infection in two to three weeks. Untreated syphilis in pregnant women may result in miscarriage, stillbirth, birth defects, or severe infection of the newborn. After treatment, have a blood test every few months for one to two years to make sure the infection has really been cured.

Trichomoniasis

Trichomoniasis vaginitis is an infection of the vagina caused by a protozoa. The incubation period is about three to twenty-one days. The Centers for Disease Control (CDC) classifies "trich" as an STD. It is diagnosed in almost 5 million men and women in the United States each year. In addition to sexual transmission, it can be contracted from an infected washcloth or towel (although rarely), or transmitted to a baby during childbirth. The CDC recommends a comprehensive STD screening following the diagnosis of trich.

Symptoms: Painful inflammation and itching of the vagina and vulva, and a profuse, yellow-green, frothy, offensive discharge. Intercourse is usually painful. There also may be pain during urination if urine flows on swollen areas. Up to 50 percent of women are asymptomatic and have never heard about this infection. Even perimenopausal and menopausal women are at risk, due to loss of normal vaginal acidity and the protection it affords to the mucous membranes. Any overestrogenic state, from using hormonal contraceptives or even breast-feeding, can make the vagina susceptible to infection.

What to Do if You Have an STD

- You can't tell by looking at someone whether or not he or she has an STD. Learn someone's sexual disease history before sleeping with a new partner.
- Tell all your sex partners that you are being treated for an STD. They also need treatment.
- Don't have sex (including oral sex) while you and your partner are being treated. After treatment, use a condom to help protect against new infection.
- Urinate immediately after intercourse.
- Wash your hands often, especially after you urinate or have a bowel movement. Don't touch your eyes with your hands.
- If you are pregnant, tell your doctor that you have a sexually transmitted disease. Your STD could spread to your unborn child.
- Wear cotton underwear or panty hose with a cotton crotch so that wetness will not be trapped in the vaginal area. Loose clothing is preferable to tight jeans or pants.
- Keep your genital area clean and dry. Don't sit around in wet bathing suits.
- Take showers instead of baths and use plain, unscented soap. Avoid too much activity, heat, and sweating.
- Avoid feminine hygiene sprays or powders. Don't douche during treatment unless your doctor recommends it. After the infection is cleared up, do not douche more than once a week.

- Applying wet tea bags (black tea) or petroleum jelly to the sores may be soothing.
- Urinating in the shower or through a tube, like a toilet paper roll (to prevent it from hitting the skin on either side), can help relieve pain. Pour a cup of warm water between the legs while urinating.
- Try to avoid stress, fatigue, and illness. They increase the chances that symptoms will return. Learn stress-reduction techniques (pages 52–58).
- Test for food allergies.
- Stop smoking: Smokers have three times the risk of nonsmokers.
- Some oral contraceptives aggravate lesions by imbalancing the body's estrogen. Consider switching methods of birth control.

Diet: High fiber, low sugar, lots of fluids.

Avoid: Refined and processed foods. Alcohol and caffeine increase acidity, which adds to inflammation and makes symptoms worse. Sugary junk foods can aggravate infections. During an outbreak of herpes, reduce or eliminate foods containing L-arginine (whole-wheat products, brown rice, raw cereals, chocolate, carob, corn, dairy, raisins, nuts, and seeds).

Nutrients
** Antibiotics are necessary to treat STDs, but they kill off the body's good bacteria and lead to an overgrowth of yeast. *Lactobacillus acidophilus* yogurt, 4–8 oz. daily for two weeks, or probiotics, one hour before or two hours after the antibiotics and two to three times a day for two weeks after stopping antibiotics. There are dairy-free probiotics for those who can't consume dairy.

** Alpha-lipoic acid, 100 mg two to three times a day for two weeks

** Vitamin A, 50,000 IU per day for a week, then 25,000 IU for another week (see doctor)

** Carotenoids, 50,000 IU per day for two weeks
** Vitamin C, 1,000 mg once or twice a day for one month
** Vitamin E, 100–400 IU per day for one month
** Zinc, 20 mg per day for one or two months
• Folic acid, 800 mcg per day for one month

For Herpes
** Lysine, 4–5 g the first two days in divided doses, and then reduce to 500–1,000 mg per day while the outbreak continues.

For Severe Acute Herpes
• Lithium succinate–zinc–vitamin E ointment
• For bad cases, ask your doctor about low-dose lithium orally with essential fatty acids and adenosine monophosphate injections.

Herbs: Cat's claw, 500 mg three times a day; echinacea, 200–500 mg; and goldenseal, 125–250 mg three or four times a day for ten days, stop for ten days, then repeat. Garlic, 500 mg three times a day; oregano, 75 mg three times a day; turmeric, 500 mg three times a day. Bayberry and barberry are used for urinary tract symptoms. After antibiotics consider sarsaparilla extract for two months, or two or three cups of calendula tea each day. If you work with a naturopathic doctor, you might try a vaginal bolus (suppository) of herbal remedies.

SHINGLES (Herpes Zoster)

A viral nerve infection that most commonly affects people over fifty years of age. The extreme pain and discomfort usually disappear when the rash is gone, anywhere from a few days to a few weeks. Some people with shingles continue to suffer pain, itching, or burning of the skin for months or even years.

Symptoms: Small fluid-filled blisters on a wide band of reddened skin on one side of the body. Other potential symptoms are chills, fever, nausea, stomach pain, diarrhea, chest and face pain. Burning pain in the skin, called *postherpetic neuralgia,* may last for months or years after an episode of shingles (especially in the elderly) and may be worse than the original attack. Those at higher risk include people with cancer, acquired immunodeficiency syndrome (AIDS), and others with impaired immune function.

Causes: The disease is caused by the varicella virus, the same virus that causes chickenpox. Once you've had chickenpox, the virus never leaves your body and can become active many years later following physical or emotional stress or immune dysfunction. Someone with shingles can give chickenpox to an individual who has not had the disease before.

Uniquely Female: Those with postherpetic neuralgia or recurrences may experience heightened pain during the last two weeks of their menstrual cycle. If so, take vitamin B_6, 25–50 mg per day; magnesium, 250 mg per day; and essential fatty acids (1–3 g per day) for one to three months.

What to Do

- Shingles can damage the cornea of the eye. If shingles develops near your eyes, have your doctor order vitamin C (usually with vitamin A) eye drops from a compounding pharmacist, which can save your vision. See an ophthalmologist right away and don't touch your eyes.
- If shingles are generalized over the entire body, it may indicate an underlying human immunodeficiency virus (HIV) infection. Get tested.
- Avoid drafts. Get sunlight on the affected area for short periods of time during the day.
- Wash the blisters gently and avoid touching or scratching them.
- Tylenol-type medication (acetaminophens) can prolong the illness.
- Learn stress-reduction techniques (page 52).
- Get enough sleep and exercise.
- Do not bandage the sores.

- Avoid persons who have never had chickenpox until you are better.

Avoid: Refined sugar and foods high in arginine, especially chocolate, peanuts, walnuts, and wheat.

Nutrients
- ** Try zinc oxide cream mixed together with plain yogurt (or yogurt alone) on the blisters. This reduces pain and hastens healing. After they have healed, apply aloe gel and vitamin E to the area twice a day for one or two weeks.
- ** Ask your doctor about vitamin B_{12} injections, daily for first week, then taper down as symptoms decrease and blisters heal. This may help pain immensely, plus decrease healing time and lower the likelihood of complications. If not available, try vitamin B_{12} sublingual.
- ** Proteolytic enzymes, 1,000 mg twice a day between meals for several weeks to help with pain
- ** Vitamin C, 1 g twice a day, plus bioflavonoids
- • Vitamin E, 1,200–1,600 IU per day, to prevent or treat postherpetic neuralgia for several months, along with vitamin E concentrate (30 IU/g) cream applied directly

Herbs: Use capsaicin cream (0.025%) four times a day for one month; burns slightly after application from first to third day. Use gloves; avoid contact with eyes. Try cat's claw, 1,000 mg three times a day for two weeks, then reduce to 500 mg two to three times a day. Or try turmeric, 300 mg three times a day.

SKIN

The skin is the body's largest organ, responsible for half its detoxification. It is the body's shield against the outer environment, and it is a mirror reflecting the state of our health.

Dry Skin

Skin thins and decreases its ability to retain moisture as we grow older, causing dry skin. Don't use strong soaps or bubble baths. Bath oil may be helpful, although excessive bathing (long baths daily) should be avoided. Cold weather can cause dry skin. Proper digestion, essential fatty acids, and associated vitamins like B complex along with alpha-hydroxy products are a good way to keep skin moist and youthful.

Scars

Any mark left on damaged tissue after it has healed. Scar tissue forms not only on the skin, but on all internal wounds. See *Adhesions*. A *keloid* is a large, irregularly shaped overgrowth of scar tissue that grows after a wound has healed. For scarring, try DMSO (dimethylsulfoxide) with 1 drop of iodine (prescription) or aloe vera or calendula gel.

Stretch Marks (Stria)

Lines on the skin caused by thinning and loss of elasticity in the underlying skin layer. They first appear as red, raised lines and later become purple, eventually flattening and fading to form shiny streaks. They are a common feature of pregnancy (see *Pregnancy*). Stretch marks are possibly caused by a deficiency or imbalance of essential fatty acids and/or zinc. Try aloe vera gel mixed with vitamin E over brand-new stretch marks, rubbed in well, twice a day for four to nine months.

Cellulite

Fatty deposits under and dimpling of the skin. The word "cellulite" was invented in Europe to make women believe that the fat on their thighs and abdomen is some special substance that can magically disappear if you buy the right product. Sorry. Cellulite is simply fat and changes in fat-to-muscle ratios caused by waning hormone levels like DHEA (dehydroepiandrosterone) and testosterone. Unfortunately, fat that is deposited on the thighs and abdomen is the last to burn up when a person diets and exercises. Eat less and exercise more (daily). And get your hormones tested and supplement them if levels are low.

What to Do for Skin in General

- The best skin comes from inside. Take essential fatty acids (like 1 Tbsp. cod liver oil a day), snack on raw nuts, make sure you digest food well (see page 468) and take multivitamins and minerals.
- Plain soap (like a mild unperfumed castile soap) and water is the best preventative against the viruses, bacteria, and fungi that can infect skin.
- The best way to help skin retain moisture is to rub on a thin layer of olive oil or alpha-hydroxy lotion while it's still wet from a bath or shower.
- For skin health, get enough sleep, early morning sunshine, and regular exercise.
- Don't smoke. It increases wrinkles, enlarges pores, and makes skin dry and leathery.
- Try food facials using the inside of papaya peels, whipped egg whites, yogurt, clay, or oatmeal.
- Try meditation and visualization. Aromatherapy, biofeed-back, and hypnosis are being studied for skin disorders.
- *Be careful in the sun* by staying indoors at midday, wearing sunglasses, and using a sunscreen with at least an SPF of 15. Sunburn doubles your risk of skin cancer, and sun damage is cumulative. Daily use of sunscreen has been found to protect against cutaneous squamous-cell carcinoma but not basal-cell carcinoma. However, 9–40 percent of Americans are deficient in vitamin D. Covering all skin surfaces every day with sunscreen completely prevents vitamin D synthesis. Expose face and arms to sun for ten to twenty minutes (before applying sunscreen) two to four times a week. Put yogurt, honey, black tea, or vinegar on burned areas for relief.
- Any skin disorder can be exacerbated by the menstrual cycle. Keep a menstrual calendar (page 328), and if symptoms are linked to your menstrual cycle, have your hormone levels tested.

Diet: Drink plenty of water, and several times a week add 1 Tbsp. liquid chlorophyll. For beautiful skin, generously use olive oil and eat olives, nuts, and seeds. Green tea may protect against some skin disorders, such as skin cancer.

Avoid: Deep-fried foods, hydrogenated oils, caffeine, excess full-fat dairy, and sugar.

Nutrients

- Jojoba, or other natural oils, on tissue or cotton, can be used to remove eye makeup.
- To prevent sun and pollutant-damaged skin, try vitamins A, C, E, zinc, selenium, and B complex from foods or supplements. Take essential fatty acids, 2–5 g per day, of various types in divided doses.
- Ask your doctor about retinoic acid. Use gel if you break out from oil forms.

Herbs

For Oily Skin: Licorice root, lemon grass, and rosebuds simmered in a pan with distilled water. Hold your face over the bowl if you can for 5 to 10 minutes with a towel over your head. Finish with a splash of cold water.

Puffiness: Splash your face with water with added drops of lavender oil.

Skin Tags

These small polyps grow on the neck, under arms, and on the torso. They have been observed by nutritional doctors to be linked to hypoglycemia or future risk of diabetes, a tendency to grow polyps in the colon and cysts in the ovaries and breasts, and to insulin resistance.

Dermatitis

An inflammation of the skin that usually causes itching, sometimes accompanied by scaling or blisters, redness, swelling, oozing, or scabbing.

There are many forms of dermatitis:

- *Atopic dermatitis* is a skin irritation that can come and go for months or years, often accompanies other allergic problems such as asthma or hay fever, and is linked to a family propensity. If you have this often, and chronically use topical corticosteroids, you are at higher risk for developing cataracts in your twenties or thirties.

- In *stasis dermatitis,* the skin on the legs of people with varicose veins and/or poor circulation may become irritated, inflamed, and discolored.

- Localized *scratch dermatitis* is a chronic, itchy inflammation caused by repeated scratching that produces dryness, scaling, and dark thick patches in oval or angular shapes. It can occur anywhere on the body, including the vagina.

- *Seborrheic dermatitis* is an inflammatory disease of the scalp, face, and occasionally other areas.

- *Contact dermatitis* is the most common. It is a reaction to some substance that comes in contact with the skin, either a direct irritation or an allergic response. Location of the initial rash may be a clue as to which substance is causing the reaction. Symptoms include mild, short-lived redness to severe swelling and blisters. The rash is confined to a particular area. It may contain tiny, itching blisters, which may ooze and form crusts. When they dry, there is residual scaling, itching, and sometimes thickening of the skin.

- In *photoallergic contact dermatitis,* the rash comes when the substance on the skin is exposed to sunlight. This can happen with sunscreens, perfumes, or oils, or when taking some antibiotics.

Uniquely Female: Always keep a calendar of symptoms and note if your skin condition (except vitiligo—areas of hypopigmentation) worsens from midcycle through the first week of your period. If so, have a saliva or twenty-four-hour urine hormone test run and get treatment to balance your hormones. Women on oral contraceptives can develop low tissue levels of vitamin B_6, which can contribute to

---

CONTACT DERMATITIS

Some substances can cause immediate skin changes; others can take up to twenty-four hours. A frequent cause is a reaction to nickel, often triggered by ear or body piercing and eyeglass frames or jewelry that contain some nickel. Wear only stainless steel or titanium posts when having piercing done. Don't wear nickel-plated jewelry; hot weather can leach nickel. If you are very sensitive to nickel, avoid apricots, canned pineapple, hydrogenated oils, chocolate, beer, tea, nuts, and other foods high in this mineral. Eight to 14 percent of women are allergic to nickel and reactions may increase in the second half of your menstrual cycle. Ask your dentist to use metals in your mouth that are absolutely nickel-free. Other common irritants are cleaning detergents, chemicals in latex gloves and condoms, chemicals used in the manufacture of clothing, certain cosmetics, plants (like poison ivy), drugs in skin creams and medications.

---

allergic conditions, especially of the skin. This may also be true for some women taking hormone replacement therapy.

What to Do

** For all chronic dermatologic conditions, identify and avoid food allergens for several months, or just try going off the most common allergens such as wheat, all dairy products, beef, corn, soy, eggs, citrus, etc. Food/inhalant/topical allergies may get worse with your menstrual cycle.

• Bathe in lukewarm water. Add ½ cup of vinegar to the water. Use olive oil soaps or oatmeal as a soap substitute.

• Baby shampoo is gentle and a good cleansing agent. Use it to clean wounds, scrapes, and cuts, and to wash away dead skin from psoriasis or eczema.

• Most cosmetics are filled with chemicals. Buy natural cosmetics.

• Try to use "green" cleaning products.

• Avoid antiperspirants. Metallic salts (aluminum chloride, aluminum sulfate, and zirconium chlorohydrate) can irritate sensitive skin.

- Avoid scented detergents and fabric softeners. Try baking soda (¼ cup per washload) to soften clothes.
- Fake nails and perfumes can cause dermatitis.
- Cold, wet dressings can relieve the itching of contact dermatitis.
- Avoid colored, scented toilet paper.
- Learn stress-reduction techniques (pages 52–58). Hypnosis has been shown to help a wide variety of chronic skin problems (*Archives of Dermatology* 136:393, 2000).

Diet: Some women get better when avoiding food additives.

Nutrients

For Chronic Dermatitis (Eczema)
- ** Zinc picolinate, 30 mg twice a day; balance with copper, 2–4 mg per day
- ** Flaxseed oil, 1 tsp. once or twice a day; balance with vitamin E, 400–800 IU. If this doesn't work in two months, switch to another kind like evening primrose oil, 3–6 g per day.
- ** Vitamin A, 25,000–50,000 IU for the first two months. Do not take if you're pregnant or have a history of liver disease; monitor for signs of toxicity and work with your doctor.
- ** Vitamin B complex, 50 mg per day, plus extra niacinamide
- ** Magnesium, 250–400 mg with multiminerals
- ** Evaluate your need for digestive enzymes (page 468).
- Use Vaseline on a rash instead of corticosteroids.

For Hives and Rashes (Chronic Urticaria):
If you have daily outbreaks for three to six weeks or more
- Identify and eliminate food allergens, hidden infections, and toxic chemicals.
- Avoid food additives like tartrazine (FD&C yellow #5), harsh detergents, synthetic clothing, yeast, and sodium benzoate.
- Evaluate your digestive enzymes (page 468).

- Vitamin C, 1,000 mg two to four times a day
- Vitamin B$_{12}$, 1,000 mcg intramuscular (IM) injections once per week for four weeks or Myer's Cocktail intravenous (IV) (see page 471)
- DHEA (dehydroepiandrosterone), 5–15 mg per day
- Ask your doctor about thyroxine treatment if you have elevated levels of thyroid antibodies.
- Test DHEA and testosterone and treat if levels are low.

Rosacea

A chronic skin disorder in which the nose and cheeks are abnormally red and may develop acne-like bumps. Most common among fair-skinned middle-aged women. Commonly begins with temporary flushing, often after drinking a hot beverage or alcohol, eating spicy food, or entering a hot environment.

What to Do
- Avoid alcohol and watch out for food allergies.
- Apply azelaic (20%) cream twice a day for three months. This may cause minor burning at first.
- Rule out low stomach acid (see page 468).
- Probiotics, once or twice a day for three to six months

Dandruff and Scaling on Face and Other Areas (Seborrheic Dermatitis)

- Biotin, 2.5–10 mg per day
- Oral vitamin B$_6$, 20 mg per day; magnesium, 250 mg per day; and essential fatty acids, several grams per day, or 1–2 Tbsp. per day of flaxseed oil. With backup vitamin E, 200–400 IU per day.
- Topical vitamin B$_6$ ointment or cream applied four times a day
- Ask your doctor about IM vitamin B$_{12}$ injections, one every three weeks for two to three injections, and sometimes requiring maintenance injections as needed.

Psoriasis

This is thickened patches of inflamed, red skin, which may be covered by silvery scales. It tends to run in families. Usually appears between the ages of ten and thirty. Can recur in attacks, triggered by emotional stress, skin damage, gluten foods like wheat, or physical illness. Most common form is discoid, or "plaque," psoriasis, in which raised patches appear on trunk and limbs, particularly the elbows, knees, and scalp.

Avoid: Foods high in gluten, especially wheat, which is a common cause in many women with psoriasis. Identify and avoid any suspected food allergies, and eliminate refined sugar and alcohol.

Nutrients
- Flaxseed oil, 1–3 Tbsp. per day, with backup vitamin E, 400 IU
- Vitamin D orally (800 IU per day) and topically as 1, 25-dihydroxy vitamin D_3 cream, calcipotriol cream, or 1-alpha-hydroxy vitamin D_3 creams, which need prescriptions from a doctor
- Antifungal medications: Some holistic doctors find these remedies to be helpful.

Scleroderma

Sclerosis is a rare chronic disease occurring four times more often in women than in men. It causes diffuse fibrosis and degeneration, affecting the skin (called scleroderma), joints, and internal organs. The cause is not known. Avoid swift increases in fiber intake, which may cause intestinal obstructions.

Nutrients
- Estriol, 2 mg taken twenty-five days per month, was shown in two cases to improve skin and joints.
- Vitamin E, 800–1,600 IU per day, improves the skin.
- PABA (para-aminobenzoic acid), 3 g four times per day, taken for years has been shown (in an uncontrolled trial) to slow down lung deterioration.
- Vitamin D_3, 800 IU improves skin.

SMOKING

Study after study has identified cigarette smoking as a major cause of serious respiratory disease, including bronchitis, emphysema (the most common form of chronic lung disease in women), and lung cancer. Smoking also increases the risk of mouth cancer, lip cancer, and throat cancer. The most harmful effect of smoking is coronary heart disease. It damages arteries, raises blood pressure, and affects the arteries of the legs, leading to peripheral vascular disease or even gangrene, which may result in amputation. The arteries of the brain can be affected, which may result in stroke. Children from homes where one or both parents smoke are more likely to suffer from asthma or other respiratory diseases, such as bronchitis and recurrent ear infections, and are more likely to become smokers themselves. Wives of smokers have a higher risk of getting lung diseases later in life. People who stop smoking before middle age avoid 90 percent of the risk of lung cancer.

> **A CIGARETTE-SHORTENED LIFE**
>
> Each cigarette smoked subtracts eight to eleven minutes from your life.
> A carton takes away 1.5 days.
> Two packs a day shortens your life span by twelve to fifteen years.

Causes: Cigarettes contain 4,000 known chemicals. *Nicotine* is the substance that causes addiction to tobacco. It acts as a tranquilizer, but also stimulates the release of the hormone epinephrine into the smoker's bloodstream, which may explain raised blood pressure. The *tar* in tobacco chronically irritates the respiratory system and is a major cause of lung disease and lung cancer. Smokers have a persistently high level of carbon monoxide in the blood, which leads to hardening of the arteries, increasing the risk of coronary thrombosis.

Uniquely Female: One in three women of reproductive age now smokes cigarettes. Lung cancer rates in women increased more than sixfold between 1950 and 1990. Women who smoke reach menopause earlier, face a greater risk of osteoporosis and a much higher risk of cancer of the cervix or uterus. They are less fertile and, during pregnancy, women who smoke more than twenty cigarettes a day are more likely to abort, to have a baby that weighs less at birth, and to have a stillbirth or malformations of the newborn. Thirty to forty percent of cases of sudden infant death (SID) are thought to be avoidable if pregnant women would stop smoking. And for those of you with my favorite sin, vanity, know that nothing ages a woman more quickly than smoking! Women who want to stop smoking should quit the day their period starts or in the two weeks afterward. Quitting in the premenstrual phase may heighten withdrawal symptoms.

How to Quit Smoking

Withdrawal from nicotine induces intense craving, nervousness, irritability, headache, difficulty concentrating, stomach cramps, tremors, disrupted sleep, and more. Here are some steps to help beat the nicotine addiction:

- The urge to smoke lasts only three to five minutes at a time. Get up and take a walk outside, exercise, or do anything that takes your mind off your craving.
- To reduce cravings, either take ½ tsp. baking soda in water two to four times a day on an empty stomach or dissolve 1 Tbsp. baking soda in 12 oz. of water and sip slowly during the day. This slows down the release of nicotine from your bloodstream and reduces cravings. Do this for only seven to ten days.
- For the same reason, you should drink green tea, Green Drinks (page 465), and fresh vegetable juices.
- Suck on a clove or chew a small piece of fresh ginger root to help reduce cravings. Plantain tea, three cups a day, can help.
- Avoid junk foods. Sugar aggravates cravings.
- Nicotine gum can help stop the headaches from withdrawal.
- Withdrawal may be worse if you are allergic to nightshade plants (potatoes, peppers, eggplant, tomatoes, paprika, and tobacco). Even if you are not allergic, not eating nightshades during the first week of withdrawal may make it easier.
- Vigorous exercise facilitates cessation and minimizes weight gain.

Nutrients to Help Stop Smoking

- ** During acute withdrawal, take ½ tsp. ascorbate vitamin C powder with bioflavonoids.
- ** Magnesium, 400 mg twice a day, and B complex, 100 mg per day
- ** Multivitamin/mineral supplement
- Lobelia, ½–1 ml tincture two to three times a day can reduce nausea. Don't use for more than a month and avoid if pregnant or breast-feeding.
- Vitamin B$_3$ (niacin) can lessen cravings; take 100–150 mg two to three times a day.
- Vitamin C, 1,000 mg three times a day
- Vitamin E, 400 IU per day while still smoking, plus selenium, 100 mcg per day
- L-glutamine, 500 mg once or twice a day on an empty stomach for several months
- Free-form amino acids, twice a day on an empty stomach in the morning and evening

If You Can't Stop Smoking

- ** Multivitamin/mineral supplement *without* beta-carotene (but keep eating colorful fruits and veggies)
- ** Pycnogenol, 100–125 mg per day, or bromelain, 2–3 g once or twice a day between meals, or baby aspirin can inhibit smoking-induced platelet stickiness.
- ** Vitamin B complex, 100 mg per day, with extra vitamin B$_{12}$ and folic acid
- ** Vitamin C, 2–3 g per day (1 g of vitamin C reduces blood lead level from smoke by 81 percent after one week). The effects of smoke go from the lung arteries to the heart and impair blood flow; vitamin C reverses this.
- Vitamin A, 25,000 IU per day
- Zinc, 20–50 mg per day, balance with copper, 2–3 mg per day
- Coenzyme Q-10, 30 mg per day
- Vitamin E, 400–800 IU per day
- Smoking may decrease folic acid levels, which increases homocysteine levels, which increases risk of coronary heart dis-

ease, heart attack, bone loss, and pregnancy problems. Take folic acid and vitamin B complex in your daily multivitamin.

SOY

Plant estrogens (called phytoestrogens) occur in soy, chickpeas, and other legumes and are similar to the female hormone estrogen, though much weaker. Soy phytoestrogens have been shown to have many protective effects:

- Studies have linked soy with lower rates of breast, ovarian, and uterine cancer in China.
- Soy lowers blood pressure and cholesterol (when eating 20 g per day).
- Soy increases the formation of the "good" metabolite of estrogen (2-hydroxyestrone), which protects against cancer.
- Soy inhibits estradiol formation from estrone (the major estrogen in postmenopausal women). Estradiol is the major form of estrogen associated (at higher levels) with health problems such as breast cancer.

The American Heart Association says that consuming 25–50 g of soy protein a day can help reduce levels of low-density lipoprotein (the "bad" cholesterol) by 4–8 percent. Soy can decrease atherosclerosis and dilate blood vessels in a similar way to estrogen and Premarin, and it helps protect bones. It also reduces the risk of heart disease, while not increasing the risk of developing hormonally dependent tumors as does conventional hormone replacement therapy.

This is all good.

However, soy may have a shadow side. Isoflavones found in soy-based infant formula may be linked to shorter menstrual cycles and infertility as these children age. One Hawaiian study suggests that soy foods decreased memory in men. Other research suggests that soy may stimulate the growth of estrogen-dependent tumors. Excess soy can lower thyroid functioning and deplete iron. Also, the studies linking soy to protective effects in Oriental women are now being criticized for their design, and their conclusions are being called inaccurate by some.

We just don't know the truth about soy at the time of writing this book. It may be protective in healthy pre- and postmenopausal women, but not in postmenopausal women with a history of hormonal cancers or unopposed estrogen and who are not taking estrogenic hormones.

Adding to the confusion, much of the research performed on animals in studying soy may be muddled by the fact that these animals are raised on foods high in soy, and rodents don't have the same clearing mechanisms for plant estrogens that humans have. This means studies that suggest soy is harmful may not be telling the whole story. The experts are perplexed, so don't be frustrated if you are. My intuition is that we will find that soy is a beneficial and protective food fairly across the board. But understand that just because something is a food doesn't mean it's always safe.

SPROUTS

Sprouts are seen as a healthy addition to salads and sandwiches, soups and stir-frys, but there are risks associated with eating raw sprouts. In 1999, a year after an outbreak of illness that was linked to sprouts, the FDA issued a warning advising anyone against eating raw sprouts. Sprouts are easily contaminated by *E. coli* and *Salmonella* bacteria, which can cause fever, stomach cramps, and diarrhea. The seeds that are used for sprouting may become contaminated by animals in the fields or from the use of animal manure. It's the potential contamination, not the sprouts themselves, that creates the problem.

STRESS

Any disturbance in a person's healthy mental and physical well-being. The body responds to stress by upping its production of hormones, such as cortisol and epinephrine, which in turn leads to changes in heart rate, blood pressure, metabolism, and physical activity. After a certain point, these responses disrupt an individual's ability to cope.

Post-traumatic stress disorder is a direct response to a specific event in which the victim relives the event over and over through vivid waking memories or constant nightmares. Flashbacks are often accompanied by constant anxiety, tension, and insomnia. If the problem surfaces soon after the trauma, it's likely to disappear on its own within six months. If the onset is delayed, the condition may drag on for years.

Symptoms: Stress can cause anxiety, tension, moodiness, skin rashes, stomach pain, diarrhea, wheezing, headaches, back pain, or trouble having sex. Continued exposure to stress can lead to anxiety and depression, dyspepsia, palpitations, and muscular aches and pains. When overstressed, a body has less resistance to illness. Specific signs of post-traumatic stress include sudden feelings of sadness, fear, or anger; nervousness, panic, irritability; poor concentration; use of alcohol or drugs to numb emotional pain; and loss of interest in friends, family, and objects of enjoyment.

Signs that too much stress needs medical help: Dizziness or blackouts, a racing pulse that won't stop, sweaty palms, chronic back and neck pain, chronic or severe headaches, trembling, hives, overwhelming anxiety, insomnia.

Causes: All major changes in life are stressful, including sickness or death of a friend or family member; conflicts with a spouse or partner; moving; having a baby; money problems; and trying to do too much. Getting fired, starting a new job, injury, and illness are all very stressful. Not getting enough sleep is a source of stress. Not having enough time to get everything done, a common problem today, is a major source of stress. What seems stressful to one person may not bother another person at all. Among the traumas most frequently at fault for post-traumatic stress are rape, family violence, child abuse, automobile crashes and accidents, natural disasters such as hurricanes, floods, fires, and tornadoes, or acts of terrorism.

Uniquely Female: Many conditions of a woman's life are very stressful, such as being a single and/or working mother or being the victim of domestic violence, sexual abuse, or rape. Stress can alter a woman's menstrual cycle. The hormonal changes of menopause, pregnancy, and puberty add stress to the body and mind. Women's hearts are more vulnerable to stress than men's. Stress is also a major cause of prolonged spotting or irregular bleeding. The hormone pro-lactin is released in response to stress; when abnormally elevated, it's associated with increased risk of female problems from premenstrual syndrome to breast cancer. The hormone cortisol is elevated during stress and binds with progesterone receptors, thus blocking proges-terone and contributing to estrogen-dominant health problems in women. High cortisol may be linked to low DHEA (dehydro-epiandrosterone) levels in some women.

What to Do

- Exercise is a great stress reducer. Try it!
- Hot baths with lavender oil work wonders. At the office, run hot water over your hands until the tension drains away.
- Don't blame yourself for everything that goes wrong in your life or in your kids' lives.
- Get help from a counselor or support group, especially for post-traumatic stress.
- Learn stress-reduction techniques (pages 52–58).
- Deal with your problems one at a time.
- Make lists. If you get all of tomorrow's "to-do's" on paper, you can safely release them from your mind and sleep better.
- Alcohol or drugs relieve stress in the short term but do not solve the underlying problems and can lead to addiction.

BALANCING BREATH

Sit comfortably. Take your hand and close off your left nostril with your left thumb, putting all your other fingers up toward the ceiling. Inhale and exhale, taking long and slow breaths, five times. Now take the right thumb and close off the right nostril and repeat the same breathing through the left nostril. Re-peat five times. This breath balances the right and left sides of your body. Now sit quietly for as long as you like. You have just used the breath to stimulate your immune and nervous system and to help combat stress.

- Reset your priorities. Don't worry if your house is a little messy, or if you can't bring about world peace.
- Take good care of yourself. Eat a balanced diet, get enough sleep, and have some fun once in a while.
- Try Hyland's Calms Forté homeopathic pills, a remedy for stress.
- Have your doctor run a DHEA hormone test, as low levels can contribute to elevated stress hormones. Supplementation decreases elevated cortisol levels.
- Laugh a lot.

Diet: Increase protein and fresh fruits and vegetables high in vitamins C and B during times of stress. Interestingly, the body makes cortisol, a stress-related hormone, out of cholesterol. Elevated cholesterol levels may contribute to higher stress-hormone levels. So when you are under stress, cut down on fatty foods, especially deep-fried items such as French fries, fried appetizers, fried chicken, etc. Eat more salmon and fresh tuna, rather than cholesterol-rich shrimp or lobster.

Avoid: Reduce caffeine and avoid foods that stress the system, such as fried and junk food, sugar, white flour, potato chips. Alcohol may seem to temporarily relieve stress, but it actually depresses the nervous system and increases stress.

Nutrients
- ** Multivitamin/mineral supplement
- ** Stress hormones cause the body to lose magnesium, so you need to supplement magnesium, 250 mg one to three times a day (cut back if stools get too loose). Use magnesium aspartate, citrate, or orotate. Aspartates are well absorbed, increase energy, and help relax stressed muscles.
- ** B complex, 100 mg two to three times a day
- ** Pantothenic acid, 1,000 mg one to five times a day, higher levels when stress is higher
- ** Vitamin C with bioflavonoids, 500 mg every four hours during acute stress. Vitamin C puts a safe blocking effect on cortisol released in response to stress.

- Put 1 Tbsp. of liquid chlorophyll in a cup of water and sip.
- Vitamin A, 5,000 IU or 10,000 IU of mixed carotenoids. The adrenal glands appear to use vitamin A to help combat stress.
- Calcium, 1,000 mg per day; extra zinc, 20–60 mg per day; and copper, 2–3 mg per day
- Adrenal glandular extract, 150–200 mg twice a day for two or three weeks of highest stress
- Zinc, 30–50 mg daily when under stress, then reduce to 20 mg for maintenance
- Ask your doctor about prescription tryptophan and about injections of vitamin B complex (1 cc) and vitamin B_6 (0.5 cc), two to three times a week for two months.
- Several grams of fish oil a day decrease moodiness and aggressiveness during stress.

Herbs: Siberian ginseng, 100 mg half an hour before breakfast (one month on, one week off); valerian, 250–300 mg half an hour before bed. Rescue Remedy, 10–15 drops under your tongue every fifteen minutes when severe stress hits, then taper down to 5–10 drops several times a day.

STROKE (Cerebrovascular Accident, or CVA)

A stroke happens when the supply of blood to the brain is suddenly interrupted by the buildup of fat or by a clot (air or blood) that gets stuck in a blood vessel. A broken blood vessel can also cause a stroke because oxygen no longer reaches part of the brain. About 20–30 percent of patients who have a stroke die, while others have some kind of permanent problems (like paralysis on one side). There are various types of strokes reflecting different causes.

A *transient ischemic attack (TIA)*, the official name for a "little stroke" or "mini-stroke," is a temporary attack with stroke symptoms that can last for several hours. About 10 percent of strokes are preceded by TIAs. A person who has had one or more TIAs is 9.5 times more likely to have a stroke than someone of the same age and sex who has not. Don't ignore a TIA—it is an important warning sign and needs immediate attention!

Symptoms: Possible symptoms of stroke include sudden numbness or weakness in the face, arm, or leg, especially on one side of the body; confusion, trouble speaking or understanding; trouble seeing in one or both eyes; trouble walking, dizziness, loss of balance or co-ordination; severe headache with no known cause. Each side of the brain controls the other side of the body, so when the right side of the brain is damaged, the left side of the body has symptoms. Symptoms may be immediate or may take hours to appear. Treatment must be started within three hours of the stroke or more permanent damage is likely.

Causes: High blood pressure, diabetes, high amounts of fat in the blood (high cholesterol), sticky platelets, excess weight, and smoking. Elevated levels of homocysteine (see *Homocysteine*) are implicated. Low calcium and magnesium intake and possibly potassium may also contribute to increased risk of TIAs in middle-aged women.

Uniquely Female: High blood pressure is the most common chronic disease in older women and one of the highest risk factors for stroke. Oral contraceptives and hormone replacement therapy in high-risk women may cause stroke. As homocysteine levels rise, so does the risk of stroke. Homocysteine levels can usually be lowered with B vitamins.

What to Do
- Reduce hypertension. See *Blood Pressure.*
- Learn stress-reduction techniques, especially meditation (page 55). If anger is a problem, consider therapy.
- Acupuncture with electrical stimulation can reverse some effects of stroke.
- Physical and speech therapy should be started as early as possible after a stroke.
- Ask your doctor about treatment in a hyperbaric oxygen chamber.

Diet: Cold-water fish (salmon and halibut are best) at least twice a week. Women who ate 4 oz. of fish two to four times a week cut their risk of clot-related stroke by 48 percent. Increasing whole grains also reduces risk. Eat lots of carrots and blue and purple fruits and vegetables. Eat foods high in L-arginine—roasted soybeans, light turkey and chicken meat, pumpkin seeds, chickpeas, tofu, hummus, and black beans. Foods inversely related to stroke are cruciferous and green leafy veggies, citrus fruit and juice. Chinese red rice lowers cholesterol and is tasty.

Alcohol: Light to moderate alcohol consumption (with as little as one drink each week) in women thirty-five years old or older reduces overall risk of stroke, second stroke after the first, and heart attack. Wine, beer, and spirits have equal effects. Increasing this to one drink a day does *not* improve the benefit. Alcohol abuse *increases* risk of stroke.

Avoid: Saturated and hydrogenated fats. Reduce salt and sugar intake.

Nutrients

After a Stroke

- ** Alpha-lipoic acid, 250 mg twice a day (take backup biotin, 3 mg per day)
- ** Magnesium, 250 mg two to three times a day (decrease if stools are loose)
- ** L-arginine, 1,500 mg twice a day
- ** Vitamin C, 500–1,000 mg three times a day
- ** Vitamin E, start at 100 IU per day and over two weeks gradually increase to 200 IU morning and evening
- Coenzyme Q-10, 30–60 mg three times a day to increase the flow of oxygen to the brain
- B complex, 25–50 mg twice a day, with extra folic acid, 800–1,000 mcg once per day
- Essential fatty acids, 2–8 g per day in divided doses, especially DHA (docosahexaenoic acid)
- Green-food supplements or Green Drinks (page 465)
- Lecithin, 1,200 mg two to three times a day with meals

To Prevent a Stroke

- ** L-arginine, 1,000 mg twice a day
- ** Pycnogenol, 100–125 mg per day, together with one enterically coated baby aspirin (81 mg) or bromelain (referred to below), can reduce platelet stickiness.
- ** Vitamin B$_6$, 50–100 mg per day
- ** Essential fatty acids, 500–1,000 mg two to three times a day, and vitamin E as recommended above
- • Bromelain, several thousand MCU once or twice between meals
- • Folic acid, 400 mcg to several mg per day
- • Vitamin B$_{12}$ and vitamin B complex, 50–100 mg per day
- • Vitamin C, 1,000 mg twice a day
- • *Make sure you take medication for high blood pressure* and insist that your doctor test homocysteine blood levels.
- • Consume lots of antioxidants by eating a variety of fruits and vegetables. Research shows that the more antioxidants in the blood, the more protection from neurological damage from a stroke.

Herbs: Ginkgo biloba, 40–80 mg three times a day; astragalus, 250 mg four times a day; cayenne, 100 mg twice a day with meals; garlic, 500 mg three times a day; and hawthorn berry, 100–200 mg two to three times a day.

SYNDROME X, see *Insulin Resistance*

T

THYROID

The thyroid gland, situated in the front of the neck, manufactures the hormones that regulate body temperature, heart rate, and body weight, and affect numerous vital functions. They are T_4 (thyroxine) and T_3 (triiodothyronine, converted in liver and other organs from T_4). The parathyroid gland is embedded in the thyroid gland and acts together with the hormone calcitonin to regulate calcium balance in the body. The thyroid acts in subtle ways to help maintain proper blood sugar and fat levels, ward off allergies, control responses to foreign substance, and is vital for brain development in fetuses and children. The thyroid and adrenal glands influence each other.

Thyroid hormone and iodine have an affinity for breast tissue and can influence cystic changes. With insufficient iodine or levels of thyroid hormone, breast tissue is more sensitive to estrogenic stimulation. Several studies suggest that low thyroid levels are associated with increased risk of breast cancer, but how and why is not known. Numerous female disorders can be linked to or made worse by thyroid problems—from painful periods, heavy bleeding, and premenstrual syndrome (PMS) to having a harder time going through menopause.

Hypothyroidism

Insufficient thyroid hormone production or inability of receptors to receive the thyroid's messages. A "sluggish" thyroid is a common hormonal disturbance in America. There are many types of underactive thyroid.

Symptoms: Fatigue, emotional instability with an emphasis on depression, fibrocystic and painful breasts, dry skin, dry elbows, hair loss, unexplained weight gain, constipation, poor resistance to infections (especially in the lungs), poor memory, and sensitivity to cold. Other signs are difficulty paying attention; forgetfulness; thick, swollen, puffy skin; constant low temperature; yellowish palms and soles of feet; hair falling out; history of chronic menstrual disorders; swelling around ankles; slow heartbeat; slow response to an Achilles heel reflex test; and tingling in the fingers and wrist such as carpal tunnel syndrome. Chronic muscular painful "trigger points" that do not respond to various therapies may be a symptom.

Muscle aches and tenderness may be thought to be fibromyalgia, weakness of shoulders and hips can be similar to polymyositis. Joint problems can be hard to distinguish from rheumatoid arthritis. If these musculoskeletal problems are due to hypothyroidism, they will improve with thyroid replacement therapy.

Hashimoto's thyroiditis, an autoimmune disorder, often first manifests with elevated thyroid levels. The levels can fluctuate wildly, eventually resulting in sluggish thyroid. Main symptoms of Hashimoto's thyroiditis are tiredness, muscle weakness, weight gain, and enlargement of the thyroid gland.

"Subclinical" hypothyroidism is a condition in which blood tests are normal although symptoms indicate a low-functioning thyroid. Numerous women may suffer with undiagnosed subclinical hypothyroidism. It contributes to impaired carbohydrate metabolism, weight gain, and problems like fatigue, depression, and allergies that generally increase in incidence as women age. Subclinical hypothyroidism

> Conditions that may mimic underactive thyroid are an imbalance in essential fatty acids, low adrenal hormones, low progesterone, or inadequate nutrients for converting T_4 to T_3.

can be caused by aging, excessive dieting, hormone resistance at the cellular level due to environmental pollutants (like polychlorinated biphenyls [PCBs] or food additives or colorings), nutrient deficiencies, oxidative or genetic damage to hormone receptors, or toxic chemicals that interfere with normal conversion of thyroid hormones. One study found that 18 percent of elderly people with normal thyroid blood tests were found to have low thyroid when more extensive tests were run.

Causes: Multiple chemical exposures, such as to lead or PCBs; radiation; environmental chemical sensitivities; immune system malfunction; damage or removal of some or all of the thyroid gland; excessive treatment for hyperthyroidism (overactive thyroid); infection of the thyroid gland; iodine deficiency (mostly in developing countries); or overuse of diet pills and other drugs. Low thyroid functioning is linked with elevated levels of homocysteine (page 269). Low thyroid tends to run in families.

Uniquely Female: Hypothyroidism affects five to eight times more women than men. Menstrual problems such as painful PMS, difficulty becoming pregnant, and miscarriage may result from hy-

---

THYROID TESTING

Overt hypothyroidism is diagnosed with low levels of serum T_3 and T_4 and an elevated level of TSH (thyroid-stimulating hormone). Low thyroid often elevates serum cholesterol. Any kind of iodine, medical or dietary, interferes with thyroid testing.

Subclinical hypothyroidism: Some cases of underactive thyroid are not picked up by basic lab tests. Suggested tests for finding subclinical low thyroid:

1. Run TSH-stimulation and transthyretrin blood test (low levels suggest low thyroid functioning).

2. "High-normal" TSH along with elevated cholesterol levels.

3. Perform a home thyroid test (from Broda O. Barnes, M.D.): Keep a basal thermometer that has been shaken down by your bedside. Before getting out of bed in the morning (even to go to the bathroom), hold the thermometer tightly under your armpit for ten minutes while lying completely still. Do this for seven days (except during the first few days of your menstrual cycle and during ovulation) and calculate your average temperature. If it is low (below 97.6°F), hypothyroid *may* be a problem. A healthy thyroid promotes 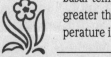 basal temperatures of 97.8–98.2. The lower the temperature, the greater the degree of possible hypothyroidism (but not all low temperature is related to thyroid problems).

pothyroidism. Low thyroid can be associated with menstrual difficulties, but especially with bleeding problems and a tendency toward ovarian cysts. Hashimoto's thyroiditis is eight times more common in women than men, and usually develops between the ages of thirty and fifty. Hormonal changes during puberty or pregnancy may cause a minor degree of *goiter* (enlargement of the thyroid gland), which usually subsides when hormone levels return to normal. Some women can develop short-lived underactive thyroid within one to six months after having a baby, which may precipitate postpartum depression. Also, it is more common for women with low thyroid to have high cholesterol.

What to Do
- Exercise. It increases energy, fights depression, reduces stress, and helps normalize thyroid function.
- Avoid sulfa drugs and antihistamines.
- Avoid chlorinated water and fluoride toothpaste. They can block iodine receptors in the thyroid gland.
- Don't take iron supplements at the same time as thyroid medication. It binds up thyroxine and makes it insoluble.
- Evaluate your need for stomach acid (studies suggest that up to 40 percent of those with overt hypothyroidism are low in stomach acid).
- Sometimes underactive thyroid is really a sign of inadequate progesterone. Have your progesterone levels tested. If low, supplement. In some women this will normalize thyroid functioning.
- Get adequate rest. Exhaustion can create and/or worsen low thyroid.
- Women who are on thyroid replacement therapy may need to adjust thyroid dose if they are also taking hormone replacement therapy or oral contraceptives.
- Have your homocysteine levels tested; they can run higher in patients with low thyroid.
- Make sure you are on a *replacement* dose of thyroid and not a *suppressive* dose. Suppressive doses show up in tests as thyroid-stimulating hormone (TSH) = 0, which means you are

THREE TYPES OF
THYROID HORMONE REPLACEMENT

1. *Synthroid* and *thyroxine,* the most common treatments, consist of one kind of thyroid hormone, T_4. The body must convert T_4 to T_3, but not every body can do this. This is why some women on thyroxine still "don't feel right."

2. *Desiccated thyroid* (like Armour) contains both T_4 and T_3 (USP-approved standards, 1 grain = 0.1 mg of L-thyroxine). Its combination of two thyroids may be more effective for some women than taking Synthroid or its generic equivalents. Women with pork allergies may have problems with this form.

3. *Hormonal glandulars* are substances available at health food stores that have most of the hormone removed. They are not as effective for overt hypothyroidism but are often fine for mild cases of subclinical hypothyroidism. If you have subclinical hypothyroidism, try thyroid glandulars for several months before moving to prescription medications. Take with essential nutrients listed at the end of this section.

 A little more than half of women treated for hypothyroidism may wean off treatment in one or two years without reexperiencing symptoms. Others need to continue supplementation indefinitely.

losing bone and may be adversely affecting your heart. Have your TSH levels run yearly while taking thyroid medication. While on thyroid therapy, watch for rapid heartbeat, a sign of overmedication.

- Excessive doses of thyroid cause jitteriness, insomnia, fast heartbeat, anxiety, and chest pain (the symptoms should go away when the dose is lowered).
- Problems (jitteriness, more fatigue, or feeling poorly) taking thyroid supplementation when you need it suggest low adrenal functioning. Correcting low adrenals may improve thyroid and vice versa (see *Adrenal Insufficiency and Adrenal Fatigue*).
- Thyroid medication blocks the absorption of calcium carbonate, so take them three hours apart. Also, antacids and laxatives (aluminum hydroxide and magnesium hydroxide) bind up thyroid medication and make it ineffective. If you use

these for heartburn or constipation, don't take them at the same time as thyroid.

- Antacids and laxatives can block absorption of thyroid hormone and lead to serious undersupplementation. Tell your doctor (*Pharmacology and Toxicology* 84:107–9, 1999).
- Some women over sixty years of age may become extremely sensitive to thyroid supplementation, which shows up as profound fatigue. These women need a lower dose. Women with low thyroid may have low levels of DHEA (dehydroepiandrosterone). Have your doctor run a blood test. Postmenopausal women with both underactive thyroid and low DHEA levels may be at higher risk of bone loss. Women taking DHEA and thyroid supplements need to be monitored, since the DHEA may lower the amount of thyroid supplement needed.

Diet: Seafood and sea vegetables (kelp, dulse, kombu, hijiki) are rich in iodine. Also beneficial are molasses, egg yolks, parsley, apricots, dates, and prunes. Drink pure water; cancer of the thyroid has been linked to water with high fluoride content. Soy foods can boost natural thyroid activity, but too much can block it.

Avoid: Raw cruciferous vegetables if consumed in excess can inhibit thyroid functioning.

Nutrients
- ** Iodine, 150 mcg per day
- ** Tyrosine, 500 mg on an empty stomach in the morning and sometimes in the evening as well. This amino acid can be converted into T_4.
- ** If perimenopausal, try hypothalamus/pituitary glandular extract

Nutrients to Help Convert T_4 to T_3
- ** Vitamin B complex, 25–50 mg once or twice a day (add more niacin if you have high blood fats)
- ** Zinc, 30–60 mg per day, balanced with copper, 2–3 mg per day, for one to two months, then reduce to 20 mg per day. Sele-

nium, 50–100 mcg per day. Check the nutrient charts for signs of deficiency (pages 35–39). Magnesium, 250 mg per day; copper, 2–3 mg per day; manganese, 2–5 mg per day; and essential fatty acids (several hundred mg to several g per day).

- Vitamin A, 5,000 IU per day
- Coenzyme Q-10, 20–60 mg per day
- Vitamin B$_{12}$ lozenges, three times a day on an empty stomach
- Vitamin C, 1,000 mg twice a day (higher doses may affect production of thyroid hormone)

Hyperthyroidism

Overproduction of thyroid hormones (thyroxine) is much less common than low thyroid. *Grave's disease* is an autoimmune disorder that produces an overactive and enlarged thyroid gland, often diagnosed by the presence of bulging eyeballs *(exophthalmos)*.

Symptoms: Insomnia, anxiety, palpitations, arrhythmias, sweating, weight loss, diarrhea, and intolerance of heat. There can be nervousness, mood swings, restlessness, trembling hands, and constant hunger or loss of appetite. Too much thyroid hormone leads to an increase in perspiration, which can cause skin rashes and sores.

Uniquely Female: Grave's disease sometimes surfaces after an infection or pregnancy. The problem is more common among young to middle-aged women and in people with a family history of hyperthyroidism.

What to Do
- Regular exercise can help stabilize metabolic function.
- Acupuncture and craniosacral therapy can be helpful.
- Rule out low stomach acid (page 469).
- In severe cases, ask your doctor about using a benzodiazepine along with conventional therapy to help reduce recurrence and stress in the beginning of treatment.
- Rule out celiac disease (have your doctor run antigliadin antibodies); and if necessary follow a gluten-restricted diet (see page 493).

Diet: Large amounts of raw cruciferous vegetables can suppress thyroid hormone production.

Avoid: Caffeine, nicotine, and alcohol. Avoid dairy for three months.

Nutrients: You must work with a doctor, as nutrients can reduce hyperactive thyroid extremely quickly and sometimes cause a transient underactive thyroid.

> Following an infection, pre-eclampsia, or a stressful event such as surgery, people with hyperthyroidism may develop a life-threatening condition called *thyroid storm*. Symptoms include extremely high temperature, severe diarrhea leading to dehydration, very rapid or irregular heartbeat, exaggerated emotional swings, and finally coma. This is a medical emergency!

- ** Lugol's iodine (with doctor's supervision), 5 drops three times a day for five days; then add lithium carbonate, 300 mg three times a day, and reduce with improvement.
- ** High-dose multivitamin/ mineral supplement
- ** Antioxidants
- ** Vitamin B complex, 25–50 mg once or twice a day
- • GABA (gamma-aminobutyric acid), 500 mg two to three times a day, one week on, one week off, especially if perimenopausal.

Herbs: Dandelion root, 500 mg, or a cup of dandelion tea twice a day for six weeks on, one month off. Valerian, 200–300 mg half an hour before bed.

TOXIC SHOCK SYNDROME (TSS)

A rare condition that occurs about once every 12 million times a tampon is inserted. At least 40 percent of menstrual TSS cases affect women thirteen to nineteen years old, who are not usually aware of the risk for TSS. There are an increasing proportion of nonmenstrual cases of TSS, particularly cases caused by postoperative infections or by infections from prosthetic devices.

Symptoms: High fever (102–105°F), vomiting, diarrhea, muscle pains, a painless sunburn-like red rash, sudden drop in blood pressure leading to shock. Extreme lethargy comes on very quickly. This is a medical emergency! One to two weeks later, the skin may peel off the palms of the hands.

Causes: Bacteria (staphylococcus) colonize the mucous membranes (such as the lining of the vagina) and release a toxin that is absorbed into the blood.

Uniquely Female: Eighty-five percent of TSS cases involve women, although the number associated with menstruation has declined to 55 percent. Diaphragm users are also at risk.

What to Do

For Prevention

- Change tampons every four to six hours during the day and use external pads at night. Never leave a tampon in longer than eight hours.
- Use the lowest-absorbency tampon possible. Always using super-high-absorbency tampons significantly alters vaginal flora and soaks up large amounts of magnesium from the body.
- Look for nonbleached all-cotton tampons. Avoid deodorant tampons.
- Don't use tampons with plastic applicators that can scratch the mucous membranes of the vagina.

Herbs: After tampon use, douche with a solution of grapefruit seed extract, 10 drops in 1 quart of water as a precautionary measure.

Cotton tampons, introduced in the 1930s, were used for nearly fifty years without a problem. Then, in the late 1970s, tampon makers started using synthetics to boost absorbency, and toxic shock syndrome appeared. Now most tampons are made of rayon or cotton/rayon blends. Rayon is much cheaper than cotton. (Rayon is made from cellulose that comes from leftovers like sawdust.) Anything that's in a tampon will go into your body, including the pesti-

cides sprayed on cotton crops and the dioxins from the bleaching process. Read my book *Hormone Deception* (Contemporary/ McGraw-Hill, 2000).

U

URINARY PROBLEMS

Urinary Frequency and Urgency

Urinary frequency is the need to urinate often. *Urinary urgency* is the sudden need to urinate. If urination is not painful, then frequency or urgency is probably due to a narrowing of the urethra (called *urethral stenosis* or *stricture*). Stricture may first show up in adolescence, develop from an infection such as gonorrhea, or begin after menopause from hormonal changes. *Cystocele,* a vaginal hernia or bulge that develops from weakened vaginal wall muscles, especially in postmenopausal women, may be another cause. Frequent urination may be due to intake of excess fluids, anxiety, bladder spasms from food allergies, alcohol, caffeine, diuretics, adrenal "burnout," or *working women's overactive bladder* (too busy to pee).

Urge Incontinence

An urgent desire to urinate when the bladder is not full, leading to uncontrollable, involuntary urination. May be caused by injury, local infection, neurologic problems, anxiety, or by prolapse of the uterus or vagina. Magnesium deficiency (and possibly vitamin B_6 and essential fatty acid deficiency) is linked to incontinence in peri- and postmenopausal women. Hormone replacement therapy can cause this.

Urinary Stress Incontinence

The involuntary escape of a small amount of urine during physical stress, such as when a person coughs, sneezes, laughs, or picks up something heavy. It is very common in women after childbirth, when the muscles around the urethra have been stretched. It particularly affects elderly women because the muscles that surround the urethra decline with age, with women over sixty who have had hysterectomies, and often accompanies uterine prolapse or chronic coughing.

What to Do

** Rub triple estrogen cream around your urethra.
• Quit smoking! Smoking lowers estrogen levels.
• Avoid or reduce sugars.
• Identify and avoid foods that trigger allergies.
• Lose weight if you are overweight.
• Exercise regularly. Do Kegel exercises (see box on page 433).
• Estriol, or low-dose vaginal estradiol rings or suppositories help restore urethral epithelium while avoiding high systemic levels of estrogens. They may even prevent uterine prolapse. They may be contraindicated in DES (diethystilbestrol) daughters with a history of cervical dysplasia or ovarian cysts.
• The four-year Heart and Estrogen/Progestin Replacement Study demonstrated that daily oral estrogen plus progestin worsened urinary incontinence in older postmenopausal women (*Obstetrics and Gynecology* 97:116–20, 2001).
• If all else fails, ask your doctor about medications like pseudoephedrine, imipramine, or prolo therapy.

Nutrients

** Magnesium, 200 mg two to three times a day for two to four weeks (cut back if you have loose stools)
** Vitamin B_6, 25 mg daily, plus B complex
• Kidney glandulars, 500 mg one to three times a day, then reduce to once a day for two to three more months

KEGEL EXERCISES

Developed by Dr. Arnold Kegel in the 1940s, these exercises strengthen the pubococcygeus muscle that surrounds the urethra, vagina, and anus. They need to be done on a daily basis.

First, identify the muscles that need to be strengthened.

1. Imagine trying to control a bout of diarrhea by tightening the muscles around the rectum. Squeeze these muscles for about four seconds.

2. Go to the toilet and start to pass urine. Try to stop the stream before your bladder is empty.

3. Insert a finger into your vagina and contract the muscles so the finger is squeezed.

Next, do the exercises.

1. Sit or stand with your legs slightly apart and contract the muscles around the rectum and vagina. Hold for a slow count of five, then relax the muscles. Repeat five times.

2. Contract the same muscles for one second, relax them, and repeat these short contractions five times quickly.

Do these exercises while sitting at your desk, watching TV, standing at the sink, in the shower, or anywhere and anytime.

A lying-down position works both the muscles and the internal organs. Lie down on your back, knees bent, with your feet on the floor. Raise your pelvis until you feel the pull and then begin squeezing.

1. Contract the muscle for three seconds, relax for three seconds, and repeat. Gradually build to ten seconds.

2. Contract and release as rapidly as you can, starting with thirty repetitions and working up to two hundred.

Herbs: Chinese herbs ("Support the Left Kidney" and "Support the Right Kidney," 500 mg of each twice a day for one month).

Urinary Tract Infection

Lower urinary tract infections (UTIs) may involve the urethra (*urethritis*), the bladder (*cystitis*), or the ureters. Bladder infections are the most common type of UTIs. Prescriptions for the treatment of bladder infections are inscribed on a 3,000-year-old Egyptian papyrus. It's possible to have repeated infections. Untreated, UTIs can cause kidney damage. *Honeymoon cystitis* may follow sexual intercourse, especially if there is not enough arousal or lubrication.

Symptoms: A frequent need to urinate with only a small amount of urine coming out, pain and burning during urination, and dribbling or leaking during the day and/or while asleep. The urine may have a foul odor or become specked with blood. If the problem is in the kidneys, you may have pain in your abdomen, back, or side accompanied by fever and nausea.

Causes: Eighty-five percent of bladder infections are due to fecal bacteria *(E. coli)* that migrate from the vagina (where it causes no problems) up the urethra to the bladder. Cystitis causes painful and sometimes bloody, frequent, or urgent urination. When a burning sensation is the only symptom, urethritis is more likely the cause. *Urethral syndrome* has painful, frequent urination with no bacteria present and no known cause. Persistent bloody urine may indicate a kidney stone or tumor in the urinary tract. Other possible causes include inadequate water intake, chlamydia or gonorrhea, candida overgrowth related to overuse of antibiotics or excessive intake of refined sugars, spermicides and some contraceptives, problems with blockage in the urethra that causes incomplete voiding of urine, an extra short or narrow urethra, a bladder or kidney stone, diabetes, a cystocele, poor diet and emotional stress, a little sac called a diverticula, or heavy-metal toxicity. Latex allergies from condoms or diaphragms can mimic or cause recurrent cystitis in some women.

Uniquely Female: UTIs are far more common among women than in men (in women twenty to fifty years of age, it is fifty times greater in occurrence), especially in women who are sexually active and who use a diaphragm and spermicide. During pregnancy, hormonal changes cause a relaxation in muscle tone of the urinary system, resulting in urine retention, which makes the woman susceptible to bacterial growth. Painful urination can also come from herpes infections, vaginal infections, and chemical irritation from vaginal medication or contraceptive products.

Cystitis is considered a female malady because it's so common due to a woman's short urethra. Fifty to 75 percent of women have at least one bladder infection at some time in their lives, and 20–30 percent have multiple infections. In pregnancy, the uterus presses against the bladder, which can result in incomplete emptying of the bladder, increasing risk of infection. In menopause, lowered estrogen levels may thin the urethra and bladder lining, causing painful urination even though no infection is present. Before doctors treat repeat UTIs, they must rule out other problems, like interstitial cystitis or bladder cancer.

Interstitial Cystitis

A nonbacterial condition that seems to be caused by scarring, ulcers in the bladder lining, or an autoimmune problem. It often accompanies endometriosis and is triggered by many of the same things that cause migraines. (Cranberry juice does not help this type of cystitis.) Rather, doctors insert dimethylsulfoxide (Rimso-50) into the bladder or stretch the bladder under anesthesia.

What to Do
- Urinate frequently during the day, at least every few hours. Go whenever you need to; don't hold in your urine.
- If urination is painful, sit in a tub of warm water to relax the muscles and dilute the urine, and take pharmaceutical painkillers or two extra-strength aspirin, Tylenol, or Advil.
- Take sitz baths several times a day, using 10 drops of essential oils such as tea tree, bergamot, or thyme. Do not use harsh bubble baths or vaginal perfumes.
- Drink a glass of water just before intercourse. Urinate immediately after making love, which will wash out any bacteria that have been transferred into the bladder, and drink a glass of water to allow further flushing.
- If you use a diaphragm and have frequent cystitis, see if you could use a smaller diaphragm.
- If you have a bladder infection when you have your period, use pads instead of tampons and change them more frequently than required.

- If you have a history of urinary tract infections and are pregnant, ask for a urine culture during prenatal urine evaluations.
- Keep your genital and anal areas clean and dry. Wipe from front to back after a bowel movement to help prevent infection.
- Avoid caffeine and alcohol during treatment; they irritate the bladder.
- Wear underwear and panty hose with a cotton crotch.
- Recurrent infections can be a sign of hidden food allergies, chronic low-grade intestinal yeast infections, and/or the need for digestive enzymes (page 468).
- A product called Dipstick can be purchased at drugstores. If the tip changes color when dipped in urine (to get a clean sample, collect the specimen in midstream), a bacterial infection is present. Check yourself weekly if you are susceptible to infections.

Diet: Drink unsweetened blueberry or cranberry juice, three 8-oz. glasses a day, or take 400 mg of concentrated cranberry extract twice a day. Cranberries and blueberries both prevent bacteria from sticking to the bladder wall and have antibiotic properties. *E. coli* bacteria populations double about every twenty minutes, so it's vital to keep flushing them out. Cranberry juice also reduces unpleasant urine odor. Drink as much pure water as possible to dilute the urine so it causes less pain when voiding. Another alternative for the acute stage is to add 1 tsp. baking soda to drinking water once an hour on an empty stomach (check with your doctor if you have high blood pressure or a heart condition). Avoid refined sugars and alcohol.

Avoid: Don't eat acid-forming foods, such as caffeine, tomatoes, citrus fruits, cooked spinach, or chocolate, and avoid excessive sugars, refined carbohydrates, and alcohol. Don't use aluminum cookware. Avoid carbonated drinks, salty and fatty foods, and refined foods.

Nutrients

** Vitamin C, 1,000 mg in calcium ascorbate form three to five times a day inhibits the growth of *E. coli*. At the first sign of symptoms, take 1 g per hour. You must work with a doctor if taking more than 3 g a day.

** Bromelain, 500 mg four times a day on an empty stomach for one to two weeks

- Acidophilus multiple formula, 2–4 capsules two to three times a day
- Vitamin A, 25,000 IU twice a day for two weeks, then reduce to once a day for one to two months. Work with your doctor.
- Multivitamin/mineral supplement
- L-arginine, 1-2 g per day

For Chronic Infections

- Alternate 1 Tbsp. cherry concentrate and 1 Tbsp. cranberry concentrate first thing in the morning and last thing at night.
- Drink corn silk water or tea, especially for urine that feels scalding. (Boil 1 handful of dried corn silks in a pot of water for fifteen minutes, or use commercial tea.) Drink two to three glasses a day.
- Green drink, two to three times a week (page 465)
- Eat alkalizing foods, including celery, watermelon juice, and umeboshi plum balls, and consume yeast-free foods as much as possible.
- Try 2 Tbsp. apple cider vinegar and 1 tsp. honey in a glass of water before each meal.
- If prone to recurrent infections, generously consume products containing live active cultures, such as yogurt, or take supplements five to seven times a week for several months and then see if you can reduce to three to four times a week.
- Urinate each time after making love.
- Drinking carrot/beet/cucumber juice every other day for several weeks may help.
- Identify and treat any thyroid problems, including "subclinical" low thyroid functioning.
- Identify and avoid foods that trigger allergies.
- Topical treatment: ½ tsp. plain yogurt around your vaginal opening after intercourse as a preventative measure until you stop having recurrences.

- Thymus polypeptides, 500 mg once or twice a day
- Drink two to five cups of parsley and/or burdock, corn silk, or watermelon seed teas throughout the day for three days.

For Interstitial Cystitis

This disorder is very painful and difficult to treat. Sulfated poly-saccharides (like hyaluronic acid, chondroitin sulfate, dermatin and keratin sulfates) help alleviate symptoms even in the most severe cases. Avoid foods that trigger allergies.

Herbs: Cranberry extract, 400–500 mg two to three times a day; grapefruit-seed extract, 100–200 mg three times a day; goldenseal, 250–500 mg three times a day for seven to fourteen days; oregano extract, 140 mg three times a day. Take only for the duration of the infection and several days afterward. Make a tea from uva-ursi leaves and drink one cup every three hours for two days.

UTERUS

The hollow muscular organ of the reproductive system situated in the pelvic cavity behind the bladder and in front of the bowel. The fertilized egg normally becomes embedded in the uterus, and the developing embryo and fetus is nourished and grows there.

Imbalance of prostaglandins may lead to painful or heavy periods. Benign tumors of the uterus include polyps and fibroids. See *Fibroids.* Cancers of the uterus include cervical and endometrial cancer (see *Cancer, Female*). Imbalances of hormones, especially estrogen dominance, can manifest as various uterine problems. Certain environmental pollutants, like dioxin, can bind to receptors within the uterus and, along with excess body weight, poor lifestyle habits, and genes, may be contributing to the rise of uterine diseases.

Prolapsed Uterus

A condition in which the uterus descends from its normal position down into the vagina, always accompanied by some amount of vaginal "relaxation." The degree of prolapse can vary from only a slight displacement to a severe condition in which the uterus can be seen outside the vulva. Your sexual partner may notice a blockage during penetration. Most common in middle-aged women who have had children, it's aggravated by obesity. There are often no symptoms, or there may be a dragging feeling in the pelvis or a sensation that something is being pushed downward. It *must* be treated to prevent ulcerations and infections. Ask your doctor about estrogen rings or pessaries.

Tipped (Retroverted) Uterus

A condition in which the uterus inclines backward rather than forward. About 20 percent of women have a tipped uterus (which is the usual position of the uterus in infancy). The uterus may tip backward after childbirth, or, less commonly, can tip because of endometriosis or pelvic inflammatory disease. Some certified hands-on practitioners can help realign the uterus in certain cases.

V

VAGINAL PROBLEMS

The vagina is the muscular passage, usually 2.5 to 4 inches long, that connects the cervix with the external genitalia. It has three functions: as a receptacle for the penis during sexual intercourse, bringing sperm closer to the egg for fertilization; as an outlet for blood shed at menstruation; and as a passage for the baby during childbirth.

Vaginal Atrophy

Thinning of the wall of the vagina that causes pain and burning with intercourse in some women after menopause. This can make sex a scary thought. There are treatments to help slow down the aging process and even rebuild the cell walls of the vagina to restore more comfortable and pleasurable lovemaking.

What to Do
- Kegel exercises, twice a day, bring more circulation into the area and may enhance cell nutrition and thickening of the vaginal wall (page 433).
- *To increase circulation*—Activities that get the blood flowing to the genitals keep them young—including intercourse, masturbation, massage, and plain old exercise. One study of fifty-two postmenopausal women indicated much less vaginal atrophy among women having intercourse more than three times per week than ladies who had sex less than ten times a

440

year. Sexual activity maintains a more optimal acidic vaginal climate, which offers plentiful protection against infection.

- *To increase vaginal lubrication* and prevent soreness during sex, you have several choices. *Lubricating creams* like Astroglide, Lubrin, and K-Y jelly work well and need to be applied either to the vagina and/or penis each time you have intercourse. *Moisturizers,* like Replens, contain polycarbophil, an insoluble compound that absorbs water and adheres to vaginal skin cells. Replens is not a sexual lubricant, but a moisturizer. It needs to be applied to the vagina two to three times a week on a regular basis, not before or during intercourse. *Estrogen treatments* can also help (see box).

ESTROGEN TREATMENTS

Estriol is the mildest estrogen, but its affinity for vaginal tissue exceeds other estrogens (estradiol and estrone). This is especially helpful for vaginal dryness when a woman is not sure she should take oral estrogen, for example, if she has a history of estrogen-sensitive breast cancer. See your doctor. Some doctors don't know about estrogen rings. Dr. Michael Moen, in Chicago at 845-825-1590, is an expert at this.

- *Estrogen Ring:* A pliable ring, impregnated with either estriol or estradiol, that easily fits into most women's vaginas. It does not need to be removed for sex or cleaning. Each ring lasts three months, does not have systemic side effects, and is safely used without progestins or if you have a history of breast cancer. Rings allow a woman on oral hormone replacement therapy to take a low systemic dose while the ring moistens the vagina. For oral estrogen replacement therapy to moisten the vagina, the dose needs be a fair bit higher.
- *Vaginal Estriol Suppositories:* One study reports that using 0.5 mg vaginal estriol for twenty-one days and then 0.5 mg twice weekly effectively got rid of dry, painful intercourse. After one year, none of the women showed signs of excess estrogen (such as thickening of the endometrium).
- *Vaginal Premarin* or *Vaginal Estrace Creams:* Applied nightly in low doses (about one eighth the usual dose needed to treat menopausal hot flashes or palpitations), these creams have been shown to help without raising serum levels of estrogens.

 It's best to use any vaginal hormone therapy for at least three months to determine its effectiveness.

Nutrients to be used without any hormones or hormone rings
 ** PABA (para-aminobenzoic acid), 300–500 mg once or twice a
    day, or hormone potentiator formulas containing PABA
 • Vitamin A orally, 10,000–25,000 IU per day. Insert 5,000 IU
    vaginally for several weeks or on the day before intercourse
    and see if that helps. Ask your doctor.

<u>Herbs:</u> Korean ginseng (panax), 100 mg three times a day.

Vaginal Odor

The vagina stays clean because of the friendly bacteria that live there,
producing secretions that normally have only a faint odor. Advertising makes women think the smell is due to poor vaginal hygiene.
Vaginal deodorants are neither hygienic nor necessary and the chemicals they contain may cause irritation. Douching also does not rid
the vagina of its natural odor, and it increases the risk of infection.
Avoid wearing tight panty hose that don't let air circulate, evaluate
your need for digestive enzymes and vitamin B complex, and sip
1 Tbsp. chlorophyll in 1 cup water daily for several weeks.

Vaginal Discharge

A mucous secretion from the walls of the vagina and neck of the
cervix is normal in a woman during the reproductive years. It varies
considerably among women and at different times in the menstrual
cycle. Sexual stimulation increases vaginal discharge. If the discharge
is abnormal, as in vaginitis, it may be excessive, offensive smelling,
yellow or green, or cause itching. *Candida albicans* causes a thick white
discharge. The parasite *Trichomonas vaginalis* causes a profuse green-
yellow discharge. A forgotten tampon may cause a plentiful and very
smelly secretion.

Vaginal Itching

Usually caused by an allergic reaction to chemicals that are present in
deodorants, spermicides, creams, and douches. Itching is also common after menopause due to low estrogen levels. Vaginal infections,
especially yeast infections, may cause itching.

Vaginal Bleeding

Bleeding may come from the uterus, the cervix, or from the vagina itself. Possible causes of nonmenstrual bleeding include endometritis and endometrial cancer. Use of hormonal therapies can result in spotting, and hormonal imbalances and deficiencies can also occur. In early pregnancy, bleeding may be a sign of threatened miscarriage; later in pregnancy, it may indicate serious fetal or maternal problems. Bleeding from the cervix may be the result of cervical erosion, cervicitis, polyps, or cervical cancer. Bleeding from the vaginal walls is rare, with the most likely cause being injury during intercourse, especially after menopause.

Vaginitis

Inflammation of the vagina.

Symptoms: Sometimes the normal bacteria of the vagina multiply and cause an offensive fishy-smelling discharge, which is called *nonspecific vaginitis* or *bacterial vaginosis*. The odor may be very unpleasant after intercourse due to the chemical reaction between the bacteria causing the infection and the alkaline semen. Other signs may be itching, redness, or swelling of the vagina and vulva (area around the vagina). *Atrophic vaginitis* results from the thinning of the vaginal tissue from a decline in estrogen after menopause. The vagina becomes dry and inflamed and there is sometimes a discharge. Before menopause, women who have had surgical removal of the ovaries may get atrophic vaginitis. Chronic vaginal infections usually result in inflammation of the cervix as well.

Causes: Most commonly caused by the fungus *Candida albicans* (see *Yeast Infections*) or the parasite *Trichomonas vaginalis*. Bacterial infection, improper douching, a vitamin B deficiency, allergic reaction, hormone deficiency associated with aging (atrophic vaginitis), or a foreign body (such as a forgotten tampon) can cause vaginitis. Some types are sexually transmitted, such as those caused by chlamydia or gonorrhea. Oral contraceptives can produce vaginal inflammation (taking vitamin B complex and vitamin B_6 concurrently may reduce this problem).

What to Do

- Get a diagnosis to find out what is causing the infection.
- Make sure your partner is treated for any infection you have.
- Clean the inside folds of the vulva where bacteria are likely to grow and keep them as dry as possible.
- Avoid nylon-crotch panty hose, tight pants, or jeans. Wear cotton underwear and loose clothing. Wash underwear in hot water with chlorine bleach to kill microorganisms.
- Use plain, unscented soap.
- Don't use feminine hygiene sprays or powders.
- Don't have sex while you are being treated. Otherwise, the infection could be passed back and forth between you and your partner(s).
- Wipe from front to back after you go to the bathroom.
- Avoid activities that make you sweaty, especially during hot, humid weather.
- Try sitz baths with added liquid calendula and goldenseal extract or tea tree and lavender oils. Or add three cups apple cider vinegar to bathwater. Soak at least twenty minutes. Remember to spread your legs.
- Open a nonsynthetic vitamin E capsule and put the oil on the inflamed area.

Diet: For recurrent infections, try an elimination or rotation diet to identify food allergies or sensitivities. Eat a diet low in carbohydrates and sweets, which may reduce the amount of yeast in your intestines.

Avoid: Refined foods, alcohol, sugar, dairy products, and simple carbohydrates.

Nutrients

- ** Vitamin C and bioflavonoids, 1,000 mg three or four times a day for three days
- ** Vitamin B complex, 25–50 mg one to three times a day
- ** Vitamin B_6, 50 mg three times a day (important if you're taking estrogen in oral contraceptives, hormone replacement therapy, or fertility drugs)

Choose One

** *L. acidophilus* orally and/or as an acidophilus douche with 1 tsp. acidophilus powder mixed with 1–3 oz. water or milk, once a day for three days, or use several teaspoons plain yogurt containing live cultures

• Vitamin E orally (800 IU per day) or topically (400 IU capsule inserted vaginally) for three to fourteen days

• Vitamin A, 5,000 IU orally and 1 vitamin A capsule per day inserted into the vagina for no more than seven days.

Herbs: Herbal douche: 40 drops each of echinacea, goldenseal, and calendula with 2 Tbsp. aloe vera gel in 16 oz. of water. Or ⅓ tea tree oil with ⅔ vitamin E, put on a tampon and use daily (leave in overnight) for four to six weeks for yeast, trichomonas, and other vaginal infections. Echinacea, 300 mg three times a day for seven to fourteen days. Goldenseal, 250–500 mg three times a day for ten to fourteen days or as needed.

Vulvitis

Inflammation of the vulva. Can be caused by infections such as candidiasis, genital herpes, and warts and infestations of pubic lice or scabies. May also result from a change in the vulval skin after menopause, known as *vulval dystrophy*. Other possible causes are allergic reactions to soap, cream, detergent; excessive vaginal discharge; urinary incontinence. Any chronic inflammation may be caused by an unidentified allergen or may be a sign of cancer or parasites.

Vulvovaginitis

Inflammation of the vulva and vagina, usually due to candidiasis or trichomoniasis, which cause vaginal discharges that affect the vulva.

VARICOSE VEINS

Twisted, swollen, distended, bluish superficial veins (just beneath the skin) that affect 10 to 20 percent of adults. Varicose veins on the inside of the legs and on the back of the calves are the most common. The problem tends to run in families. (Hemorrhoids are varicose veins of the anus.)

Spider veins, common after pregnancy, are clusters of very tiny blood vessels seen as thin blue lines just under the skin, usually on the thighs and legs. They are not early varicosities, are not dangerous, and can be easily removed by a plastic surgeon.

Symptoms: Some may have no symptoms, but others experience a severe aching in the affected area, swollen feet and ankles, and persistent itching of the skin. If backflow of blood is severe enough to cause tissues to become oxygen-starved, the skin can become thin, hard, dry, scaly, and discolored, and ulcers may form.

Causes: The veins in the legs pump the blood upward, back to the heart. Valves in the veins prevent blood from draining back down the leg under the force of gravity. If the valves become defective, pooling blood makes the superficial veins become swollen and distorted. Contributing factors include pregnancy, obesity, standing for long periods, diets deficient in bioflavonoids, and genetics. Veins become more fragile with age. Inflammation and clotting of blood in the veins *(thrombophlebitis)* or clotting in the deeper veins *(deep vein thrombosis)* may be associated with varicosities. See *Phlebitis*. Varicose veins are not caused by crossing your legs.

Uniquely Female: Four times more women than men have varicose veins. Hormonal changes during pregnancy or at menopause, or pressure on pelvic veins during pregnancy, can cause varicose veins. Symptoms are often worse just before menstruation and/or menopause.

What to Do
- Do not wear tight clothing. And wear sensible shoes.
- Try elastic support hose (put them on before you get out of bed). Don't wear knee-high hosiery; it blocks circulation.
- Stay off your feet as much as possible.
- Rest your legs often by propping them up above the level of your heart.
- To keep from getting varicose veins, exercise regularly and lose weight if necessary.

- Don't stand or sit in one position for long periods of time.
- Walk as much as possible to increase blood flow. Swimming is excellent for legs.
- Massage feet and legs with diluted myrrh oil (5 drops in ⅓ cup massage oil) in the morning and evening.
- Raise the foot of your bed with two-inch blocks.
- Effective compresses include white oak bark; witch hazel; or cider vinegar and water.

Diet: Blueberries and grapes contain flavonoids that help prevent varicose veins.

Avoid: Salty, sugary, and caffeinated foods and drinks. Reduce saturated fats.

Nutrients
- ** Bromelain, 500 mg four times a day on an empty stomach
- Mix ¼ tsp. vitamin E oil and 2 Tbsp. liquid lecithin and apply to veins before bed for one or two months.

Herbs: Horse chestnut, 300 mg three times a day; bilberry, 20–40 mg two to three times a day; butcher's broom, 300–500 mg per day; gotu kola, 200 mg three times a day.

VIRILIZATION

Usually, women produce small amounts of androgens (male hormones) in their adrenal glands. A woman who develops a tumor of the adrenal gland or a particular ovarian tumor, either of which may secrete androgens, may develop changes called *virilization:* the clitoris grows larger, hair may appear on her face, her voice may deepen, and her breasts may become smaller. When the tumor is removed, the virilization regresses.

VULVODYNIA

Chronic vulvar pain. Women who experience vulvodynia may be so uncomfortable that they can barely sit, can't wear jeans or panty hose, and find sex out of the question. It's a greatly underdiagnosed problem because there are usually no visible signs and many women are reluctant to talk about it. Emotional stress from being with the wrong relationship partner or job can be linked to this condition.

Symptoms: Constant or intermittent pain, usually described as a burning, irritation, or rawness of a woman's genitals. The pain may be localized or diffuse and can last for months or years. It can stop as suddenly as it started. Women with *vulvar vestibulitis*, a type of vulvodynia, experience pain only when pressure is applied to the area surrounding the entrance to the vagina.

Causes: Theories include injury to or irritation of the nerves surrounding the vulva, allergies or a localized hypersensitivity to yeast, or spasms in the pelvic muscles. Many women with vulvodynia have a history of treatment for recurrent vaginal fungal infections, use of birth control pills, or celiac disease. There's no evidence that vulvodynia is sexually transmitted or related to cancer.

What to Do
- Biofeedback therapy helps you to learn to relax your pelvic muscles, which can sometimes constrict in anticipation of pain, thereby increasing the pain.
- Hook up with a support group or seek counseling to help you cope.
- Reduce stress (pages 52–58) or change whatever isn't working in your life.
- Test for celiac disease (antigliadin antibody blood test); if result is high, avoid gluten foods (see page 493).

W

WEIGHT

In healthy adults, weight remains more or less stable because calorie intake from the diet matches calorie expenditure. Weight loss or gain occurs if the balance is disturbed. Losing and gaining weight after age twenty-five may increase your risk of a variety of ills, including osteoporosis, certain cancers, and exposure to various pollutants stored in fat and released with yo-yoing weight loss.

Weight Loss and Underweight

A decrease in weight may be due to deliberate weight reduction, a change in diet, or change in your level of activity. However, weight loss is also a symptom of a wide range of disorders, from intestinal parasites to chronic illnesses such as cystic fibrosis, celiac disease, or heart disease. Persistent digestive disorders, such as gastroenteritis, and cancer of the esophagus, stomach, or colon cause weight loss, as does malabsorption of nutrients from disorders of the intestine or pancreas. Some disorders increase the rate of metabolic activity, thereby causing weight loss, such as any type of cancer, chronic infection, and hyperthyroidism. Untreated diabetes mellitus causes weight loss, as does wasting syndrome in those with AIDS (acquired immunodeficiency syndrome). Any unex-

> Loss of appetite in senior citizens is often caused by undiagnosed infection with a bug *(H. pylori)*. Have a blood test, not an endoscopic test, for diagnosis.

plained weight loss—10 percent or more of your usual weight over three to six months—should always be checked by a physician.

What to Do

- Red-colored plates are said to stimulate the appetite.
- Eliminate caffeine.
- Eat small, frequent meals.
- Moderate exercise is important.
- Don't eat when you're upset or nervous.
- Exercise in moderation—walk, for instance—to help trigger your appetite.

Diet: Don't drink excess liquids before or during meals to avoid appetite suppression.

Nutrients

- ** Zinc, 20 mg three to four times a day (reduce if nauseated); balance with 2–3 mg per day of copper
- ** Glutamine, 1,000 mg two to three times a day
- ** Multivitamin/mineral supplement
- ** Free-form amino acids, twice a day on an empty stomach in the morning and evening
- Evaluate your need for digestive enzymes (page 468).
- Vitamin B complex, 25–50 mg two to three times a day
- *Protein drink:* Protein powder (whey, rice, or soy), 25 g, blended with ground flaxseed (⅛ tsp.) or flaxseed oil and water with a little added diluted fruit juice or nondairy milk (multigrain, rice, almond). Drink once or twice a day. Optional: Add some fruit, like blueberries.
- Acidophilus and bifidobacteria, 2–3 capsules twice a day for several weeks

Herbs: Gentian root, 500 mg three times a day with meals; fenugreek is an appetite stimulant and aids digestion.

Overweight and Obesity

Americans are getting fatter despite all the available diet books and pills. A person is considered obese when she weighs 20 percent or more over the maximum desirable weight for her height and age. Forty percent of adult American women are trying to lose weight, and these numbers are higher among very overweight women. Getting down to an optimal weight has many benefits, from improving memory to enhancing sexuality. Excess fat (especially fat that infiltrates muscle and makes it unhealthy), particularly around the abdomen (and some studies add the upper thighs) is associated with increased insulin resistance, which is linked to numerous diseases. It is estimated that 280,000 deaths a year occur due to obesity in the United States. Severely overweight people show symptoms of low-grade, chronic inflammation, which may increase their risk of heart and other diseases.

Causes: Basically, obesity is usually the result of taking in more energy (calories from food and drink) than is being used for maintaining body functions, for body repair, and for exercise. The excess energy is converted into fat. Emotional tension, poor eating habits,

---

TO HELP CONQUER FOOD CRAVINGS

1. Glucomannan, 1.5 g half an hour before breakfast and dinner with a large glass of water

2. Chromium, 100–200 mcg twice a day

3. Magnesium, 500 mg, for chocolate cravings

4. *Garcinia cambogia* reduces sweet cravings; 500 mg twice a day

5. Homeopathic lycopodium, 30C, for sweet cravings

6. Flaxseed oil, 1 Tbsp., for fat cravings. Balance with vitamin E.

7. Kelp powder as a salt substitute for salt cravings

8. Cut down on carbohydrates to reduce fat cravings.

9. For compulsive eating: Tyrosine, 500 mg twice a day; free-form amino acids in morning on empty stomach; arginine and ornithine, 1,000 mg of each at bedtime; and zinc, 30 mg each day

overconsumption of carbohydrates, especially refined and processed oils, and love of food can all contribute to overweight. However, fat isn't fair and isn't always about calories. Sometimes weight control problems can come from genetics, cravings caused by body sugar imbalances or food allergies and/or inadequate digestive enzymes, sluggish thyroid, liver malfunction, exposure to pollutants that mimic hormones in the womb, or poor elimination/maldigestion. Another cause is stress, which influences the nervous system and hormones in ways that encourage fat to accumulate around the waist. Hormone disruptors may also be a contributing factor.

Uniquely Female: Heavier women get more breast, uterine, and cervical cancers. Osteoarthritis may be aggravated by obesity. Heart disease, high blood pressure, stroke, and adult-onset diabetes occur more in overweight women. Extra weight places undue strain on the hip, knee, and back joints and wallops self-esteem. Obesity in women has almost doubled in the last twenty years. Three key times when a woman is likely to gain weight are at the beginning of the menstrual cycle, after pregnancy, and after menopause. Earlier menarche may cause plumper girls, and vice versa, who may become heavier women later in life. Environmental pollutants may play a role.

What to Do

There are no magic pills or miracle formulas that will make you lose weight and keep it off. Eat less, exercise more, find dietary/lifestyle improvements you can live with, and reduce stress, because stress hormones add pounds to the waists of susceptible women.

** Lose weight slowly by finding a lifelong diet that appeals and works for you. Sudden weight losses are associated with various health problems and even death. Be moderate!

** Take calcium! Dieters are often susceptible to losing bone mass. Also, studies show that women consuming high amounts of calcium lose the most weight. Calcium helps burn fat.

** Test for food allergies and intolerances, which may contribute to weight gain.

** Evaluate your need for digestive enzymes (page 468).

- Bright lights decrease winter bingeing, especially in women with bulimia. Try full-spectrum lightbulbs.
- Avoid over-the-counter weight loss or appetite suppressant drugs. They can be dangerous. In particular, phenyl-propanolamine has been recalled.
- Chewing increases the appetite, although some women say that chewing slowly helps them eat less. Do whatever works for you.
- Don't grocery shop on an empty stomach.
- Exercise, exercise, exercise, a minimum of twenty minutes each day. Heavier women get better fitness even if they do not lose weight. Vary your exercise regime.
- Get emotional support.
- Try visualization.
- Put one serving of each food on your plate. As soon as you finish eating, leave the table and wash your plate. Your satiety center takes about ten minutes to kick in. Don't get seconds during these first ten minutes.
- Diets that focus on proteins and fats, and almost banish carbohydrates, are hard on the kidneys and bones. Very few people who lose weight this way maintain the loss. However, focusing less on low-fat, high-carbohydrate foods, especially refined ones, and more on lean protein, vegetables, fruits, and grains appears to help some women achieve permanent weight loss.
- Consume less sodium, which is linked to increased risk of death from all causes in overweight people.

Diet

- Don't go on a crash or starvation diet. The more you starve, the better your overweight body gets at storing fat and lowering the rate at which you burn off fat. If you have been overeating, start by consuming 500–1,000 calories less a day for a one- to two-pound weight loss per week. If, however, you have been starving yourself for years, with no results or yo-yoing your weight, you may actually need to increase your metabolism. Do this by slowly increasing your caloric intake in a sensible manner (avoiding excess carbohydrates, especially refined)—grazing throughout the day—adding several hundred calories every week or so until you are eating 1,500–1,800 healthy calories daily, accompanied by regular, "must do" aerobic daily exercise of at least twenty minutes. For example, do stretching and then ride the exercise bike for a half hour; then for breakfast eat scrambled egg whites (with one yolk added for every three or four whites), natural turkey sausage, and sprouted bread or half a bagel with a little olive oil, pepper, and salt. At lunch and dinner, eat lean protein and vegetables (nothing fried). For snacks have fruit, small amounts of nuts, or 1 tsp. of peanut butter.

- Rotate foods, eating a wide variety.
- Try going off dairy and wheat for two months. Avoid sweet foods and undiluted juices.
- Eat enough fiber to avoid constipation, such as whole grains, seeds, and nuts.
- If you are insulin resistant, the best diet is higher protein/lower carbohydrate. (If any member of your family has type 2 diabetes, be sure to test for insulin resistance.) If you are not insulin resistant and have been eating a high protein diet but not losing weight, eat more vegetarian meals with high-fiber, complex-carbohydrate foods. If you have been eating a vegetarian diet and not losing weight, consume more quality proteins, don't overdo the carbohydrates, and graze throughout the day. Learn about the glycemic index (pages 129, 300).
- Ask a trainer about "internal" training.
- Drink plenty of water. Avoid sweet drinks and fruit juices.
- Try barley malt or stevia sweeteners instead of sugar.
- Red pepper, caffeine, and the fiber in whole foods help increase satiety and decrease hunger.

Avoid: Additives, preservatives, sugar, caffeine, and sweets. Avoid eating heavy meals or large snacks late at night.

Nutrients

- ** CLA (conjugated linoleic acid), 1,000 mg three times a day before meals
- ** Calcium, 800–1,200 mg per day in divided doses
- ** Multivitamin/mineral supplement
- ** Chromium, 200 mcg with meals two or three times a day
- ** Fiber Cocktail (page 464), once or twice a day, no matter which diet you use
- Carnitine, 500 mg two to three times a day
- Magnesium, 250 mg twice a day
- Vitamin B complex, 25–50 mg per day
- Pyruvate, 22–44 g per day, for short-term use
- Have your doctor run a DHEA (dehydroepiandrosterone) test, and supplement if necessary (especially for weight gain that happens with getting older).
- 5-hydroxytryptophan (5-HTP) 600 mg per day in divided doses, may help, but you should work with your doctor and use reputable sources as some extreme health problems have been linked to contaminated products in isolated cases.
- *For night-eating syndrome:* People with this syndrome lack appetite in the morning, overeat at night, and often suffer from insomnia. Ask your doctor about melatonin, 1–3 mg before bed, and leptins, along with stress reduction. Excess carbohydrate consumption is another form of self-medication.
- Red pepper capsules, 5–6 taken with fatty meals, may help increase weight loss during the first two weeks of a diet. Up to 10 g per day of pantothenic acid also appears to enhance weight loss. Work with a doctor.

Note: Women whose stomachs have been surgically reduced to treat morbid obesity may develop elevated levels of homocysteine a year later. Take folic acid, vitamin B_6, vitamin B_{12}, and B complex.

WINE and ALCOHOLIC BEVERAGES

Wine seems to protect the heart by acting as an antioxidant. It also widens and softens arteries and decreases clot formation even in someone consuming a high-fat diet. However, more is not better. Light to moderate drinkers who report occasional heavy bouts of drinking—four to eight drinks at one time, or getting drunk once a month—have been shown to have higher death rates at earlier ages, even if they've quit drinking. Women should not have more than one or two alcoholic beverages a day.

Wine has high levels of phenolic compounds that have many favorable effects, such as elevating good cholesterol, making platelets less sticky, and increasing nitric oxide, which is good for arteries. But berry juices without the alcohol have many of these same positive benefits. Even though red and white wines and grape juice all have high antioxidant activity, white wine does not appear to be as heart-friendly as red. Look for organic wines if you have trouble with nitrites. Moderate wine drinkers seem to have less death from heart disease and cancer. Wine may protect against colon cancer, even in smokers.

Forty studies have shown that moderate alcohol intake (one to two drinks a day in women) may create a 10–40 percent lower risk of coronary heart disease than in women who abstain (*British Medical Journal* 319:1523–8, 1999). Even one drink per week has a positive benefit. However, *excess* alcoholic intake increases the risk of many diseases, such as osteoporosis and cancer. Women with lifetime exposure to excess estrogen (see *Estrogen Dominance*) may be adversely affected by alcohol. Alcoholic consumption in excess can increase estrogenic signaling and lower progesterone signaling. It is so estrogenic in some women who regularly consume three or four drinks a day can delay onset of menopause by two years.

Y

YEAST INFECTIONS
(Candidiasis, Thrush, or Monilia)

Infection by the fungus *Candida albicans*, usually within the vagina but sometimes inside the bowel or on moist skin. The fungus is present in the vagina of 5–25 percent of women between the ages of fifteen and fifty. For candida-related complex syndrome (yeast infection in intestinal lining) read my book *Healthy Digestion the Natural Way* (John Wiley, 2000).

Symptoms: Intense itching of the external genitalia, which may also be red and sore. May have painful urination or pain during intercourse. Monilia causes a white discharge that looks like cottage cheese and may have a bad smell. Chronic monilia may be a woman's first sign of diabetes; chronic yeast infections that also involve oral thrush may be the first sign of AIDS (acquired immunodeficiency syndrome). Some women have no symptoms.

Causes: Impaired immune function, diabetes, HIV (human immunodeficiency virus), pregnancy, and food allergies may encourage growth of the fungus; eating refined sugar on a daily basis; heavy consumption of commercially raised meats; several rounds of antibiotics close together; using steroids on a regular basis; regular use of Tagamet, Zantac, or other antacids or asthma medications.

Uniquely Female: More common during pregnancy and in women taking hormones, including birth control pills. May be linked

WHEN TAKING ANTIBIOTICS

Antibiotics kill off friendly bacteria as well as the infection you're treating. To avoid yeast infections, take probiotics several times a day one hour away from antibiotics and for seven to fourteen days after finishing the course. If you are prone to yeast infections, take oil of oregano or grapeseed extract, 2–3 capsules twice a day after meals for one week after antibiotics. Consume cultured food generously, but always finish the entire round of antibiotics.

to premenstrual syndrome, menstrual irregularities, and chronic vaginitis.

What to Do
- Don't wear tight jeans.
- Keep your vaginal area clean and dry. Wipe from front to back.
- Wear cotton underpants or panty hose with a cotton crotch.
- Don't use dusting powders. Most have a starch base, and starch is the perfect medium for growing fungus cultures.
- Use unscented tampons and pads and white unscented toilet paper.
- Don't have sex until your symptoms are gone. Afterward, to prevent reinfection, avoid chemical douches, contraceptive foams and sprays, and feminine deodorants. Use natural lubricants, such as oils and plain yogurt. Your sexual partner may need to be treated, too.
- Don't take antibiotics unless you absolutely must.
- Add ½ cup vinegar to a warm sitz bath to help rebalance vaginal pH.
- For chronic vaginitis, try boric acid capsules inserted into the vagina twice a day for two to four weeks as needed. Don't use if pregnant. Work with your doctor.

Diet: Yeast doesn't like quality fats, so include olive oil in your diet. Drink plenty of water to flush toxins from your body.

Avoid: Yeast-based foods and sugar. Yeast thrives on sugar, including artificial sweeteners and too much lactose from dairy products. Alcohol is an immediate sugar in the body. If you must drink, vodka has the least impact on candidiasis.

Nutrients
- See the section on vaginitis under *Vaginal Problems* for nutrients.
- Garlic, 450 mg twice a day

For Chronic Infections
- Evening primrose oil or flaxseed oil, 2–5 g per day for three to six months
- Thymus glandular, 1–3 capsules at breakfast and lunch
- Vitamin B_6, 50 mg once a day, plus vitamin B complex
- Oil of oregano, 2–5 capsules after meals twice a day for one to two weeks

Herbs: Pau d'arco, 500 mg twice a day for four to six weeks, or a bath with five pau d'arco tea bags (put bags in cheesecloth and run under the hot water), soak for twenty minutes several nights a week; use extremely diluted tea tree oil as a douche or as a coconut oil–based suppository (with 2 percent tea tree oil).

APPENDIX A
Hormone Testing

Whenever we say to check or run hormone levels, we're inferring that if the test results are low or borderline low–normal, your doctor should consider your individual situation in deciding whether or not to give you supplements. If you do take supplemental hormones, in most cases the doctor should prescribe *physiologic doses* (equal to the dose your body should naturally make). Sometimes higher doses are required.

Three estrogens, progesterone, luteinizing hormone (LH), follicle-stimulating hormone (FSH), dehydroepiandrosterone (DHEA), testosterone, cortisol, melatonin, adrenal hormones, and thyroid can all be tested. However, there is disagreement among the experts about the best way to measure hormone levels. Women were given hormones for decades with virtually no testing. Now that the safety of hormonal supplementation and dosages of therapeutic treatment is more in question, no one seems to know what method is most accurate—blood, saliva, or twenty-four-hour urine-catch tests.

Blood tests for hormones (except DHEA or testosterone) are notoriously inaccurate, especially for estrogen and progesterone. Most hormones in serum are bound to blood proteins and are not available to tissues and cells, and blood tests are a one-time random spot-check, when in reality hormone levels vary greatly throughout the day. Saliva tests measure the free (bioavailable) form of hormones circulating in tissues and cells, are relatively inexpensive, are easy to do at home, and are considered by many to be an accurate measurement of various hormones. Saliva tests can do spot measurements, but they can also easily be obtained for several levels at various times during a day, or, what's really nice, throughout an entire month. The problem with saliva testing is that some doctors say that once you use topical creams, you no longer can use saliva tests. One company says not to use its saliva test until you have stopped using topical hormones for up to four months. But according to Dr. John Lee, inaccuracies in testing and controversies have arisen from women taking saliva measurements at inappropriate times. Dr. Lee says proper saliva testing should be done eight to ten hours after the last application of cream.

Some doctors prefer twenty-four-hour urine tests. Since hormones fluctuate greatly over the course of a day, a twenty-four-hour urine hormone assessment gives the average of your hormone levels over an entire day.

It's obvious that there are disagreements about testing hormones. Most doctors agree that it is necessary to get a baseline measurement and then follow up by testing how a woman feels along with a repeat test. Currently, most holistic practitioners test first with saliva and/or twenty-four-hour urine hormone panels. Ask your doctors which tests they like working with and why.

Some labs that do such testing are:

- AAL Reference Laboratories (800-522-2611)—Twenty-four-hour-urine hormone screens and tests for estrogen metabolites and ratios
- Aeron Lifecycles (800-631-7900)—Saliva tests
- Diagnos-Techs (800-878-3787)—Saliva tests
- Great Smokies Diagnostic Laboratory (800-522-4762)—Saliva tests
- Life Extension (800-544-4440)—Hormone and blood testing
- Meridian Valley Laboratories (253-859-8700)—Twenty-four-hour urine hormone screens and tests for estrogen metabolites and estrogen ratios
- Nutraceutical Labs Inc. (888-999-7440)—Saliva tests
- ZRT Laboratory (503-466-2445)—Saliva tests

APPENDIX B
Compounding Pharmacies

To order natural hormone supplementation, contact *compounding pharmacies*, which make natural hormones out of molecules that look exactly like our body's hormones. Natural hormones do not contain nonhuman substances, such as the horse's urine in Premarin. They often are prescribed in physiologic doses and can be customized to your unique needs. Ask your doctor to call one of the pharmacies below or one like them.

Apothecure (800-969-6601)

College Pharmacy (800-888-9358)

Key Pharmacy (800-878-1322)

Professional Arts Pharmacy (800-832-9285)

APPENDIX C
Fiber Cocktail

Add one heaping teaspoon of bran (psyllium or oat, soy, or rice bran) to an 8-oz. glass of water or diluted fruit juice. Stir briskly and drink quickly. Follow with another glass of plain water. Or swallow two to four fiber tablets followed by one to two large glasses of water. Start once a day, build to twice a day if no problems, then reduce as symptoms and evacuation normalize. Rotate your sources of bran, as you can become allergic to *anything* you eat daily, even fiber. Contraindicated with diseases that should avoid sudden increases in fiber, like scleroderma.

APPENDIX D
Green Drink

Basic

Pour a glass of pineapple juice or half water and half pineapple juice into a blender. Add four or five well-washed leaves of romaine lettuce and a handful of parsley (stuff a fairly large amount of greens into the pineapple liquid). Blend extremely well and drink immediately. Delicious. Great way to get *live* absorbable greens, chlorophyll, and magnesium. Parsley is high in apigenin, a flavone that fights cancer and inflammation. Avoid using large amounts of parsley when breast-feeding.

Options:

1. Add some raw spinach leaves once or twice a week, but not daily.
2. Add 1 Tbsp. flaxseed oil or ⅛ tsp. ground flaxseeds (don't use more; too many raw ground flaxseeds can be hard on the liver). Yellow flaxseeds have more lignins than dark ones, but both are healthy.
3. Add mixed salad greens instead of romaine.

Green Drink Variations

Protein Green Drink: Add one scoop of quality protein powder.
Anticancer Green Drink: Add a few florets of raw broccoli. Don't do daily, especially if you have an underactive thyroid.

Liver Detox: In season, add a few (not too many) dandelion greens.

Essential Oil Green Drink: Add varied nuts to your Green Drink, like hazelnuts, walnuts, or almonds. Add them raw, or soaked overnight (changing the water several times) for a creamier taste.

Calcium Booster: Add 1–2 Tbsp. yogurt with live cultures—one of the best-absorbed forms of calcium.

APPENDIX E
Coffee Enemas

Coffee enemas are useful tools for detoxing harmful substances from the liver. Brew a pot of organic coffee with filtered water, cool down until room temperature. Fill an enema bag. With clean hands, lubricate the enema tip with olive oil. Lie on your right side and empty as much of the bag as possible (you may need to get up and go much more quickly when you first start doing this). Remove the tip and go into head-down/rear-end-up position for a few minutes or until you must get up and go.

APPENDIX F
Digestive Enzymes

A healthy stomach makes the digestive enzymes *stomach acid* (hydro-chloric acid—HCl) and *pepsin.* These are necessary for the body to be able to absorb nutrients from proteins and minerals (calcium, copper, iron, zinc) and certain B vitamins (folic acid and others). According to the studies performed at the Mayo Clinic, healthy people can make one hundred to two hundred different levels of stomach acid. This means that even if your stomach secretes HCl within the normal range, it may not be enough for digesting many of your nutrients. Also, just as your skin ages, so does the lining of your intestinal tract, where many of the digestive enzymes are made. It is thus sensible to evaluate your need for digestive enzymes to get your digestion and any health problems back on track.

The pancreas secretes three kinds of digestive enzymes: *proteolytic enzymes* to digest protein, *lipases* to digest fat, and *amylases* to digest carbohydrates. *Pancreatin* contains all three digestive enzymes from the pancreas and is rated according to a standard established by the United States Pharmacopeia (USP). A typical dose of 3–4 g of 4X pancreatin taken with each meal usually helps those who do not make adequate amounts of digestive enzymes to digest food better. Pancreatic enzymes should be taken at the end of meals away from stomach acid. Contraindicated if you have any ulcerated intestinal condition or if you are allergic to the source of enzymes, *i.e.,* pork.

Digestive Enzymes

Stomach Acidity: Symptoms of inadequate levels include belching and/or bloating, stomach discomfort, or vague pain behind the breastbone *immediately after or up to one half hour after meals*, gallbladder problems, loose stools in the morning, chronically coated tongue and bad breath, recurrent nausea* for no reason or associated with meals, painful dentures, and using herbs and nutrients and not benefiting from them. Other signs of low HCl include chronic abnormal changes in the mouth (particularly a sore tongue or mouth soreness, burning, or dryness); nails that crack, break, and peel; brittle hair or hair loss; childhood asthma; severe childhood eczema; or autoimmune diseases (such as lupus and multiple sclerosis). There may be no *outright* signs until disease shows up. Health disorders linked in the scientific literature to low stomach acid are bone loss, Addison's disease, arthritis (all types), asthma, celiac disease, diabetes, eczema, gallbladder problems, periodontal disease, lupus erythematosus, and vitiligo.

A doctor with a Heidelberg Gastric Analysis machine can directly measure your stomach acid.

How to Take Stomach Acid: Take one 500–650 mg capsule containing hydrochloric acid and pepsin after several bites of food (not on an empty stomach). If you have no discomfort, add one capsule per meal, working up to about 1–3 g per meal. Take throughout the meal to mimic natural secretions. Always take a bite of food first. Some people do better with glutamic acid form rather than betaine. Never take with nonsteroidal anti-inflammatory drugs (NSAIDs), aspirin, or cortisone.

Pancreatic Enzymes: Symptoms of inadequate levels include belching and/or bloating or intestinal discomfort *several hours* after meals, chronic intestinal gas, undigested food in stools, recurrent bubbles and grease in stools, chronic constipation or diarrhea or alter-

---

* *Chronic* nausea can also come from taking more enzymes than you need, food allergies, a bacterial infection with *H. pylori*, emotional stress, or reaction to progestins.

nating between the two, fat-soluble deficiencies (vitamins A, E, D, and K), and not benefiting from a good diet, herbs, or nutrients.

How to Take Pancreatic Enzymes: Start with one pancreatic enzyme supplement after meals and see how you feel. If necessary, slowly increase to a higher dose, 2 or more grams per day.

Never take digestive enzymes if you have ulcers or inflammatory or active bowel disease, or without a doctor's supervision. Only take for several months while improving digestive symptoms, while seeing an overall reduction of health problems, or while still seeing signs of nutrient deficiencies (pages 35–39). Then see if you can maintain gains while reducing doses. Enzymes may inhibit folic acid absorption, so make sure you take vitamin B complex with folic acid at different times than enzymes.

APPENDIX G
IV Protocols

Myer's Cocktail*—A slow intravenous (IV) push of nutrients (in one syringe):

Nutrient	Amount
Magnesium chloride hexahydrate (20 percent)	2–5 ml
Calcium gluconate (10 percent)	2–3 ml
Hydroxycobalamin (1,000 mcg per ml)	1 ml
Pyridoxine hydrochloride (100 mg per ml)	1 ml
Dexpanthenol (250 mg per ml)	1 ml
B complex 100	1 ml
Vitamin C (222 mg per ml)	1–20 ml

Add 10–20 ml of sterile water. Must be administered slowly, from five to fifteen minutes, through a 25G butterfly needle. Ask your doctor to order the preservative-free form.

There are very specific instructions and warnings regarding this protocol. Have your doctor check with an experienced practitioner. Theo Gerontinos, a registered nurse specializing in nutrient IVs and integrative medicine (with years of experience working with top doctors in the field) is available to train medical office staff in these procedures. Call 858-793-2634.

---

* This technique has been taught to thousands of doctors by Drs. Alan R. Gaby and Jonathan B. Wright.

APPENDIX H
Detoxify Yourself

Pantethine

Taking pantethine, 300 mg two to three times a day, helps detoxify aldehydes. This reduces toxicity and symptoms from hangovers, working in fabric and carpet stores, living in mobile homes, or for medical and chiropractic students working in cadaver labs (they need to take 600–900 mg before dissection laboratory).

Liver and Lung Helper—Glutathione

This complex of three amino acids is a natural detoxifier and antioxidant important for liver and lung function. It is found in cruciferous vegetables (cabbage, broccoli, cauliflower, radish sprouts, mustard greens, kohlrabi), allium vegetables (garlic, onions, leeks, asparagus, and chives), and nuts. Most forms of cooking except for freezing harm glutathione. Vitamin C and N-acetyl-cysteine help the body make glutathione. Regular use of alcohol and acetaminophen deplete the body of it.

APPENDIX I
Supplement and Drug Interactions

Review this section before taking nutrients, to avoid potentially harmful nutrient and drug interactions.

Alpha-Lipoic Acid

This antioxidant can have toxic effects on your system if you are deficient in vitamin B_1 and vitamin B complex. Take backup B vitamins. If you are taking 100 mg or more per day, add 2–3 mg of biotin per day.

Antacids

Pharmaceutical antacids inhibit folic acid absorption; used for long periods, like a year, they can inhibit absorption of calcium. Long-term use of antacids has been associated with an increased risk of stomach and esophageal cancers. Aluminum-containing antacids have been linked to certain kinds of Parkinson's disease, and aluminum from high-aluminum antacids accumulates in bones, promoting bone loss, and in brain tissues, where it *may* increase the risk of dementia.

Aspirin

Regular use of aspirin can aggravate asthma and other chronic lung conditions. It also decreases the body's ability to absorb vitamin C, so regular users of aspirin need more supplementation with C. Aspirin in low-dose form or with enteric coating still increases your risk of upper gastrointestinal bleeding, and the risk is even higher when aspirin is combined with nonsteroidal anti-inflammatory drugs (NSAIDs). Bleeding problems may offset its benefits. Long-term use is linked to hemorrhage. Many practitioners are not aware of this (*American Journal of Gastroenterology* 95:2218–24, 2000). Long-term use of aspirin also lowers melatonin hormone levels. If you are taking aspirin prophylactically for your heart concerns, a natural alternative is to take 1 Tbsp. cod liver oil (do not take cod liver oil if you are on Coumadin) or bromelain daily. Aspirin can act like an antioxidant.

Beta-Blockers

These heart medications can block melatonin release.

Blood Thinners

Bromelain should not be taken if you have arrthymias, extra heartbeats, are on blood thinners, or two weeks before surgery.

Capsules

When purchasing vitamin capsules, request veggie sources when possible.

Diuretics

Chronic use of diuretics calls for supplementation with vitamins B_1 and B_{12}, magnesium, and potassium. Diuretics drain the body of these nutrients, which can then elevate homocysteine levels.

Flavonoids

Either citrus (600 mg per day) or rutin (500 mg per day) for several months can be used to treat venous insufficiency, food allergies, easy bruising, heavy bleeding during menses, and hemorrhoids.

Folic Acid

Folic acid may interfere with cancer treatments that use methotrexate. People with rheumatoid arthritis or severe psoriatic arthritis taking methotrexate need large amounts of folic acid. They and anyone on 1,000 mcg or more require a doctor's supervision.

Glucocorticoids

Long-term use of glucocorticoids (for conditions such as rheumatoid arthritis, lupus, etc.) is associated with decreased production of DHEA (dehydroepiandrosterone), which contributes to bone loss. Ask your doctor about DHEA testing and supplementation when on these drugs.

Grapefruit Juice

Grapefruit can inhibit certain liver detoxifying enzymes and thus *increase* the action of certain drugs like benzodiazepines, cyclosporine, felodipine, nifedipine, and nisoldipine.

Melatonin

Melatonin may interfere with nifedipine in hypertensives.

Monoamine Oxidase Inhibitors

Monoamine oxidase (MAO) inhibitors, such as Nardil and Parnate, can have adverse effects if mixed with foods containing tyramine—yogurt, liver, pickled herring, wine, beer, aged cheese, and chocolate. If you have been on a tricyclic or selective serotonin-reuptake inhibitor (SSRI) antidepressant, wait two weeks after stopping medication before beginning an MAO inhibitor. *Fatal reactions can occur when the two are mixed.* Also, certain SSRIs can contribute to upper intestinal bleeding, which worsens when given with nonsteroidal anti-inflammatory drugs (NSAIDs). Some studies suggest that antidepressants may increase the risk of cardiac events like heart attacks.

Try natural therapies first if you have a history of heart disease or are on synthetic hormones, which can also increase adverse cardiac events.

Nonsteroidal Anti-inflammatory Drugs

Nonsteroidal anti-inflammatory drugs, like Advil and aspirin, when consumed over long periods of time, can contribute to bone loss (osteoporosis), copper deficiencies, and inadequate levels of the hormone melatonin. They can also, over time, worsen cartilage damage.

Oral Contraceptives

The effectiveness of oral contraceptives is decreased by barbiturates, carbamazepine, phenytoin, rifabutin, and rifampin, and combining these drugs may result in unwanted pregnancies.

PABA (Para-Aminobenzoic Acid)

Very large dosages (over 12 g per day) can cause fever, rash, hypoglycemia, and some rare fatalities. It is contraindicated in women on sulfonamide medications.

Phenytoin

Folic acid and the anticonvulsive phenytoin affect each other. Only take them together with a doctor's supervision.

Proteolytic Enzymes

Pancreatic enzymes and bromelain inhibit folic acid absorption and should only be taken for several months, along with extra folic acid. Don't take if you have ulcers or any ulcerative condition.

Vitamin B_6

Treatment with vitamin B_6 may inhibit depression, headaches, and fluid retention from estrogen/oral contraceptives; drug-induced lupus from hydralazine drugs; and neuropathies from isoniazid. Vitamin B_6 may interfere with levodopa while enhancing Sinemet's effect (levodopa plus carbidopa). Certain drugs and chemicals can cause imbalances or deficiencies of B_6, including oral contraceptives, cigarette smoke, FD&C yellow dye #5 (tartrazine), hydralazine, phenelzine, isoniazid, theophylline, and pesticides similar in structure to hydrazine.

Vitamin B_{12}

Certain drugs can inhibit absorption of vitamin B_{12} (and may necessitate sublingual and B_{12} injections), such as antacids, colchicine, potassium chloride, potassium citrate, and some oral hypoglycemic agents.

APPENDIX J
Vitamin Interactions

N-Acetyl-Cysteine

N-acetyl-cysteine (NAC) may, over time, increase your body's need for calcium, iron, magnesium, and zinc. Avoid it if you have a history of liver disease.

Essential Fatty Acids

The dose of omega-3 and omega-6 oils depends on the type of oil and the condition that is to be treated. Common therapeutic doses include evening primrose oil (2–6 g per day), borage oil (1–6 g per day), cod liver oil (5–15 ml per day), MaxEPA (3–12 g per day), flaxseed (5–30 ml per day), and black currant seed (2–10 g per day). One Tbsp. cod liver oil contains 15 g of essential fatty acids. Taking essential oils increases your body's need for vitamin E, and large doses over time increase your need for more antioxidants. Keep oils in airtight containers in the refrigerator and squeeze in a vitamin E capsule when you open the container for the first time to avoid harmful oxidation of oils.

Folic Acid

Large doses of folic acid can deplete zinc and vitamin B_{12}, may interfere with the diagnosis of pernicious anemia, and may cause seizures in epileptics. Large dosages of vitamin B_6, vitamin B_{12}, or zinc may increase your need for folic acid. Take with backup vitamin B complex. It is best absorbed on an empty stomach. Folic acid is required during the first two to three weeks of pregnancy to avoid many birth defects such as neural tube problems, and birth control pills (BCPs) rinse the body of folic acid, so you must supplement with this and other B vitamins when on BCPs. Do not take high dosages if you are also taking Dilantin (anti-epileptic medication). It may interfere with methotrexate when used for treating cancer, but it's okay when used in treating arthritis.

Indol-3-Carbinol

Indol-3-carbinol (I3C) is a constituent of cruciferous vegetables that has been shown in animal and human studies to have anticarcinogenic properties. The active component of I3C, formed in the stomach, is called diindolylmethane (DIM) and blocks the effects of estrogen via the AH receptor. I3C favorably alters estrogen metabolism, inhibits carcinogen-induced mammary tumor growth in rodents, and regresses precancerous lesions in women. Adequate stomach acid is necessary to make DIM.

Niacin (Vitamin B_3)

This vitamin can cause short-term flushing, redness, and discomfort. Large dosages of niacin can decrease blood sugar in some diabetics, elevate liver enzymes, and in rare cases cause hepatitis. Do not take more than several hundred milligrams per day without a doctor's supervision and never go over 3 g per day. Niacinamide and inositol hexanicotinate are forms of niacin that do not cause liver problems or flushing, although niacinamide can still elevate liver enzymes. Sustained-release niacin can be more toxic to the liver than regular niacin. Niacin can elevate homocysteine levels, so always take it with folic acid and vitamin B complex. Get your liver enzymes checked if you are taking higher dosages (500 mg or more per day). The first sign of liver toxicity is nausea. It is a sign that your liver enzymes may be elevating. When you feel nauseated, stop niacin for several days, get your enzymes tested, and restart at a lower dose.

Pantothenic Acid (Vitamin B$_5$)

You can use large dosages without toxicity.

Vitamin A

Five thousand IU per day is the recommended dose. Some do better with up to 25,000 IU daily, or even short-term higher therapeutic dosages, both of which require medical supervision. Higher dosages are not safe for most people with a history of liver disease. Women over sixty-five should not take more than 15,000 IU per day without being under a doctor's supervision. Adverse reactions from high dosages may be: headaches; fatigue; bone pain; skin and nail pitting; dry and flaking skin, especially on fingers and toes; joint and muscle pain; and nausea; all of these side effects reverse upon stopping the nutrient. Liver damage is a later effect. If a doctor recommends high levels of the vitamin, tests for liver and calcium should be run every several weeks. Whenever taking short-term high dosages of vitamin A or prescriptions for 13-cis-retinoic acid, also take vitamin E. *Beta-carotene* can be safely taken in high dosages, but it should be avoided by smokers and those with lung cancer.

Vitamin B$_1$

Large levels can deplete vitamin B$_6$ or magnesium.

Vitamin B$_2$

Drugs such as Dilantin, phenothiazines, and the chemotherapy drug Adriamycin can affect vitamin B$_2$, so extra should be taken after discussion with your doctor.

Vitamin B$_6$

The safest range is 50–100 mg per day. Signs of deficiency are poor dream recall, and reactions to monosodium glutamate (MSG) in Chinese food (feeling spacey or wired, and finger swelling in the morning). Taking B$_6$ before a meal usually reduces this reaction, but it's best to avoid MSG. Several hundred milligrams per day may cause insomnia or anxiety, which can be prevented by taking magnesium at the same time. Large dosages may also increase your need for other B vitamins, zinc, or essential fatty acids. Five hundred mg per day or more may cause tingling in your hands and feet, and dosages over 600 mg per day may suppress lactation. Pyridoxal-5'-phosphate is a predigested form, but it's not as easily absorbed as pyridoxal phosphate which is cheaper. Avoid more than 25 mg per day while pregnant or nursing, as higher levels can inhibit milk production.

Vitamin B$_{12}$

Large dosages may increase your need for folic acid. Low-normal blood levels of vitamin B$_{12}$ often indicate mild deficiency states that require supplementation. This is especially important for women on birth control pills, hormone replacement therapy, or at risk for pregnancy, blood pressure, and heart problems. Do not use nasal gel forms of B$_{12}$, as the cobalt in these forms is toxic to nasal membranes.

Vitamin C

Do not take more than 3 g a day unless working with a doctor. Excess dosages for your body will cause gas, abdominal pain, bloating, and diarrhea, which will go away when the dose is subsequently reduced. Rare folks with a genetic defect in oxalate metabolism may not do well with more than 1,500 mg of vitamin C. Don't stop taking large doses of vitamin C abruptly, as this can cause *rebound scurvy*, which may show up as spontaneous bruises and/or gum or nosebleeds. Vitamin C enhances uptake of iron, so individuals predisposed to iron overload should be monitored. Large dosages of vitamin C can alter stool tests for blood, urine tests for blood sugar, and scratch tests for allergies. Inadequate levels of vitamin C and bioflavonoids will manifest as multiple bruises that occur without any trauma. You can take larger amounts of oral vitamin C when you are also receiving vitamin C intravenously, often avoiding annoying bowel side effects.

Do not regularly use chewable C, as it is not good for your teeth.

Vitamin D

Dosages of 2,000–3,000 IU per day an extended time may increase calcification of soft tissues and may increase risk of plaque formation in the arteries. However, vitamin D deficiencies (overt and subclinical) are being linked to a wide variety of illnesses from colon cancer to unusual muscular problems such as fibromyalgia and chronic fatigue syndrome. Five patients in wheelchairs with severe muscular disorders of unknown origin all got out of wheelchairs in six weeks after taking high dosages of vitamin D (50,000 IU per day). Anyone contemplating megadoses of vitamin D must work with a doctor and should be tested. Vitamin D *resistance* (there is adequate D in the bloodstream but the body can't use it) may be on the rise, secondary to environmental pollutants. It may be contributing to the increased incidences of illnesses like osteoporosis.

Vitamin E

It is best to take mixed tocopherols. Supplementing with omega-6 and omega-3 oils and vitamin B_6 may increase your body's need for vitamin E. Large amounts may increase the risk of eye hemorrhage in diabetics. In cases of rheumatic heart disease or history of it, start vitamin E supplementation at 100 IU per day and increase slowly. Vitamin E does not raise blood pressure, except on rare occasions. Vitamin E can make blood thinners more potent; tell your doctor you are taking it. Avoid for two weeks before surgery.

APPENDIX K
Mineral and Amino Acid Interactions

Some minerals can be tested by blood intracellular tests or an EXA (elemental X-ray analysis) test.

Amino Acids

These are best absorbed on an empty stomach and taken with some diluted fruit juice.

L-Arginine

This amino acid is usually well tolerated, but can cause nausea and diarrhea in some people. It may raise blood sugar in diabetics, which may increase their need for medication.

Calcium

Large dosages interfere with absorption of many minerals. Take with magnesium, zinc, iron, manganese, and multiminerals. Take in capsules, as many women cannot break down tablets. Safest taken with food. When taken between meals, it can promote the risk of kidney stones.

Copper

Copper taken with aspirin and nonsteroidal anti-inflammatory drugs (NSAIDs) greatly enhances the anti-inflammatory action and often lowers the dosage necessary to reduce pain. Long-term use of aspirin and NSAIDs can adversely raise blood levels of copper. Large dosages of zinc and vitamin C can cause low copper. Copper supplements can cause nausea. Copper water pipes in the home and copper supplementation in those with liver disease can cause an excess of copper, which has been linked to certain psychiatric disorders. NSAIDs and penicillamine can cause copper depletion.

Glandulars

Try to obtain organic sources from isolated herds.

Iron

Vitamin C increases iron absorption. Coffee, tea, soy, calcium, and calcium-rich foods inhibit iron absorption, and iron inhibits absorption of zinc and vitamin E when taken at the same time. Excess iron can contribute to cancer, heart disease, liver disease, and diabetes and can worsen inflammation in rheumatoid arthritis. Iron supplements should be used only when tested iron and ferritin blood levels reveal a deficiency.

Magnesium

Excess magnesium can cause loose stools, and large dosages of calcium and vitamin B_6 can increase your body's need for magnesium. Use cautiously and work with a doctor if you have had kidney failure. Many women are deficient in magnesium, because it is rinsed out of the body by stress, excessive noise, and junk-food diets and in those with type A personality. Refined flour and grain has lost 80 percent of its magnesium. Take magnesium in capsules, as many women cannot absorb tablets. Magnesium is a natural pain reliever for cramps, headaches, fibromyalgia syndrome, and even works in some cases of bone pain from cancer.

Melatonin

Those with Hodgkin's disease, lymphoma, leukemia, and rheumatoid arthritis should not take melatonin until more is known about it. Because of its hormonal effects, pregnant or nursing mothers should also avoid using melatonin. Melatonin aids sleep, lowers estrogen levels, and may help reduce abdominal fat. It is poorly absorbed and sometimes requires higher doses for effectiveness. Nonsteroidal anti-inflammatory drugs, even aspirin, with long-term use, lower melatonin levels, as does working night-shift jobs.

Potassium

Large dosages can cause diarrhea. Contraindicated in cases of kidney failure or for diabetics with potassium metabolism problems. A potassium deficiency will increase digitalis toxicity. Potassium is best obtained in food, except for women on potassium-depleting diuretics who may need high dosages. Must be monitored by a doctor.

SAMe

S-adenosyl-methionine is contraindicated in bipolar conditions, must not be taken with antidepressants, should be discussed with your doctor first, and must be taken with B vitamins to enhance proper metabolic pathways. Make sure to purchase enterically coated tablets from reputable companies, as this supplement is hard to manufacture properly. Take this on an empty stomach.

Selenium

Vitamin C inactivates sodium selenite (one form of selenium) when they are taken together on an empty stomach. Selenium enhances the effects of vitamin E. Alcohol abuse depletes selenium. Excess selenium causes brittle and mottled nails, hair loss, rashes, garlic breath, and neurologic problems.

Tryptophan

Available by prescription, tryptophan is often very helpful for depression, addictive problems, and rare cases of premenstrual syndrome. Higher doses are often less effective than optimal dosages, which are 1,000–1,500 mg per day.

Tyramine

May exacerbate hypertension, asthma, epilepsy, angina, or diabetes.s

Zinc

Eighty percent of zinc is lost in refined flour and grains. Zinc is lower in modern soils, so zinc deficiencies are becoming more common. Best absorbed forms: picolinate, citrate, monomethionine. Zinc lozenges do shorten the duration of a common cold, but you must use zinc acetate or gluconate; other forms don't work. Additives, like hydrogenated oils, decrease efficacy. Well-made lozenges work; poorly made ones don't. Zinc nasal gels are better absorbed, though they can irritate nasal membranes. Excess zinc causes nausea. Large dosages over time deplete copper and folic acid. Some diuretics increase the body's need for zinc. Zinc deficiency is associated with poor taste acuity, especially of sweets (which means you use more as you can't taste it as well), delayed healing, and with prolonged gestation, slowed labor, atonic bleeding, increased risk to the fetus, stomach pain, nausea (can get if low or too high), vomiting, diarrhea, dizziness, poor immunity, and low levels of good cholesterol. Prolonged large doses of zinc must be monitored, as they can cause anemia. Work with a doctor.

APPENDIX L
Important Herb Considerations and Drug Interactions

Herbs are usually considered to be safe. However, they are still powerful agents and should not be used indiscriminately. Most herbs should be taken on an empty stomach away from meals or twenty minutes before.

- Do not take American ginseng if you have a fever. Avoid astragalus if you have a fever or acute inflammation.
- Do not use black cohosh if you are allergic to aspirin or are pregnant.
- Do not use bilberry, red clover, or garlic if you have bleeding problems or are on anticoagulants.
- Do not take cat's claw if you are pregnant, nursing, an organ-transplant recipient, or are on blood thinners.
- Do not use chamomile if you are allergic to ragweed.
- Dong quai may interfere with anticoagulants due to its high natural warfarin components. It also binds to estrogen receptors, and it is not yet known whether or not it blocks or stimulates growth of fibroids or estrogen-receptor-positive breast cancer.
- Echinacea is not a preventative and works well only for acute cases of flu, upper respiratory tract infections, and sinusitis. It reduces recurrences of candidiasis infections if taken with the first infection. Do not take echinacea on an

ongoing basis, and do not take if you have fertility problems. Do not have your male partner take ginkgo biloba or St. John's wort if you are trying to conceive. Echinacea cross-reacts with ragweed, so do not take if you have a history of grass allergies.

- Do not take false unicorn without the supervision of a professional.
- Do not take more than 500–1,000 mg per day of ginger if you are pregnant.
- Ginseng is contraindicated with monoamine oxidase inhibitors and certain psychiatric medications, and should not to be taken along with estrogen replacement therapy.
- Do not use goldenseal or any herbs when pregnant without a discussion with your doctor. Take goldenseal only three weeks at a time, then go off it for at least two-week rest intervals.
- Drink green tea when on antibiotics, and take probiotics several times a day for two weeks afterward. However, green tea in large quantities (½ gallon or more a day) may interfere with anticoagulants such as Coumadin or warfarin. Tell your doctor you drink green tea before she prescribes certain medications.
- High dosages of certain herbs (rosemary, sage, wormwood, eucalyptus, etc.) can induce seizures. Do not take these herbs if you are an epileptic or have had a seizure.
- Do not use peppermint, menthol, or camphor if taking homeopathic medications.
- Kava is contraindicated with Parkinson's disease and should not be used with benzodiazepines and/or alcohol. There have been more than sixty reports of adverse effects, mainly affecting the skin (rashes) and nervous system. These side effects go away after stopping the herb.
- Do not use licorice if you suffer with unopposed estrogen disorders, have high blood pressure or a family history of it, have heart disease, or are pregnant.
- If you have liver disease, use milk thistle only under a doctor's care. Certain herbs have caused hepatitis in some

people, so if you have a history of any liver disease, don't take chaparral, scullcap, senna, valerian root, and some Chinese herbs.

- Do not use ginkgo biloba or turmeric if you are on non-steroidal anti-inflammatory drugs (NSAIDs). Do not take turmeric if you are sensitive to aspirin-like substances (salicylates). Avoid ginkgo if you are pregnant.
- Oil of oregano can cause *die-off* of bacteria and viruses (it's so effective at killing foreign organisms that you may feel sick for several days). Don't take if you are pregnant or nursing.
- Large amounts of parsley or sage during pregnancy can inhibit milk production.
- Passionflower should not be used with alcohol or when you are driving or using heavy machinery, and it may affect drugs for insomnia and anxiety.
- St. John's wort may interact with a variety of drugs and the enzymes that metabolize them. It may reduce the efficacy of digoxin and turn women into nonresponders. St. John's wort has been associated with mania and has caused problems with blood thinners, cyclosporine, antiretroviral drugs, and even with thyroid medication. Do not take if you have high blood pressure or are a transplant patient. Check with your pharmacist and doctor. Do not use herbs for depression along with drugs for depression, although you can slowly wean off the medication and onto the therapeutic dose of the herb over a month-long period under a doctor's supervision. Interactions with other medications, like birth control pills, antiepileptics, antibiotics, antifungals, etc., still need to be studied.
- Valerian should not be used with benzodiazepines or barbiturates and can cause tremors, headache, and cardiac problems in some people when taken in large doses for prolonged times.
- Do not take vitex if you are pregnant or nursing. Do not use vitex with progesterone. Some doctors do not recommend using it longer than three months. Work with a doctor.

GLOSSARY

Acetaminophen: Pain relievers such as Tylenol, Datril, and others.

Adhesions: Fibrous bands of scar tissue that can make tissues and organs stick together, sometimes causing limitation of movement and pain.

Allergens: Substances that provoke allergic reactions.

Amino Acid: One of thousands of known organic nitrogen-containing acids acting as building blocks of proteins.

Antihistamine: A compound that blocks the action of the histamines (substances released during immediate allergic reactions) that cause allergic symptoms.

Antioxidants: Substances that prevent adverse oxidative reactions (reactions that take place in the presence of oxygen), such as vitamins C and E, selenium, glutathione (an amino acid), and alpha-lipoic acid.

Autoimmunity: Condition in which the body attacks its own tissues.

Ayurveda: A system of healing techniques practiced for thousands of years on the Indian subcontinent (adjective, Ayurvedic).

Bacteria: Single-celled microorganisms that can promote health or cause disease. More than four hundred species of beneficial "friendly" organisms and harmful "unfriendly" microorganisms inhabit the human intestinal tract simultaneously. When the ecology of the gastrointestinal tract becomes disturbed or otherwise altered, the balance becomes disrupted—called dysbiosis—and serious health problems can occur.

Bowel Detoxification: Bowel cleansing. Various programs using fiber, herbs, water, exercise, etc., can be used to cleanse and rebuild the intestinal tract.

Carbohydrates: The chief source of energy for all bodily functions, found in sugars, starches, and cellulose.

Carcinogenic: Causing cancer.

Carotenoids: Substances found in yellow and red plants that have beneficial antioxidant properties.

Colostrum: The substance that precedes breast milk and is rich in immune enhancers, including *transfer factor*.

Comprehensive Stool Exam: Various stool analyses performed with purge techniques or samples taken over several days to identify parasites, microbes, yeast infection, etc. Other comprehensive stool panels evaluate digestive function and bacterial balance.

Corticosteroids: An adrenal hormone or a synthetic substitute, often used to treat inflammation.

Crucifers: A family of vegetables (often called brassica) that includes cabbage, broccoli, brussels sprouts, cauliflower, turnips, bok choy, mustard, and rutabagas. These vegetables contain substances that help maintain optimal estrogen metabolism. Stomach acid increases production of these healthful substances.

Cultured Products: Foods with live beneficial bacteria such as yogurt or kefir.

Cyclic: Recurring at regular intervals, as in a twenty-eight-day menstrual cycle.

Desensitization: A treatment using gradually increasing amounts of diluted allergens, which are injected into the skin. This encourages the body to overcome allergic reactions.

Detoxification: The process of assisting the body in removal of toxic substances.

DIM (Diindolylmethane): A powerful metabolite of cruciferous vegetables that promotes optimal estrogen metabolism.

Dyspepsia: Indigestion.

Enzyme: A protein that acts as a catalyst in various chemical reactions.

Fiber: The part of plant food that moves through the digestive tract undigested.

Flavonoids: Colorful substances found in more than four thousand plants that have many beneficial effects. They protect the heart and act as antioxidants.

Free Radicals: Highly reactive compounds created inside the body by normal metabolism or introduced by the environment. They are thought to play a role in numerous diseases, such as heart disease, cancer, arthritis, and aging. The body produces several enzymes to neutralize, or *scavenge*, these substances.

Genetic Glitches: Inherited predispositions to health problems.

Glandulars: Preparations of gland extracts that contain enzymes, minute amounts of hormones, and other essential substances.

Glucose: A simple sugar that is the main source of energy for all the body's cells.

Gluten: A protein occurring in barley, rye, and wheat. Oats used to be thought to contain gluten, but now are considered safe on a gluten-free diet for *most* people. Intolerance is tested by anti-endomesial and anti-gliadin antibodies.

Homocysteine: An amino acid that is a natural by-product of protein metabolism.

Hormone Disruptors: Environmental pollutants and certain plant foods that can mimic natural hormones and cause altered hormonal responses in some individuals, especially when exposure occurs in the womb, to infants and children, or to the elderly.

HRT: Hormone replacement therapy with synthetic hormones (patented by drug companies and containing nonhuman hormone molecules).

Hypersensitivity Reactions: Inappropriate reactions of inflammation, swelling, or attacking the body's own tissues rather than foreign invaders.

Ibuprofen: A nonsteroidal anti-inflammatory drug.

IM: Injection into a muscle.

Immune Dysfunction: The immune system not doing its proper job of fighting off foreign invaders, like viruses and bacteria.

In Utero: Occurring in the womb.

Inflammation: A reaction to illness, injury, or stress characterized by redness and swelling of tissues.

Ischemia: Lack of blood due to constriction or blockage.

IV: Injection into a vein.

Leaky Gut (Syndrome): The intestinal lining normally acts as a barrier that allows proper substances into the body and keeps undigested or toxic ones out. An intestinal tract with faulty barrier mechanisms is called a "leaky gut."

Lycopenes: Substances found mainly in tomatoes that have beneficial antioxidant properties.

MAO: Monoamine oxidase inhibitors, a family of antidepressants.

Metabolite: A breakdown product formed from a parent compound during metabolism.

Metabolize: The body takes substances and breaks them down into smaller units.

Mutagenic: Causing genetic alterations, usually in a single gene.

Myofascial: Referring to muscles and overlying tissues called *fascia*.

Natural Therapies: Treatments utilizing nutrients, herbs, hands-on therapies, and body-mind techniques.

Neuritis: Inflammation of a nerve.

Neurotransmitters: Chemicals that deliver important messages, mostly in the brain.

NHRT (Natural Hormone Replacement Therapy): Compounded hormones (molecules made by pharmacists) that have exactly the same structure as human hormones.

Nightshade Foods: A family of foods containing solanine: tomatoes, white potatoes, all peppers except black, eggplant, and tobacco.

NSAIDs: Nonsteroidal anti-inflammatory drugs, such as aspirin, ibuprofen, and others.

Overt: Obvious.

Ovulation: The release of the egg, usually between days ten and fifteen of the menstrual cycle, accompanied by a rise in body temperature.

Oxalic Acid: A substance found in raw spinach, rhubarb, coffee, peanuts, green peppers, some beans, and chocolate; may promote kidney stones. Calcium-rich foods protect against this.

Oxidation: A chemical reaction between oxygen and a substance that often causes adverse effects.

Palliative: Gives pain relief but isn't a complete cure.

Parasite: An organism that feeds on or lives within a host organism.

Phosphoric Acid: Acid added to colas to improve taste, but it enhances bone loss.

Physician's Desk Reference: A book of FDA-approved drugs and side effects, widely available in bookstores.

Premenstrual Phase: The two weeks prior to the menstrual period.

Probiotics: Beneficial bacteria like *Lactobacillus acidophilus* and *Bifidobacterium bifidum.* Can be purchased singly or in multiple formulas, and/or with FOS (fructooligosaccharides), which support the growth of certain strains.

Prostaglandins: Substances that occur in the body in very low concentrations that act like powerful hormones affecting various organs. There are good and bad prostaglandins, and the health of numerous tissues is affected by their ratios. Types of dietary fats influence which prostaglandins are produced.

Protein: A nitrogen-containing compound that is the major source of building and repairing material for muscles, blood, skin, hair, nails, and internal organs.

Proteolytic Enzymes: Enzymes that digest protein. Animal-based trypsin and chymotrypsin, and bromelain from pineapple, assist digestion as well as having anti-inflammatory and positive immune effects.

Purine: A by-product of certain foods that can raise uric acid levels in the body. Restricting purine foods lowers the risk of gout attack. Purine-rich foods include seafood (mackerel, scallops, sardines, herring, anchovies), organ meats, spinach, lentils and peas, red meats, turkey, and alcohol (especially beer).

RDA: Recommended dietary allowance.

Receptors: Proteins that act as receiving stations for messages sent by hormones or neurotransmitters.

Salicyclates: Aspirin-like chemicals found in certain foods (page 112).

SAMe (S-Adenosyl-Methionine): A naturally occurring compound that has been shown to help depression, osteoarthritis, liver conditions, fibromyalgia, migraine, and aging. Use the pharmaceutical-grade tablet form imported from Europe or from reputable companies in the United States. Dosage is 200–1,600 mg per day depending on the severity of the condition. Women tend to respond to low doses.

Serotonin: A neurotransmitter that affects mood, sleep, and appetite.

Sputum: Material from the lungs coming out through the mouth.

SSRI: Selective serotonin-reuptake inhibitors: a group of drugs to treat depression.

Steroids: A group of fat-soluble substances such as hormones, environmental chemicals, cholesterol, drugs, and others. There are two types of steroid hormones: anabolic (increase cell production, such as estrogen and testosterone), and catabolic (lessen cell production).

Subclinical: Not severe enough to be considered an outright disease, although the organ is stressed and not working optimally.

Sublingual: Taken under the tongue.

Sulfite: A toxic natural metabolite and also a food additive used frequently on items at salad bars and many other foods. Some women are more sensitive than others to sulfites.

Thrombus: A blood clot that can cause obstruction anywhere in the vascular system.

Toxicity: Amount of a substance that is poisonous to the body.

Triggers: Causes a reaction.

Tryptophan: An amino acid that is converted into serotonin and is used in the treatment of depression.

Uric Acid: An acid that can form the crystals that cause gout and is the by-product of protein foods high in purines.